End-of-Life Care
ETHICS AND LAW

Joan McCarthy

Mary Donnelly

Dolores Dooley

Louise Campbell

David Smith

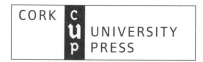
CORK UNIVERSITY PRESS

First published in 2011 by
Cork University Press
Youngline Industrial Estate
Pouladuff Road, Togher,
Cork, Ireland.

Text © The authors 2011

British Library Cataloguing in Publication Data.
A CIP catalogue record for this book is available from the British Library.

ISBN: 978 1859184813

Book Design and Typesetting: Fergus O'Neill for the Public Communications Centre.
Printed in the UK by MPG Books.

www.corkuniversitypress.com

Contents

**'Neither to hasten nor postpone . . .
an ethical and legal framework for healthcare
at the end of life'**

Foreword

In recent years in this country there has been an increasing interest in what are generally described as end-of-life issues. While many surveys have shown that the majority of people would prefer to die in their own homes, the fact is that most of us die in hospital or other centres of institutional care such as nursing homes or hospices. At times the circumstances surrounding the terminally ill at the time of their death are far from ideal. While this is, of course, not intentional, it is understandable that in the context of a busy and overcrowded hospital ward a dying person may be denied privacy and dignity. The hospice movement, and in particular the Irish Hospice Foundation, has for long emphasised the importance of a 'good death', and has worked for the creation of 'hospice-friendly hospitals', where careful planning and understanding of the relevant issues can enable the best palliative and other care to be provided for the patient at the time of death. As is articulated by the UK General Medical Council, good end-of-life care is that which 'helps patients with life-limiting conditions to live as well as possible until they die, and to die with dignity'.

The circumstances surrounding the end of our lives, whether at home or elsewhere, give rise to wider issues than those of purely medical care. Both ethical and legal issues are also of vital importance. This most welcome book deals clearly and comprehensively with just such questions. It offers an Ethical Framework of eight modules of learning which has been developed in online form by a consortium from University College Cork (UCC) and the Royal College of Surgeons of Ireland (RCSI) as part of the Hospice Friendly Hospitals Programme. The online Framework and the book draw on a significant body of research specifically addressing ethical issues in relation to end-of-life care in Irish hospitals. It is also informed by reviews and studies involving hospice, palliative and acute care services. In the course of the collaborative process between UCC and RCSI there were contributions from ethicists, legal experts, theologians, sociologists and clinicians.

It is clear, as pointed out in this book, that health professionals, patients and families must often make difficult decisions in tense, demanding, emotionally fraught and constrained circumstances. The Ethical Framework gives an opportunity to take a second look at our intuitive responses to ethically challenging situations and to examine received values, general norms and professional codes. In its general explanation of ethics, the authors point out that 'ethics may share common ground with the law, religious beliefs, popular opinion, professional codes, hospital policies and the dictates of authority figures, but it is also broader than all of these and offers a set of tools and values against which their appropriateness can be evaluated.'

The book is produced in the format of eight modules, each dealing with a specific aspect of the subject. In the context of the work in which I was previously involved with the Law Reform Commission concerning Advance Care Directives and general issues of patient autonomy and mental capacity, I was particularly interested in the modules on Patient Autonomy in Law and Practice, and on The Ethics of Life-Prolonging Treatments. Patient autonomy is well defined in the book as 'the capacity of self-determination, a person's ability to make choices about their own life based on their own beliefs and values'. It is rightly stressed that this is not just about the right to refuse treatment or procedures, but about the positive right to be involved in decisions about treatment. The module entitled The Ethics of Breaking Bad News reflects valuable research into the contrast between a theoretical belief in telling the truth to the patient and the actual practice that generally prevails in our hospitals.

All aspects of the book, however, are of great interest to the general reader as well as to the healthcare professional and to the lawyer. The issues dealt with are not simple, but the book is written in clear, elegant and readily understood language, so that the reader is encouraged to think further about what is said, and its relevance to our own lives. The end of life comes to all of us, and the bringing into practice of the principles set out in this book will benefit us all.

Catherine McGuinness
Chair, National Council of the Forum on End of Life in Ireland
Former President Law Reform Commission
Justice of the Supreme Court 2000–2006

Developed for the Hospice-Friendly Hospitals Programme of the Irish Hospice Foundation by

Authors:

Dr Joan McCarthy,
MA, PhD, Lecturer, Healthcare Ethics, School of Nursing and Midwifery, UCC

Dr Mary Donnelly,
BCL, MA, MLitt, PhD, Solicitor, Senior Lecturer, Faculty of Law, UCC

Dr Dolores Dooley,
MA, PhD, Lecturer, Healthcare Ethics, Department of General Practice, RCSI

Dr Louise Campbell,
MA, PhD, Clinical Ethicist, Clinical Ethics Ireland

Dr David Smith,
MSc, BPhil, MA, STL, PhD, Assoc. Prof. Healthcare Ethics, Department of General Practice, RCSI

Lead Researchers (empirical studies):

Ms Catherine O'Neill, Lecturer, Health Care Ethics, Faculty of Nursing and Midwifery, RCSI; Dr Christina Quinlan, Department of General Practice, RCSI; Mr. John Weafer, Weafer Research Associates

Research Assistants:

Mr Mark Loughrey, School of Nursing and Midwifery, UCC; Ms Anna O'Riordan, School of Nursing and Midwifery, UCC

Project Management:

Dr Joan McCarthy (UCC–RCSI) & Mr Mervyn Taylor, Hospice-Friendly Hospitals Programme

Special Consultants:

Dr Deirdre Madden, Senior Lecturer, Faculty of Law, UCC; Prof. Nigel Biggar, Regius Professor of Moral and Pastoral Theology, University of Oxford; Prof. Muiris FitzGerald, Board Member, Irish Hospice Foundation; Ms Orla Keegan, Head of Education, Research and Bereavement Services, Irish Hospice Foundation

Special thanks to:

Shelagh Twomey, Joanne Carr, Denise Robinson, Helen Donovan (HFH Programme) and Bob Carroll, Research Consultant, for their feedback on early drafts of the modules and research reports; Professor Geraldine McCarthy, Head of School of Nursing and Midwifery, UCC and Claire Breen, Learning Consultant and Coach, FiBre Skills, for their guidance and ongoing support.

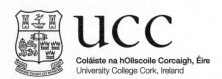

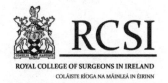

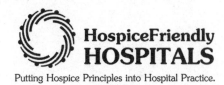

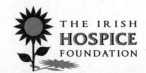

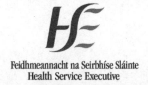

Introduction

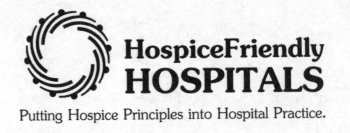

HospiceFriendly **HOSPITALS**

Putting Hospice Principles into Hospital Practice.

Introduction Contents   Page

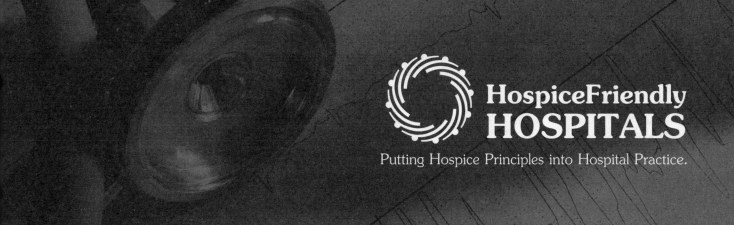

1. Background

This book offers an Ethical Framework for end-of-life decision making in healthcare settings. It is also available in online form at: http://www.hospicefriendlyhospitals.net/ethics.

The Ethical Framework for End-of-Life Care is part of a national programme, the Hospice Friendly Hospitals Programme (HfH) of the Irish Hospice Foundation, which is intended to improve the culture of care and organisation regarding dying, death and bereavement in Irish hospitals. The Framework is an educational resource that consists of eight Modules of Learning for health professionals, patients, families and the general public.

The Framework is the outcome of a unique collaboration between University College Cork, the Royal College of Surgeons in Ireland and the Irish Hospice Foundation, with contributions from ethicists, legal experts, theologians, sociologists and clinicians. It draws on a range of values and principles that have been identified as important considerations in end-of-life decision making by international experts in bioethics and by professional codes of conduct, policy documents and laws. It is also informed by extensive international research on patients' and families' experiences of death and dying and the contribution of health professionals and organisations to quality end-of-life care.

In order to ensure that the Framework addresses the concerns of the Irish public and that it is relevant and useful to the work of health professionals involved in end-of-life care in Irish hospitals, the Framework is informed by reviews and studies involving hospice, palliative and acute care services especially commissioned by the Irish Hospice Foundation in the last decade. It also draws on a significant body of research, undertaken in 2007/8, which specifically addresses ethical issues in relation to end-of-life care in Irish hospitals.

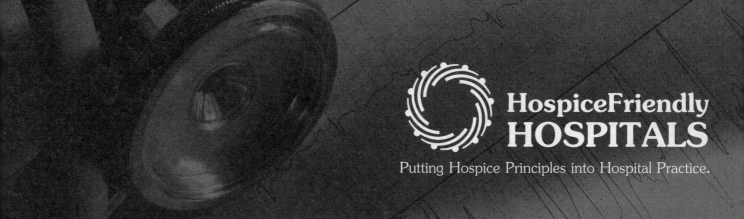

2. National Research

Reports of the national research undertaken in 2007/8 include:

- Focus group interviews with members of the general public to identify issues of concern at the end of life (Weafer, 2009a).

- A national survey of the public's understanding of, and concerns about, dying, death and bereavement (Weafer, McCarthy and Loughrey, 2009).

- Interviews with public representatives in relation to ethical and legislative issues that arise at the end of life (Weafer, 2009b).

- A literature review to explore the concept of autonomy in theory and in hospital practice and to consider a range of initiatives and interventions to support dying patients' decision-making capacity (Quinlan, 2009b).

- An analysis of Irish and UK newspapers, television and radio treatment of issues arising in relation to death and dying in Irish society (Quinlan, 2009a).

- Individual and focus group interviews conducted with healthcare practitioners working in fifteen Irish hospitals, in order to gain an understanding of their experiences of caring for dying patients and their families (Quinlan and O'Neill, 2009).

Evidence from the national research indicates the following:

- The general public and Irish legislators are largely unfamiliar with, or have little understanding of, terms associated with end-of-life treatment and care, such as do not resuscitate orders, advance directives, artificial nutrition and hydration (Weafer, 2009a, 2009b; Weafer, McCarthy and Loughrey, 2009).

- Most people want to be informed if they have a terminal condition (Weafer, 2009a; Weafer, McCarthy and Loughrey, 2009).

- Information about diagnoses and prognoses is often shared with families instead of patients (particularly older patients) at the end of life (Quinlan and O'Neill, 2009).

- If they are unable to make decisions for themselves, most people prefer their families and/or loved ones (often, in conjunction with doctors) to make decisions about starting or stopping treatment for them (Weafer, 2009a; Weafer, McCarthy and Loughrey, 2009).

- One in five people have told someone how they would like to be treated if they were terminally ill and dying. One in twenty people have written a Living Will (Weafer, McCarthy and Loughrey, 2009).

Most people believe that
- If they were severely ill with no hope of recovery, the quality of their life would be more important than how long it lasted.
- Spiritual or religious support is important to them.
- Every competent person has the right to refuse medical treatment even if such refusal could lead to their death (Weafer, McCarthy and Loughrey, 2009).

- Patients who are dying have medical concerns; but they are also concerned about other things such as family relationships (Quinlan, 2009b).

- Patients who are dying value their autonomy but they also value other things such as the well-being of others (Quinlan, 2009b, Quinlan and O'Neill, 2009).

- The notion of patient autonomy is not well understood by many health professionals working in Irish hospitals (Quinlan and O'Neill, 2009).

- Health professionals face communication challenges in sharing decision making with patients and families in end-of-life situations (Quinlan and O'Neill, 2009).

The eight modules of The Ethical Framework for End-of-Life Care address the concerns that have been highlighted in the research outlined above and consider a number of the narratives that have emerged from interviews and focus groups with health professionals.

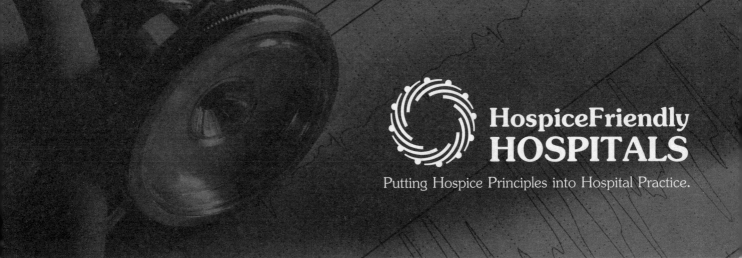

3. Aim and Objectives

Aim: The Ethical Framework for End-of-Life Care is an educational resource that aims to foster and support ethically and legally sound clinical practice in end-of-life treatment and care in Irish hospitals.

Objectives

1. A key objective of the Ethical Framework is to enhance the reflective, critical and communicative skills of health professionals, hospital staff and hospital administrators so that they become more informed, confident and collaborative in addressing ethical and legal challenges that arise in the treatment and care of dying patients and their families.

2. A second objective is to provide patients, families and the general public with easily accessible information and opportunities for learning which will deepen their ethical and legal understanding of the issues that arise in relation to death and dying and enhance their decision-making capacity in relation to their own deaths and those of their loved ones.

3. A third objective is to increase the capacity of Irish healthcare organisations
- to support health professionals to do their work and patients to receive their care in an ethically healthy climate
- to create safe spaces where individuals feel free to raise ethical, professional and legal concerns and to express nagging doubts and fears
- to encourage open, inclusive and respectful dialogue about ethical, professional and legal concerns.

13

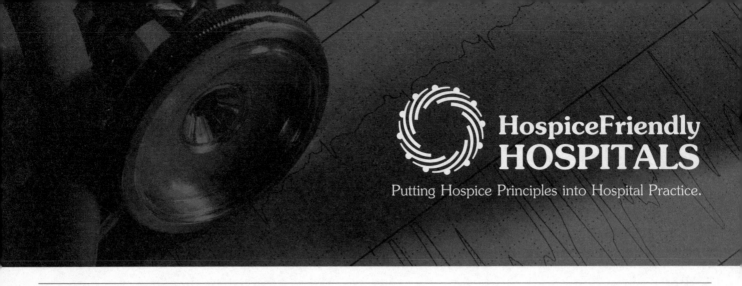

4. Educational Philosophy

Research evidence clearly indicates that health professionals, patients and families must often make difficult decisions in tense, demanding, emotionally fraught and constrained circumstances. The Ethical Framework for End-of-Life Care offers an opportunity to readers to take a reflective step back from their intuitive responses to ethically challenging situations and to examine received values, assumptions and emotional responses in light of general norms, professional codes and laws.

The philosophy underpinning the development of the Ethical Framework is one that views ethical work as a critically engaged process whose object is to negotiate, rather than eliminate, ethical uncertainty. The assumption is that it is precisely the experience of moral uncertainty, disagreement and diversity that forces us to critically reflect on our moral viewpoints: difference creates the need for moralising to begin with.

The educational aim of the Ethical Framework, therefore, is not to tell people what to do, but to offer tools for thinking about difficult problems. The educational task is to foster a range of ethical skills and competencies to ensure that ethical decisions are arrived at in the most reasonable, sensitive and collaborative way possible. These include skills of reflection and analysis as well as the critical ability to evaluate the adequacy of reasons and arguments that support different positions and courses of action. To this end, the Framework modules employ different moral perspectives – traditional and contemporary – to draw out different ethical features of each of the situations considered (See Module 1 for an account of different moral perspectives). In addition, Modules 3 and 4 have a particularly legal focus, which serves to illustrate the way in which very deeply held moral values have been enshrined and expressed in laws and court decisions.

Readers are also introduced to the process of ethical reasoning and resolution through interactive learning and reflection on case studies drawn from practice. These bring into sharper focus the need for sensitivity to the unique stories and circumstances of individual patients and families. This is all the more important given the multicultural and socially diverse world that health professionals, healthcare staff, patients and families belong to.

5. Ethical Framework Summary

The Framework is divided into eight distinct Modules of Learning which:

(1) Identify relevant considerations in situations at the end of life that may be ethically and/or legally challenging;

(2) Explore and explain the ethical and legal issues at stake, and;

(3) Offer reasonable and well-supported approaches to addressing these issues.

Module 1:
Explaining Ethics

Discusses one key notion that is linked with death and dying; the meaning of a 'good death'. Describes a range of different approaches to moral problems and distinguishes ethics from other perspectives such as religion and the law.

Module 2:
The Ethics of Breaking Bad News

Explains why telling patients the truth about their condition is important and reflects on the challenges that diverse cultural perspectives on patient and family relationships present to health professionals when they are considering breaking bad news. Presents arguments for and arguments against breaking bad news.

Module 3:
Healthcare Decision-making and the Role of Rights

Considers the way in which deeply-held moral values in relation to dying and death have been enshrined and expressed in laws and court decisions. Explains the relationship between moral and legal rights and discusses the advantages and the limits of taking a rights-based approach to the decision-making process at end of life.

Module 4:
Patient Autonomy in Law and Practice

Explains the legal right of patients to refuse treatment as well as the positive right of patients to control and direct how their treatment and care proceeds. Evaluates the contribution of an autonomy-based model of decision making and the limits of patient autonomy. Outlines the legal test of capacity, and the health professional's obligation to facilitate the participation of patients who lack capacity.

Module 5:
The Ethics of Managing Pain

Describes the different kinds of pain and suffering that patients may endure and considers reasons why adequate pain relief may not be provided to different patient groups. Explains the challenge of determining adequate and proportionate responses to patients' pain and ethically evaluates palliative measures that are sometimes provided to alleviate extreme and intractable suffering.

Module 6:
The Ethics of Life Prolonging Treatments (LPTs)

Explains the ethical and legal concerns that arise in relation to decisions not to start or to discontinue the use of life-prolonging treatments. Presents and considers different positions on the ethical and legal status of euthanasia and assisted suicide.

Module 7:
The Ethics of Confidentiality and Privacy

Describes the onus on health professionals to protect the confidentiality and privacy of patients who are dying and deceased. Discusses exceptions to the ethical and legal requirement of confidentiality and the relevant interests of others such as patients' families.

Module 8:
Ethical Governance in Clinical Care and Research

Outlines and considers the role of clinical ethics committees and the process of ethics consultation in clinical practice. Charts the emergence of research ethics committees and their contribution to the regulation of research and the protection of research participants.

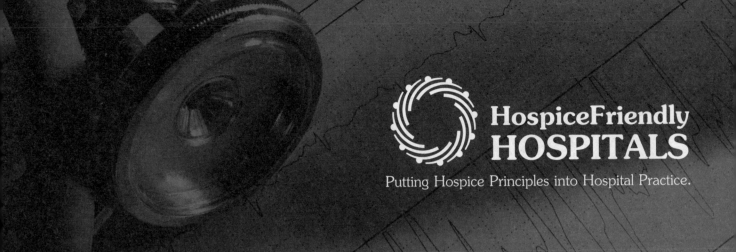

6. Module Format

Each of the modules is formatted in a similar way; it is divided into distinct sections that offer Key Points, Definitions, Background, Main Topics, Cases and Suggested Professional Responsibilities,[1] Further Discussion, Summary Learning Guides, Activities, References and Further Reading.

The uniform presentation of the modules enables readers to take or leave parts or all of any module. In addition, individual case studies are linked to specific activities and learning guides so that these can be considered independently of the rest of the module.

1. Key points

Offers a brief summary of each of the main points that arise in the module. These points are discussed more extensively in the main body of the module.

2. Definitions

Explains the meaning of key terms used in the module. Readers may find it useful to return to it when, in the course of their reading, they come across terms that they are unfamiliar with.

3. Background

Introduces the reader to the main topic of the module and indicates the key ethical and legal challenges that it presents.

---

1   Module 1 provides an overview of the task of ethical reasoning and does not consider individual cases.

4/5. Key Topics

Explains and explores the main ethical and legal issues that the module is concerned with.

6. Cases

Describe situations from practice which give rise to ethical challenges for health professionals, patients and their families, e.g. decisions about pain relief and starting or stopping medical treatments. Many of the cases are concrete narratives drawn from the everyday experiences of patients, families, health and allied professionals in Irish hospital wards, operating theatres, clinics and other healthcare settings. Where relevant, cases are drawn from other countries. The narratives highlight a number of ethical and legal questions and issues that are then explained and discussed in the text. This section suggests some of the **Professional Responsibilities** that might arise in relation to each case for readers to consider.

7. Further Discussion

This material discusses in more detail the ethical and legal issues that are addressed in the module.

8. Summary Learning Guides

Provide brief synopses of the key points that are made in the module. These are presented in boxed format in order to facilitate a revision of concepts, definitions and arguments.

9. Activities

Questions for reflection or comments are offered to readers at the end of the module to encourage them to tease out the ethical and legal questions raised in the discussion, the cases and the analyses that follow.

10. References and Further Reading

Includes a list of texts referred to in the body of the module as well as additional reading relevant to the topic. Where possible, web sources and links are provided.

7. References

Quinlan, C. *Media Messages on Death and Dying* (Dublin: Irish Hospice Foundation, 2009a)

Quinlan, C. *Patient Autonomy at End of Life: Literature Review* (Dublin: Irish Hospice Foundation, 2009b)

Quinlan, C. and O'Neill, C. *Practitioners' Perspectives on Patient Autonomy at End of Life* (Dublin: Irish Hospice Foundation, 2009)

Weafer, J. *A Qualitative Study of Public Perceptions of End-of-Life Issues* (Dublin: Irish Hospice Foundation, 2009a)

Weafer, J. *The Views of Political Representatives* (Dublin: Irish Hospice Foundation, 2009b)

Weafer, J. and Associates, *A Nationwide Survey of Public Attitudes and Experiences Regarding Death and Dying* (Dublin: Irish Hospice Foundation, 2004)

Weafer, J., McCarthy, J. and Loughrey M. *Exploring Death and Dying: The Views of the Irish General Public* (Dublin: Irish Hospice Foundation, 2009)

Note: Quinlan 2009a; Quinlan 2009b; Quinlan and O'Neill 2009; Weafer 2009a; and Weafer, McCarthy and Loughrey 2009 were sourced from http://hospicefriendlyhospitals. net/ethical-framework?start=8 [accessed 8 July 2011]

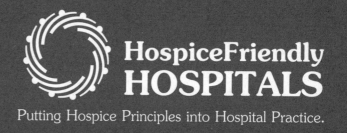

HospiceFriendly
HOSPITALS
Putting Hospice Principles into Hospital Practice.

Module 1

Explaining Ethics

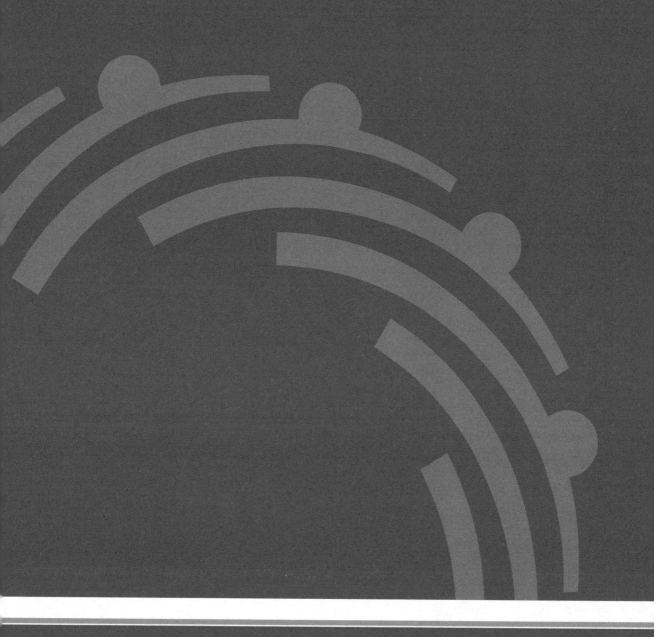

Module 1 Contents

1. Module 1 Key Points

1.1 Ethics, or moral philosophy:

considers theories about what human beings are capable of doing, alongside accounts of what they ought to do if they are to live an ethically good life. Ethics may share common ground with the law, religious belief, popular opinion, professional codes, hospital policies and the dictates of authority figures, but it is also broader than all of these and offers a set of tools and values against which their appropriateness can be evaluated.

1.2 Healthcare ethics:

is a domain of inquiry which focuses on the moral, or ethical, problems and challenges that arise in healthcare settings. While healthcare professionals may differ in relation to these issues because of their different roles and responsibilities, they nevertheless share much common ground. For example, in end-of-life situations, different professionals have different functions: consultants and doctors are, generally, the lead decision-makers in relation to treatment or nontreatment decisions, while nurses and allied professionals have much of the responsibility for caring for patients and their families through the dying process. However, these functions may also overlap in both directions; nurses and other professionals contribute to decision making, consultants and doctors contribute to care.

1.3 A Good Death and Dying:

The diversity of individual values and cultural differences tells us that an agreed consensus on what makes for a 'good death' may not be within our easy reach. But although there may be no universal agreement about what a 'good death' consists of, there is some consensus as to the core features of the care that needs to be provided to those who are dying and their families and loved ones. For example, drawing on long-established ethical principles, the UK General Medical Council (GMC) describes good end-of-life care as that which 'helps patients with life-limiting conditions to live as well as possible until they die, and to die with dignity' (GMC, 2009, p.3).

2. Module 1 Definitions

2.1 Values:

things that matter to us; that we care about; goals or ideals we aspire to, e.g. health and happiness. Ethical or moral values express ideals of conduct and character that we expect of ourselves and each other, e.g. honesty, loyalty and justice.

2.2 Family:

may include the immediate biological family and/or other relatives, spouses, partners (including same sex and de facto partners) or friends. They may have a close, ongoing, personal relationship with the patient, be chosen by the patient to be involved in treatment decisions, and have themselves indicated that they are ready to be involved in such decisions.

2.3 Harm Principle:

stipulates that individual freedom can only be limited on the basis of harm to others, i.e. when an individual, in exercising their autonomy, limits the autonomy or threatens the welfare and safety of others.

2.4 Objective Perspective:

a view that is independent of any particular person's or group's perspective.

2.5 Subjective Perspective:

a personal point of view.

3. Module 1 Background

3.1 What is Ethics?

Ethics is a branch of philosophy that attempts to understand people's moral beliefs and actions (these modules use the terms 'ethics' and 'morality'; 'ethical' and 'moral' interchangeably, although traditionally 'ethics' described the process of thinking about people's morality). Ethics, or moral philosophy, considers theories about what human beings are capable of doing, alongside accounts of what they ought to do if they are to live an ethically good life. Ethics also explores the meaning and the ranking of different ethical values, such as honesty, autonomy, equality and justice, and it considers ethical quandaries that human beings face in the course of living their own independent but, also, socially interdependent lives.

One of the key tasks of ethical reasoning, generally, is to analyse and critically consider the values we hold and the claims we make in relation to the perceived obligations that we might have towards one another. Applied to the processes of death and dying and the care provided at end of life, key values that arise include sanctity of life (the fact of being alive is itself deeply valued), quality of life (the fact of having positive experiences and avoiding negative experiences is considered deeply morally significant), autonomy (respecting someone's preferences in relation to where, how and when they die is, increasingly, considered to be deeply morally significant and challenging).

A second key task of ethics is to evaluate the adequacy of reasons that we give for our actions: it considers, for example, whether the reasons offered to support a particular course of action are based on sound evidence and/or logical argument. Applied to the processes of death and dying, reasons that are evaluated might be the arguments a health professional offers in support of resuscitating an incompetent terminally ill patient or a parent's reasons for refusing medical treatment for a severely disabled neonate.

The tasks of weighing ethical values and evaluating different ethical arguments are unlike many other kinds of human tasks. Ethical values are usually not as easy to understand as other kinds of values, e.g. it is probably easier to explain the (mainly) practical value of energy than it is to explain the ethical value of courage. In turn, it is easier to test a person's blood pressure than it is to determine whether or not they are virtuous.

Moreover, ethical problems are often not as clear as other kinds of problems and resolving ethical problems as definitively is not always possible. The aim of ethics then, is not, despite popular opinion, to take the high moral ground and tell people what to do, but, rather, to offer tools for thinking about difficult problems. Good ethical thinking purposefully seeks out the grey in questions and concerns in order to acknowledge the diversity and complexity of roles, situations and circumstances that arise in human life and relationships.

As complex as ethical situations may be, however, there is still an onus on everyone involved in ethically challenging situations to resolve any problems that arise in the most sincere, reasonable and collaborative way possible. This means that they must be prepared to review and revise their position in the light of reflection, discussion and changing circumstances. (See Further Discussion for more detail on traditional and contemporary ethical theories).

3.2 What is Healthcare Ethics?

Healthcare ethics is a domain of inquiry which focuses on the moral, or ethical, problems and challenges that arise in healthcare settings. Healthcare ethics addresses these concerns, largely from the perspective of different professional groups, including doctors and nurses, as well as occupational therapists and dentists. It can be further subdivided into medical ethics, nursing ethics, dentistry ethics, etc., but for the purposes of these modules the broader term 'healthcare ethics' is used. This is because all health professionals and some allied professionals share common ethical concerns about how best to care for patients at the end of life. These concerns arise in all patient/professional relationships, and include worries about breaking bad news, obtaining informed consent and respecting confidentiality. All health professionals also have similar experiences of dealing with challenges in relation to distributing scarce resources, addressing social injustice and dealing with incompetent or immoral colleagues (Holm, 1997).

While healthcare professionals may differ in relation to these issues as a result of their different roles and responsibilities, they nevertheless share much common ground. For example, in end-of-life situations, different professionals have different functions: consultants and doctors are, generally, the lead decision makers in relation to treatment or nontreatment decisions, while nurses and allied professionals have much of the responsibility for caring for patients and their families through the dying process. However, these functions may also overlap in both directions; nurses and other professionals contribute to decision making, consultants and doctors contribute to care.

In the past twenty years, the field of healthcare ethics in general has rapidly expanded in an effort to address the seismic moral and metaphysical shifts that have occurred as a result of technological advances at the beginning and end of life. Today, human beings can create life, modify life and prolong life in ways that make the wildest of science fiction stories sound tame. Clinical ethics committees, research ethics committees and commissions are being instituted to attend to the moral uncertainty and moral challenges that accompany such rapid changes. Similarly, the evolution of healthcare ethics can be seen as part of a process of development that involves confronting and addressing these challenges.

Where the healthcare ethics literature has traditionally addressed the ethical challenges which health professionals face during the course of their work, the focus, in recent years, has been on good judgement, collaborative decision making and professional and personal accountability. In addition, because of the particular nature of this work, human relationships, and the ethical bonds and obligations that they give rise to, are at the heart of the moral realm of healthcare provision. Storch captures this in the following quotation, in which she claims that the ethical life is one that is most deeply lived in relationship with others:

> [Healthcare] ethics is about being in relationship to persons in care. The enactment of healthcare ethics is a constant readiness to engage one's moral agency. Almost every [healthcare] action and situation involves ethics. To raise questions about ethics is to ask about the good in our practice. Are we doing the right thing for this patient? Are we listening to this person's need for pain relief? Are we respecting a family's grief over their dying child as they struggle to squeeze out a few extra days or hours for the child through alternative therapies? Are we ready to stand up for what we know to be right when we face a situation requiring us to perform a procedure that we are confident is not appropriate and that violates the dignity of another human being? Are we willing to find time to debrief after complex situations to determine how we could have done better, with a commitment to doing everything in our power to prevent similar situations from occurring in the future? (Storch, 2004, p.7)

Echoing Storch's emphasis on human relationships, Arthur Frank, author of the internationally acclaimed book *The Wounded Storyteller* has posed the question of how health professionals can remain generous in the middle of expanding needs and demands on them and the pressure to deliver treatments as commodities. Frank describes fundamental medicine as:

> [F]ace-to-face encounters between people who are suffering bodily ills and other people who need both the skills to relieve the suffering and the grace to welcome those who suffer […] Before and after fundamental medicine offers diagnoses, drugs, and surgery to those who suffer, it should offer consolation. Consolation is a gift. Consolation comforts when loss occurs or is inevitable. This comfort may be one person's promise not to abandon another. […][T]hose who make medicine their work are to find their consolation in being the kind of people who offer such hospitality.
>
> (Frank, 2004, pp.1–3)

4. A Good Death and Dying: A Spectrum of Views

4.1 Defining 'Death'

When the question is posed, 'what is death'?, it seems a straightforward question with a simple answer – the cessation of all life functions. But that's simply a biological definition and it is disputed, i.e. does death occur when the heart stops? when the brain partially or wholly stops functioning? When the question is posed, 'what is the meaning of death'?, it becomes even more apparent that death cannot be directly apprehended in straightforward scientific terms.

Death is a fact of life, but how one thinks about mortality and the limits of earthly life reflects social, not biological, realities (Kliever, 2004). This means that beliefs about death and its significance and value are 'socially constructed'. Depending on the society in which we grow up, we learn much about dying. We acquire emotions about death and dying and, along with our memories of others who have died, we accumulate anxieties or develop a sense of acceptance, dread or detachment about dying. Our 'society' is the sum of our unique environmental space, our geography, our culture, our religious traditions and family influences. Because the beliefs and attitudes towards dying are 'socially constructed' in the sense just explained, a culturally diverse society, such as Ireland is now, reveals a similar diversity of 'death perceptions and values'.

4.2 Cultural Differences

Culture provides the key medium for comprehending the final boundary between our existence as living beings and the eventual end of that existence. If one is a religious person, he or she might believe that death means the end of existence 'at least in this mortal sphere'. For example, the beliefs of Muslims hold a promise that death is not the end. 'They believe that dying is part of living and an entrance to the next life, a transformation from one life to another, a part of a journey, and a contract and part of their faith in God' (Our Lady of Lourdes Hospital, 2005, p.11).

Similarly, belief in the Catholic religion frames the way in which death is negotiated for many Irish people. As Quinlan (2009a) observes in relation to her research of media representations of death and dying in Ireland:

The Catholic nature of much of Irish spirituality was evident. It was evident in the response of one mother to the prognostication of terminal cancer in her young daughter Rachel (Tubridy: 04.02.2008). She spoke of trips to Lourdes, to Medjugorje, to Rome for a meeting with the Pope, in search of a miracle that would save her daughter's life. She said that they had not discussed

death with Rachel. Rachel was five years old when she died. Her mother said that when Rachel's siblings asked if Rachel was going to die, her response was: 'we hope not. She is very sick but we are praying to holy God. We are praying to him to make her well again'.
(Quinlan, 2009a, p.7-8)

The reality of cultural diversity is a recurring theme of the Ethical Framework for End-of-Life Care precisely because recognition of this diversity means recognition of, and respect for, the differing values of patients in the illness and dying processes. Some illustrative examples show what this may mean in practice. In Middle-Eastern societies, it is common to support a borderline existence for patients suffering from persistent vegetative state, maintaining their biological lives in specialised ventilatory-care units. It is as if death must be resisted at all costs. But the Wari people, native inhabitants of the Amazon, do not shrink from the reality of dying but employ customs that might be shocking to many Western value systems. Wari people show respect for their dead and salve their grief by engaging in ritual mortuary cannibalism. Western onlookers might be aghast at such behaviour that looks like profound disrespect for the deceased loved ones. However, the value of 'respect' is pronounced among the Wari people.

Cultural differences may also challenge some basic assumptions in hospice philosophy, making it more difficult for hospice carers to respect these differences. For example, home death is often considered an ideal in hospice philosophy, and a 'good death' is characterised as taking place at home, surrounded by family and/or friends with symptoms and pain under control and spiritual needs identified and met following appropriate goodbyes. At variance with this hospice goal, home death (or 'Hogan' death to use the Navajo term for 'home') may not always be valued in diverse ethnic groups, for whom it is deemed dangerous or polluting to be around the dead. Among traditional Navajo, dying persons were removed from the Hogan dwelling to a separate shed-like room through a special door to avoid the travesty of a death happening in the Hogan, because the Hogan would then have to be destroyed. To ensure that ghosts could not find their way back to the Hogan, family members did not touch the body (Koenig and Marshall, 2004). This task was assigned to outsiders. The Navajo Indian likewise considers advance care planning a violation of their traditional values (Carrese and Rhodes, 1995).

Quinlan's account of the views of some Irish Travellers indicate that there are culturally different attitudes to death and dying among Irish people also – some Irish Travellers, for example, find common ground with the US Navajo Indians in their view of the place of dying:

The multicultural nature of Irish society was also evident. It was evident in Regina McQuillan's discussion of Irish Travellers and their experience of hospice. Professor McQuillan said that Irish Travellers, unlike Irish people generally, did not like to die at home. She talked about how Travellers would traditionally leave a place where one of their community died. She detailed how they would burn all of the person's belongings, even burn the dead person's trailer. She said that in the history of The Irish Hospice only two Travellers had died in a hospice, both in 1999 and none since. She quoted one Traveller as saying: 'Now that we know what kind of place it is, we wouldn't want anyone to go there. It's a place without hope, and Travellers can't live without hope.' (Quinlan, 2009a, p.8)

4.3 Individual Differences

In addition to cultural differences, there are also individual differences in the way in which dying is negotiated. For some, 'a good death' may seem a contradiction, especially if one does not have the possible comfort and solace of religious belief in an afterlife. Death may signal the end of all that is loved, all that is experienced and all that is possible.

The sentiments that reject the very notion of a 'good death' are voiced by Dylan Thomas (1945/2003). Expressing a sense of frustration that his father might not resist the illness that beset him, Thomas wrote these words to his father as a moving plea not to give in to 'the dying of the light'.

> *Do not go gentle into that good night,*
> *Old age should burn and rave at close of day;*
> *Rage, rage against the dying of the light.* (p. 239)

Dylan Thomas stressed the importance of affirming life, of fighting the 'dying of the light' up until the last breath, and refusing the call to accept death quietly. An opposed view is that of Elizabeth Kubler-Ross (1975), who urges us to move through a number of stages: denial, anger, bargaining, depression and a final detachment which is an 'acceptance' facilitating a peaceful demise. On Kubler-Ross's view, health professionals would be facilitators helping the dying person with the journey through these stages. 'Since the dawn of humankind, the human mind has pondered death, searching for the answer to its mysteries. The key to the question of death unlocks the door of life' (1975, p.1).

Recent research on dying and death in Ireland also gives us some indication of the variety of responses of people living in Ireland when queried about their understanding of a 'good death'. The following features were highlighted by members of the focus groups convened in the course of Weafer's qualitative research for the Irish Hospice Foundation (Weafer, 2009):

- Fast and peaceful / to die in your sleep.
- To have your family with you when you die.
- To have control over the time and circumstances of your death.
- To be cared for at home, with adequate medical support.
- No pain or suffering involved.
- To die with dignity and all that entails.
- Your children to be reared and independent.
- When you are old; in accordance with the natural life-cycle.
- With enough time to get your affairs in order.
- With a pint of Guinness in one hand and a model in the other!

In addition, the top three concerns of the respondents in a national survey (n = 667) on the public's reported concerns at the end of life related to family/friends, pain/violent death, and actually dying (Weafer, McCarthy and Loughrey, 2009). This echoes an earlier study on the same theme, in which the three most important aspects of care cited by respondents if they were dying or in the last stages of a terminal illness were: to be surrounded by loved ones, to be free from pain, to be conscious and able to communicate (Weafer, 2004).

Quinlan claims that there is evidence of a culturally specific Irish attitude to death in Professor McQuillan's observation that 'there is a frankness about death in the UK and the US that is absent in Ireland'. 'We are not,' she said, 'so open about death here' (Quinlan 2009a, p.7). Indicating that this Irish reluctance to talk about death may be changing, Emma Doyle's recent research describes the now famous interview by Marian Finucane with Irish author and broadcaster Nuala O'Faoláin during which O'Faoláin shared her experience and subsequent struggle on learning of her diagnosis of terminal cancer. Doyle terms the interview a 'critical event' which sparked a 'national conversation about death':

On a Saturday morning in April, many Irish people stopped what they were doing and listened to the voice of a person who was talking about dying. People who missed the interview heard about it from others and listened to it later on the internet or read the transcript in the next day's papers. This voice moved many to reflect on their own feelings about dying or the deaths of their loved ones and started a national conversation about death. The emotional response of so many people to the narrative of a dying woman serves to highlight how unusual it has become to speak out publicly about death, and the belief of over half the population that death is not discussed enough shows that Irish people were ready to have this conversation. By drawing attention to the lived experience of dying, O'Faoláin began a discussion where previously there had been silence. (Doyle, 2008, p.25)

Doyle refers to one participant in this 'national conversation', Terence Cosgrave, whose editorial in the *Irish Medical Times* points out:

[I]f Nuala O'Faoláin has taught us anything, it is that we should put the person who is experiencing the trauma of terminal illness at the forefront […] Their interests should be paramount and we should not let ideology blind us to their wishes – and their rights […] Doctors know if they treat any patient long enough, it will […] end in failure. But the failure to keep a patient alive forever is acceptable – that is the nature of life. An undignified death – and needless suffering – is a much more catastrophic failure, and one that should be consigned to history. (Cosgrave, 2008)

Cosgrave's editorial is of interest not just because it underlines the inescapability of death but also because it focuses on the obligations of health professionals to accompany the dying well. Murray and Jennings (2005) support this commitment to addressing the issue not of death but of dying badly. They suggest that in the past, end-of-life care reform in the US has been excessively driven by the law and that it is time to turn the lens on the need for culture to catch up.

The next decades should be, we believe, a time of education and soul-searching discussions in communities and at kitchen tables, as well as in health care settings. […] We must talk about what we dare not name, and look at what we dare not see. We shall never get end-of-life care 'right' because death is not a puzzle to be solved. Death is an inevitable aspect of the human condition. But let us never forget: while death is inevitable, dying badly is not. (Murray and Jennings, 2005, p. S57)

Speaking of death and dying, commentators such as Murray and Jennings agree that we have witnessed a basic change in the way we die. With this change has come a rethinking of the goals of medicine and the roles of health professionals. If one accepts that dying and practices surrounding death vary within Irish culture and across many other cultures, then engagement in and awareness of these cultural realities need to be encouraged. Persons who are not members of a society's dominant cultural group cannot simply be seen as a challenging 'other'. Ethnic, social and cultural differences that reveal meaning through end-of-life rituals generally deserve professionals' respect, in the form of efforts to become informed and through efforts to avoid harmful stereotyping. The caveat on giving this respect would be if a certain practice sought was clearly limiting another individual's autonomy or putting another's welfare at risk (see discussion on Autonomy in Module 4).

Finally, recent years I have witnessed intense public debates in many Western societies in relation to the moral and/or legal permissibility of euthanasia and assisted suicide. In countries such as the Netherlands and Switzerland, the notion of a 'good death' is linked by some with the notion of a 'right to die', i.e. the right to have active steps taken to end a person's life (euthanasia) or to assist a person in ending his or her own life (assisted suicide). Some of the ethical and legal challenges to which these issues give rise are discussed in more detail in Modules 4 and 7. For present purposes, one important point to note is that neither is permissible under Irish law. Under Irish law, any person who deliberately ends the life of another person is potentially guilty of murder. It makes no difference that the person consented to the ending of his or her life or even that he or she requested that this should happen.

A second point to note is that the focus of the Irish Hospice Foundation, through the HfH programme, is to work assiduously to get a 'right to die' understood, not as a right to euthanasia or assisted suicide, but as a claim or expectation on state and institutional provisions to facilitate the most appropriate care and treatment at the end of life. A central objective of the HfH programme is to draw attention to the obligation on state institutions and the Department of Health and Children to assume the responsibility to make resources, policies and physical environments consistent with a 'good end-of-life care'.

4.4 Elements of Good End-of-Life Care

As illustrated, the diversity of individual values and cultural differences tells us that an agreed consensus on what makes for a good dying may not be within our easy reach.
However, if there is no universal agreement about what a 'good death' consists of, there is, fortunately, some consensus as to the core features of the care that needs to be provided to those who are dying and their families and loved ones. Drawing on long-established ethical principles, the UK General Medical Council (GMC) articulates good end-of-life care as that which 'helps patients with life-limiting conditions to live as well as possible until they die, and to die with dignity' (GMC, 2009, p.3). Many documents have been published that address the elements of such end-of-life care (The College & Association of Registered Nurses of Alberta, 2005; German National Ethics Council, 2006; Medical Council, 2009; National Consensus Project for Quality Palliative Care, 2009; NCEPOD 2009; New South Wales

Department of Health, 2005; Sisters of Bon Secours, 2000). Ten general features that recur in these documents are listed below. They apply equally to those in the end stages of life as well as those suffering from chronic, long-term illnesses.

Elements of Good End-of-Life Care

1. Health professionals with communication skills and sensitivity towards the beliefs and practices of diverse cultures and individuals in their understandings of a 'good dying'

2. Respectful opportunities for the patient's voice to be heard concerning their dying

3. Provisions for comfort and relief of pain and suffering

4. Due regard for, and provisions made to ensure, patient privacy

5. Respect for the right to refuse treatment or the request for withdrawal of treatment

6. Respect for health professionals' responsibility not to start, or to discontinue some treatments when appropriate, with consideration for both patient and family preferences

7. A collaborative approach to care: families and the healthcare team work together for patients who lack capacity, taking into account their previously expressed wishes

8. Non-discriminatory care: decisions are dependent only on factors relevant to the patient's medical condition, values and wishes

9. Transparency and accountability: decisions are fairly made and the decision-making process is clear to all concerned and accurately recorded

10. Hope for the one suffering and loved ones, sustained by reassurances from health professionals that all that can be done to achieve a peaceful end of life will be done

5. What Ethics is Not

5.1 Ethics is More than the Law

Laws are rules that govern certain human activities which are prescribed by a constitution (in Ireland), legislators and courts and the court system. They are binding on everyone and are enforced by penalties, such as fines or imprisonment. Law and ethics overlap because many illegal actions are, often, also unethical, e.g. killing the innocent or stealing. In turn, many ethical actions are also obligatory in law, e.g. paying taxes.

But there are also important differences between the law and ethics. For example, there are many actions, such as infidelity, lying and cheating, which would be considered unethical but are not usually enforced by law. Equally, there are many ethically praiseworthy actions such as being kind, saving a drowning person and working for charity that we are not legally obliged to perform.

Laws and ethics may also conflict: people might judge laws such as those permitting euthanasia to be unethical, while they might view legally prohibited actions, such as abortion, as ethically acceptable. The law can also lag behind the moral standards of a society, or it may be used as a tool by a ruling class or dictator – for example, in some societies, laws may enshrine racism or discriminate against women. When this happens, social reformers usually appeal to more general ethical standards of equality or justice in order to have such laws repealed. In short, ethics and law overlap, but ethics offers a set of tools and values against which the appropriateness of laws can be evaluated.

5.2 Ethics is More than Religion

Different religions offer moral training, e.g. the Sermon on the Mount or the teachings of Confucius. In addition, religious leaders remind their followers of values, such as generosity and compassion, and sometimes provide good role models, e.g. Gandhi or Christ. Moreover, many eminent moral thinkers (such as Immanuel Kant [eighteenth-century German philosopher] and Charles Taylor [contemporary Canadian philosopher]) are also theists who critically explore the faultline between ethical theory and moral theology.

However, the texts and teachings of the various religions are ambiguous and the interpretations of their leaders often differ on important issues such as war, family planning and the role of women in society. As such, judgements have to be made as to what weight to assign them. This is all the more apparent in pluralist societies where individuals, not simply Catholics, Protestants, Hindus or Jews, must share more commonly held values that appeal to people of different and no religious persuasion. In short, ethics and religion overlap, but ethics appeals to more general rules and values than are expressed by religion and does not rely for sanction or legitimacy on the existence of a deity or transcendent being.

5.3 Ethics is More than Popular Opinion

Popular opinion is the view that is perceived to be generally held in a society. It is determined by the media and/or social analysts on the basis of surveys, polls, and interviews or the responses to radio or television programmes. Ethics and popular opinion may overlap, in that popular opinion expresses views on moral issues and it may be a useful indicator of important social concerns

But there is also much disagreement. Popular opinion is considered to be unsatisfactory as a means of determining what the right thing to do is in any circumstance, for a number of reasons. The main one of these is that popular opinion is often volatile, reactionary and unreflective, e.g. the majority of people who are polled immediately after a harrowing case of child abuse and murder may call for the, arguably unethical, death penalty. A second reason why popular opinion is not a satisfactory determination of right action is that determining popular opinion is fraught with difficulties – which poll/survey/interview counts as truly representative? In short, popular opinion and ethics may overlap, but ethics is more reflective and critical and appeals to more general rules and values than are expressed by popular opinion.

5.4 Ethics is More than Professional Codes

Professional codes, such as the Medical Council's (2009) *Guide to Professional Conduct and Ethics for Registered Medical Practitioners* and the An Bord Altranais (2000) *Code of Professional Conduct for Each Nurse and Midwife*, express the ethical and professional standards of professionals, such as doctors and nurses. They are inherently ethical in that they express the aims of these professions and they enumerate the ethical obligations that these bodies of health professionals expect of their members. Ideally, codes function to help professionals in deciding what is the ethically acceptable course of action to take when ethically worrying challenges arise (e.g. issues concerning patients' rights or safety). In turn, these professional bodies, through their Fitness to Practice Committees, may penalise any member who is deemed to have failed in their professional duties.

However, while codes are themselves ethical in nature, they are inevitably incomplete; they cannot provide precise guidance for every single situation that may arise. Moreover, some professionals and patients may disagree with the duties imposed in certain circumstances (see Module 4 and 6 for a discussion of the views of the Irish Medical Council and An Bord Altranais and the Irish Supreme Court in relation to the status of Artificial Nutrition and

Hydration). In short, ethics and codes of ethics overlap, but ethics takes a broader view and offers tools that enable individuals to critically consider the aims, duties and implications for practice of their professional codes.

5.5 Ethics is More than Hospital Policy

Hospitals and other clinical settings usually have a range of policies on issues such as patient confidentiality, informed consent, resuscitation and the allocation of resources. Like professional codes, it is reasonable to assume that these policies are ethically sound, but this is not always the case. For example, hospitals may have policies which deny access to certain procedures, such as heart transplants and infertility treatment, to groups of people on the basis of their age or family status, and this might be considered ethically dubious or, at least, debatable. In short, while hospital policies may be ethical in general, health professionals need to take a critical stance in relation to the obligations and constraints these policies place on them as employees.

5.6 Ethics is More than Authority

Doing what you are told just because you have been told to do it has always been viewed as ethically suspect. This is because, while people in authority may often mean well and often give ethically sound orders and requests, this is not always the case. That obedience is not an excuse for harmful actions was confirmed in law in the Nuremberg trials, when doctors, nurses, guards and collaborators were found culpable for their part in Nazi war crimes. Similarly, health professionals are ethically, professionally and legally obliged to question instructions and requests that put patient safety and/or rights at risk. No matter the source of authority, individual health professionals are responsible, and held accountable, for their own actions. In short, while figures in authority, such as managers, consultants and directors of nursing may mean well and may direct health professionals to do the right thing most of the time, individuals are, nevertheless, accountable for what they do themselves.

6. Ethical Theories

An ethical (or moral) theory is an effort to interpret moral life and moral intuitions in a more or less formalised way.

6.1 Traditional Ethical Theories

Traditional ethical theories, such as Utilitarianism, Deontology and Virtue Theory, are termed 'traditional' because they have been part of the canon of moral philosophy for many centuries.

6.1.1 Utilitarianism

Utilitarianism – sometimes referred to as 'consequentialism' – is a moral theory which emphasises the consequences or outcomes of an act rather than the act itself. Good outcomes or consequences are those that yield overall benefits, pleasures and happiness for the greatest number of persons affected by an action. Good outcomes of actions also diminish overall suffering or harm. Any action that produces benefit, pleasure or well-being is a 'useful' action – useful as conducive to the greater good.

The choices or actions that contribute to maximal happiness or well-being have instrumental value. Instrumental values refer to something useful or important for achieving some goal or purpose or as a means to some end.

The utilitarian goals of maximising pleasure, happiness or well-being are contentious. There is no consensus about the meanings of these valued goals or human ends. It seems clear that different people view pleasure, happiness and well-being with considerable disagreement. Diverse cultures might disagree even more profoundly. The nineteenth-century philosopher, John Stuart Mill, defined in his 'happiness theory' an understanding of happiness which he believed would be universally accepted :

> *According to the Greatest Happiness Principle, the ultimate end, with reference to and for the sake of which all other things are desirable (whether our own good or that of other people), is an existence exempt as far as possible from pain, and as rich as possible in enjoyments, both in point of quantity and quality* (J.S. Mill, [1859], 1991, p.142)

The ultimate end sought by the utilitarian is a life described by Mill, rich in many pleasures of intellect, emotion and sensibility, and spared in terms of suffering and pain. Both quantity of rich experiences and quality (range and depth) of experiences mattered in Mill's account of utilitarianism.

Utilitarians do not focus on the importance of motives for choosing when locating the moral quality of an action. Almost any motive is acceptable for a choice which delivers a positive outcome and best overall results. Saving a drowning man is always good, whatever the motivation of the rescuer. I might be doing this to get my picture in the paper and maybe get some reward from the man I save, yet this doesn't take away from the good result. Feeding starving people who have no subsistence is a good act, and it matters not whether one's motive is primarily to get nominated for the Nobel Peace Prize or whether it arises from a deep obligation to suffering humanity.

Utilitarian theory is a prospective moral theory. It is forward-looking, going beyond the choices of the individual to the outcomes of those choices. Utilitarians think that the consequences of an action are the effects which the individual could have reasonably foreseen, on the basis of information or understandings available to him or her.

Three-Step Action Formula

Utilitarianism might be construed as offering a three-step action formula for action:

1. On the basis of what I know, I must project the consequences of each alternative option open to me (e.g. taking different kinds of actions or taking no action).

2. Calculate how much happiness, or balance of happiness over unhappiness, is likely to be produced by anticipated consequences of each action or none.

3. Select that action which, on balance, will produce the greatest amount of happiness for the greatest number of people affected (see Yeo and Moorhouse,1996, p.45).

6.1.2 Deontology

What makes a 'right' act right? The utilitarian or consequentialist answer to this question is that it is the good outcome of an act which makes it right. Moral rightness or wrongness is calculated by determining the extent to which the action promotes values such as pleasure, well-being, happiness, etc. To this extent, the end justifies the means. In many respects, deontological moral theory is diametrically the opposite of utilitarianism.

The German philosopher Immanuel Kant (1724–1804) is identified with the moral theory known as deontology. Kant was adamantly opposed to the idea that the outcome of an action could determine its moral worth. For deontologists, it is not consequences which determine the rightness or wrongness of an act but, rather, the intention of the person who carries out the act. The emphasis is on the correctness of the action, regardless of the possible benefits or harm it might produce. Deontologists maintain that there are some moral obligations which are absolutely binding, no matter what consequences are produced.

As a 'rationalist', Kant believed that we can use our reason to work out a consistent set of moral principles which apply in all possible situations and cannot be over-ridden. One way of describing these deontological moral principles is to say that they are 'non-negotiable' and cannot be argued away by persuasion or counter-reasons.

Unlike utilitarianism, according to which the value of moral actions is determined by their instrumentality for achieving the greatest overall benefit, deontology regards good choices as intrinsically valuable, that is, valuable in and of themselves. Whether or not they bring about good consequences is not essential to their moral quality. Kant aimed to establish a fundamental point about morality: that there is such a thing as non-negotiable morality; in other words, there is a domain of laws which apply to our conduct and from which we cannot exempt ourselves. The laws governing our conduct are derived from a supreme or highest principle, which Kant calls the categorical imperative; this is a command that admits of no exceptions and must be obeyed by all of us, insofar as we consider ourselves rational beings.

One Step Action Formula

Kant formulates the categorical imperative in different ways but it is easiest understood as a universal rule which tells us how we ought to live if we are to live an ethically good life:

1. Act in such a way that I could imagine all other persons doing the same thing in the same circumstances.

The challenging test for us when we choose to do something is that we are required to act, not out of self-interest, but because we believe it is the right act to do for anyone in the same situation. So if we are deciding to lie in order to escape a difficult task, then we must be ready to allow everyone else to lie for the same reason. If we are stealing rare lilies from our neighbour's garden to bring to a friend in hospital, we need to be ready for our neighbour in turn to steal rare roses from our garden for her friend. Kant believed that this requirement of universality places necessary constraints on our conduct.

Here it is clear that Kant does not entirely ignore consequences. We take them into account in order to consider our choices. We ask: what would be the consequences if everyone acted on the principle I want to follow? So to answer that, we need to imagine the consequences for our world if everyone acted in a manner which is contrary to the duties spelled out above. We cannot discount consequences, but good outcomes will never make an immoral action moral. Our motives – whether we act with a 'good will' according to the categorical imperative – determine whether we are persons of moral character or not.

Deontological morality is grounded in human motivation, and not merely in consequences. Even a person with a mean and bitter disposition who has to work hard to be sympathetic towards suffering people can, nevertheless, with effort, exercise their will and do the right thing in spite of their negative inclinations. They do the right thing, not because they will be praised or rewarded or gain immortal life, but simply because it is the right thing to do. A Kantian deontologist cautions us to be wary of our natural inclinations – whether they are negative or positive. Because we are kindly or compassionate by temperament does not give us an edge on being moral. It may make it easier to do good for other people, but that is not the yardstick Kant uses. People who have negative inclinations by temperament are considered much more praiseworthy if they succeed in doing the right thing!

Kant was a rigorous moralist and a religious believer. However, he argued that religion and the possible rewards of immortality could not form part of his argument that morally praiseworthy actions must have universal worth. We cannot presuppose that the presence of certain religious beliefs will make people moral. Nor can we rely on the presence of good inclinations, feelings or sentiments in people to make them moral. We need to look to the disciplined will.

Before concluding this discussion of deontology, it is important to note that deontologists are alive and well today. Religious believers would often consider themselves as deontologists, in their acceptance of some actions as categorically right and others wrong. The religious belief might, additionally, appeal to revelation for an understanding of which actions are right and which are to be avoided. The often uncompromising positions held by religious believers may not reflect stubbornness or closed-mindedness, but may instead demonstrate the Kantian conviction that consequences – no matter how good – cannot make evil actions good. A review of some of the positions presented in Modules 2 and 5 illustrate the contemporary deontological perspective most clearly.

6.1.3 Virtue Theory

The ancient Greek philosopher Aristotle (384–322 BC) first wrote a detailed discussion of virtue morality in the Nichomachean Ethics. 'Virtus' he understood as strength. Correspondingly, specific virtues are seen as strengths of character. But many years after Aristotle's death, virtue theory came to be over-shadowed by the development of utilitarianism and deontology.

In the past fifty years, however, virtue theory has resurfaced as a major moral theory. But why is that so? Virtue ethics has been restated and reinvigorated in the years since 1958 by philosophers such as Philippa Foot, Alasdair MacIntyre and Elizabeth Anscombe. They and many others became disillusioned with the promises of mainstream theories.

They argue that how we ought to live could be much more adequately answered by a virtue-based theory than in terms of calculating consequences or obeying rules.

Moral Virtue: Centrality of motives

A virtue is a trait of character which is socially valued and a moral virtue is a trait which is morally valued. Courage might be a socially valued trait, but it only becomes moral courage if the context is a moral one. Moral virtue is a disposition to act, or a habit of acting in accordance with moral ideals, principles or obligations (Pence, 1991).

Aristotle distinguished between external performance and internal state. This is the difference between right action and proper motive. An action can be right without being virtuous, he said, but the action can be virtuous only if performed on the basis of the right state of mind of the person.

Virtue, then, is closely aligned with motives. We do care how persons are motivated. Someone who gives donations to mental health research and is motivated by personal concern or sympathy for suffering people meets with approval, while someone acting the same way in order to be able to proclaim generosity as a feature of their character would not obtain our endorsement. Persons who are properly motivated – not just in carrying out a single action but by disposition or habit, persons of virtue – don't simply follow rules, but have a morally relevant motive and desire to act as they do. Virtue theorists think that basic instruction and an emphasis on the right motives and desires will guide us not only in terms of what to do but who to be (Frankena, 1998, pp.291–6).

The person of morally good disposition is properly motivated. To be properly motivated, says Aristotle, one must experience appropriate feelings. Aristotle explains:

> *We may even go so far as to state that the man [woman] who does not enjoy performing noble actions is not a good man [woman] at all. Nobody would call a person just who does not enjoy acting justly, nor generous who does not enjoy generous actions, and so on.*
> (Aristotle, 1955, p.42)

Aristotelian virtue theory cautions us away from a negative view of morality that mainly requires us to do what we really don't feel like doing. Anne Thomson speaks of the critical role of emotions in developing a moral disposition of fair-mindedness. This focus on the centrality of cultivating proper feelings and emotions as ingredients of virtuous action stands in stark contrast to the suspiciousness about feelings associated with Kantian deontology (see Thomson, 1999, pp.143–52).

Character is More Important than Conformity to Rules

Virtue theorists think that their views supplement deontology and utilitarianism by offering a more comprehensive moral theory, which acknowledges our common intuitions that motives do make a difference to the quality of our actions and that appropriate feelings facilitate virtuous behaviour.

Writers in the field of healthcare ethics suggest that efforts to replace the virtuous judgements of professionals with rules, codes or procedures will not result in better decisions and actions. For example, some believe that, rather than always appealing to government regulations or international conventions to protect subjects in research, the most reliable protection is a researcher with a character marked by informed conscientiousness, responsible sensibility, and compassion. The thesis is that good habits of character are more important than conformity to rules, and that such good habits are most likely to lead to behaviour consistent with rules.

The position is that virtues should be inculcated and cultivated over time through educational interactions, role modelling, moral mentoring, and the like. Gregory Pence contends that the right kinds of desires, feelings and motives are the best protectors of patient well-being (Pence, 1991). Almost any healthcare professional can successfully evade a system of rules. Pence argues that we should create a climate in which healthcare professionals desire by virtue of strong habit not to abuse their subjects. The educational process for healthcare professionals provides a context for modelling the virtues of good nurses, good doctors and good allied health professionals. Where adequate role models are lacking, little progress can be made by further exhortations to become a 'good (virtuous) nurse', or a 'good (virtuous) doctor'.

This last point stresses the argument that we do not make moral decisions as isolated persons in a social vacuum. It is rather in families, schools or communities that natural affection, shared concerns, spontaneous sympathies and expectations for the virtues arise.

6.1.4 Compatibility of Virtues and Principles

The rule-governed theories of utilitarianism and deontology are not at odds with virtue theory; rather, they are compatible and mutually reinforcing. Persons of good moral character sometimes have difficulty discerning what is right and recognise that they need principles, rules and ideals to help them choose right or good acts.

One often cannot act virtuously unless one makes judgements about the best ways to manifest sympathy, desire and the like. The virtues need principles and rules to regulate and supplement them. As Aristotle suggests, ethics involves judgements like those in medicine: Principles guide us to actions, but we still need to assess a situation and formulate an appropriate response. This assessment and response flows from character and training as much as from principles.

(Beauchamp and Childress, 1994, p.67)

If we are to progress as moral agents and justify our actions in the eyes of those affected, this need to explain and justify requires that we translate our virtuous claims into an explanation of the values, duties or principles on which we base those claims. To do this, we may need to say why we consider it compassionate behaviour to lie, why we believe that it is fair to break the confidence of patients, or why we think it is loyal to keep silent when speaking out would correct wrong-doing. This requirement to justify our moral decisions reveals the intricate connection between virtue theory and the rule-governed theories discussed earlier.

6.2 Contemporary Ethical Theories

While utilitarianism, deontology and virtue theory have been in place in the canon of moral philosophy for centuries, they have not remained fixed and static as theories. Volumes have been written which critique elements of these theories, sharpening them for greater clarity and attuning them more to the fullness of human living. In addition, insights into moral living come in fresh forms, breathing new life into the traditional moral canon. This is the case with contemporary ethical theories such as principlism, narrative ethics and feminist ethics. In these we find new insights that attempt a number of tasks:

1. To offer developments of, and improvements on, essential features of traditional theories.

2. To fill in the dimensions of human living that were often omitted or understated in traditional theorising.

3. To acknowledge that the challenges of moral development require that we move from a realm of moral abstractions to concrete situations. This allows us to see whether or how much the resources of moral theory help to guide our decision making.

6.2.1 Principlism

What is known as the principlist approach to ethical decision making has dominated Western healthcare ethics for the last twenty years. It emerged with the publication of several well-known texts in the 1970s and '80s. One of these was the Belmont Report which identified basic principles that would underlie and guide the regulation of research involving human subjects (National Commission for the Protection of Human Subjects of Biomedical and Behavioral Research, 1979). Three books published around the same time outlined and defended a principlist ethical framework, written by Tom Beauchamp and James Childress (1979), Robert Veatch (1981) and H. Tristram Engelhardt (1986).

Of these three, the account developed by Beauchamp and Childress in their book *Principles of Biomedical Ethics* is the best known. This principlist model (hereafter called the PBE model) is an ethical decision-making process which negotiates between fundamental principles on the one hand and the unique nature of specific moral situations on the other.

These principles oblige the healthcare professionals to behave in certain ways in relation to patients.

1. The principle of autonomy obliges healthcare professionals to respect the views, choices and actions of the individuals in their care. (See Module 4)

2. The principle of nonmaleficence obliges healthcare professionals not to harm patients. (See Modules 5 and 6)

3. The principle of beneficence obliges healthcare professionals to act for the benefit of, or in the interests of, patients. (See Modules 5 and 6)

4. The principle of justice obliges healthcare professionals to treat people in their care equally and to ensure that resources are distributed fairly.

A good deal of the *Principles of Biomedical Ethics* text is taken up with an analysis and discussion of each of the four principles in terms of their nature and scope. In particular, the specific rules which are supported by these principles and which permit, prohibit or require particular kinds of action are delineated. These include rules governing truth-telling, confidentiality and informed consent (Beauchamp and Childress, 2001, pp.57–112).

What is special about the four principles, according to Beauchamp and Childress, is their universal or objective nature. These principles, according to Beauchamp and Childress, have been drawn from a 'common morality', beyond tradition, and beyond the vagaries of individual character and culture, the set of norms that 'all morally serious persons share' (2001, p.3). This common morality 'contains moral norms that bind all persons in all places; no norms are more basic in the moral life', and the notion of international human rights is invoked as an example of such universal norms (2001, p.3). Having grounded their four principles, they justify their particular choice of principles by pointing out that these four have been presupposed by traditional ethical theories and medical codes throughout history.

The most immediate way to decide on the merits of a proposed course of action, on the Principles of Biomedical Ethics (PBE) model, is to determine whether or not that course of action obeys the moral rules derived from the four principles. For example, on this view, a healthcare professional might consider that it is, generally, morally required to provide a patient with information about their illness because this action obeys the moral rule 'Tell the truth' which is, in turn, derived from the principle 'Respect patient autonomy'.

In morally difficult situations, however, where there is a conflict between principles or between principles and particular judgements, the PBE model stipulates that none of the principles is privileged. In any given situation, each principle must be specified and weighed relative to the particular context in which it is applied, and informed by generally accepted background theories of human nature and moral life. Following John Rawls, this weighing and balancing is described as a process of reflective equilibrium and the principles are described as *prima facie* rather than absolute (Beauchamp and Childress, 2001, p.398). This expresses the idea that any principle is, *on first impression*, morally obligatory, but that it may be modified or overridden in certain situations.

In the case of Joanna, the patient with Alzheimer's in Case 5 of Module 2, for example, a nurse might initially believe that telling Joanna the truth about the death of her son might be the morally correct thing to do. However, on consideration of the concrete circumstances of the patient, she might reconsider. In this case, it could be argued that it is her particular judgement in relation to what Joanna might find meaningful which prompts her to reconsider whether the principle of autonomy, or some other rule, such as nonmaleficence, should be the focus here.

On this understanding, the processes of moral deliberation are akin to scientific processes: plausible beliefs and possible decisions are considered and accepted, rejected and modified on the basis of reflection and experience. Also, analogous to the scientific goal of achieving theoretical consistency and unity, the aim of reflective equilibrium is to unify all one's moral beliefs and background commitments.

In positive terms, the PBE model provides a method of supporting ethical decisions that has a strong justificatory force. Put simply, on this view, the force of the imperative 'Respect autonomy' derives from its grounding in universally accepted norms and not in the subjective viewpoint or intuition of the individual professional.

Moreover, even in situations of doubt and uncertainty, such as in the case of Joanna in Module 2, the deliberative process which comes into play appeals to reasoning strategies and goals which are also considered objective, not intuitive or subjective. In addition, the course of action that would be considered the most successful, on this view, would be one which manages to meet as many of the relevant principles as possible.

The challenge in Joanna's case is to respect her autonomy, while at the same time acting in her best interests.

6.2.2 Narrative ethics

While different shades of principlism have dominated the healthcare landscape in the last twenty years, an increasing number of theorists have begun to turn their attention to alternative approaches to describing and understanding the various elements of moral life (McCarthy, 2003). One such approach deploys narrative concepts and methodologies drawn from literary criticism and philosophy as tools of moral understanding and assessment. In common with contemporary thinkers in other disciplines (e.g. anthropology, philosophy, cognitive psychology and history) who have turned their attention to narratives, narrativists in the healthcare arena argue that the first person narrative, or personal story, is a rich medium for qualitative data about the unique lives of individual people. Further, for some of these theorists, the narrative is not only an important form of communication, it is also a means of making human life, and specifically the moral life, intelligible. While they deploy narrative tools in different ways, all of these thinkers are engaged in 'narrative ethics'.

Martha Nussbaum (1992), for example, views literature as a vast resource of moral knowledge and a means of sensitising people to the responsibilities, obligations and challenges of a full moral life.

Alternatively, the narrative approaches of Albert Jonsen and Stephen Toulmin (1988) and John Arras (1991) take a casuistic turn and resolve ethical dilemmas by comparing each new situation with others and with paradigm cases. These authors argue that local, contingent moral rules and maxims to guide action can be derived from paying attention to the morally relevant similarities and differences between cases.

More recently, Rita Charon (1994) has suggested that our understanding of healthcare situations will be greatly enhanced if we pay attention to their narrative elements, e.g. the function of the narrator – who tells the story? – the development of plot – how the story unfolds – and the relationship with the audience – who hears and interprets the story? In addition to supporting Charon's view, Tod Chambers (1999) has sparked a lively debate in the healthcare ethics community by arguing that the task of reporting cases is, itself, not a neutral enterprise. This is because, he argues, the process of describing any set of events involves making decisions about which pieces of information to include or exclude and making choices about the way different facts are presented. For example, take any of the modules in this framework and consider how the case scenarios are narrated: from the patient's, professional's or family's point of view? Or from an observer point of view? Consider the difference that this might make to what is left in and left out of the story that is told. Because narrative ethics is in the early stages of development, there is, as yet, no ready-to-hand canonical position that best expresses its central tenets. Even so, what follows is a rough sketch of a plausible and defensible account of narrative ethics. It is also one which highlights the tensions between narrative ethics and principlism and exposes the congruities and incongruities between these supposedly competing positions.

On the narrative view, when ethically challenging situations arise, it is the whole journey of an individual's life as he or she conceives it which is privileged (Nelson 1997, p.2001). Howard Brody, for example, sees the practice of healthcare as in part 'a storytelling enterprise' (Brody, 1987, p.xiii). For Brody, actions are made meaningful in the context of an individual life story. As such, it is difficult to isolate any given decision or choice, to uncouple it from the whole person who acts and evaluates it in terms of abstract and general rules. In healthcare settings, this means that the patient's own account, where it is possible to hear it – of their illness, their preferences, their needs – is considered profoundly important. However, not any tall tale will do and personal stories are tested against various criteria, such as the stories of others and the medical chart.

This idea of testing personal narratives against various criteria can be likened to the way in which the principlist model tests its principles through the application of the process of reflective equilibrium. In the case of the PBE model, the four principles are *prima facie* privileged, but may be subsequently modified. On the narrative view, it is first-person narratives which are *prima facie* privileged; however, like principles, they can be challenged and modified in the process of a 'narrative reflective equilibrium'. Recalling the Socratic ideal, Paul Ricoeur describes the final story or account of a life that emerges from such evaluation as 'the fruit of an examined life' (1988, pp.246–47).

In recent years, a narrative approach of this kind has contributed to discussion and debate in relation to surrogate decision making in end-of-life situations. For example, it informs one of the recent recommendations of the US Council on Ethical and Judicial Affairs, which suggests that, when it comes to making decisions for incompetent patients, one of the tasks of a surrogate decision maker is to consider 'how the patient constructed his or her identity or life story' in order to enable a decision about a proposed course of treatment which continues the story 'in a manner that is meaningful and consistent with the patient's self-conception' (Council on Ethical and Judicial Affairs, 2001). In addition, the Council argues that it is precisely the fact that a number of different options might be consistent with a person's life story which makes the narrative approach so attractive, because it avoids having to predict only a single course of action as compatible and, therefore, morally acceptable.

Finally, the task of moral justification for narrative ethics is not, primarily, a unifying one. Rather, its focus is on acknowledging and embracing the multiplicity of – often contested

– meanings that are available in any given situation. What is key for this narrativist account is the idea that many different voices and readings of moral situations and individual lives are possible. And, generally, narrativists focus less on trying to reduce competing perspectives to a commonly shared view and more on involving as many people as possible in the dialogue. Anne Hudson Jones summarises this view as:

In ideal form, narrative ethics recognizes the primacy of the patient's story but encourages multiple voices to be heard and multiple stories to be brought forth by all those whose lives will be involved in the resolution of a case. Patient, physician, family, healthcare professionals, friend, and social worker, for example, may all share their stories in a dialogical chorus that can offer the best chance of respecting all the persons involved in a case. (Hudson Jones, 1998, p.222)

In turn, for narrativists, relational virtues such as empathetic listening and support are privileged. In the course of such privileging, these virtues are reworked to acknowledge and accommodate the narrative view that, in some senses, difference is irreducible. For example, Howard Brody radically reconceives the moral demands of 'empathy' in the following passage:

In a culture that prizes autonomy and independence, we may fondly imagine that most people are whole and intact, unlike those who suffer from disease […] Charity tends to assume that I start off whole and remain whole while I offer aid to the suffering. Empathy and testimony require a full awareness of my own vulnerability and radical incompleteness; to be with the suffering as a cohuman presence will require that I change […] Today I listen to the testimony of someone's suffering; tomorrow that person (or someone else) will be listening to my testimony of my own. Today I help to heal the sufferer by listening to and validating her story; tomorrow that sufferer will have helped to heal me, as her testimony becomes a model I can use to better make sense of and deal with my own suffering (Brody, 1987, pp.21–2)

On Brody's view, the demand of empathy does not require us to 'step into another's shoes' in order to understand their pain. It does not presuppose that it is ever possible to fully understand another's pain. The other person is always 'other' to us, their difference persists, resisting assimilation under the umbrella of mutual understanding. Instead, empathy demands that we bear witness to our own vulnerability and lack so that we stand, not as whole to part, or healthy to ill, but as a 'cohuman presence'. On this view, the healthcare professional cannot offer patients the reassurance that they know and understand them, only the acknowledgement that they have listened and heard. On this view too, they cannot be untouched by a patient's pain and vulnerability, there is professional engagement, not detachment.

6.2.3 Feminist Ethics

Feminist ethics considers the impact of gender roles and gendered understandings on the moral lives of individual human beings and draws attention to the power and power differentials inherent in moral relationships at individual, societal and organisational levels. Feminist ethics, in short, is the application of feminist theory to understanding the ethical realm: it critiques traditional ethical frameworks from a feminist perspective such as those already discussed: deontology, utilitarianism and principlism. (McCarthy, Murphy & Loughrey, 2008).

The diversity of theoretical starting points when tackling the subject of ethics makes it difficult to identify or talk about a single 'feminist perspective' in ethics. However, what each of these approaches share is a common concern with the marginalisation and disempowerment of women in sexist societies and a transformative concern to change those societies for the better (Murphy, 2004). In addition, as Sharon Murphy points out:

Given their sensitivity to the oppression of women, feminist perspectives also often share a sensitivity to the oppression and marginalisation of other social groupings based on age, race, class, sexual orientation, etc. With this sensitivity comes an interest in feminist ethics in analysing how moral authority and the status and power that goes with it has traditionally been constructed, aligned and divvied out, moral authority and moral agency having traditionally been inequitably distributed among different social groups, with women in particular being deemed less morally capable than men. (Murphy, 2004)

In general, feminist ethics has widened the scope of healthcare ethics to include consideration of the social, cultural and political dimensions of moral decision making in healthcare settings. Susan Sherwin makes this point in the following way:

[M]edical and other health care practices should be reviewed not just with regard to their effects on the patients who are directly involved but also with respect to the patterns of discrimination, exploitation, and dominance that surround them. (Sherwin, 1992, pp.4–5)

Contemporary moral philosopher Margaret Urban Walker (1997, 1998) critiques ethical frameworks such as deontology and principlism, which, in her view, represent morality as a set of compact codes of impersonal statements guiding the actions of individuals. She replaces these with a moral framework that represents morality as a process rather than a set of prescriptions or outcomes. For Walker, morality and politics cannot be pulled apart and individuals are not the bounded integrated decision makers that traditional moral approaches seem to presuppose. Rather, who we are and how we decide upon a course of action at any given time must be understood contextually. Morality, for Walker, is a socially embedded process which determines what is morally significant, who is assigned responsibility for decision making and who is permitted and enabled to participate (Walker, 1998).

In short, feminist ethics:

- recognises human interdependency and vulnerability
- pays attention to the needs of concrete particular individuals in their specific situations
- validates traditionally feminine virtues such as nurturance and empathy
- affirms the importance of being actively concerned with the welfare of others
- widens the scope of healthcare ethics to include consideration of the social, cultural and political dimensions of moral decision making in healthcare settings. (See discussion on Relational Autonomy in Module 4)

7. Module 1 Further Discussion

7.1 The ethical map

The subject of ethics can be divided into three broad categories:

7.1.1 Meta-ethics:

- Examines the meaning of moral terms and concepts and the relationships between these concepts.

- Explores where moral values, such as 'personhood' and 'autonomy', come from.

- Considers the difference between moral values and other kinds of values.

- Examines the way in which moral claims are justified.

Meta-ethics poses questions of the following kind: What do we mean by the claim 'life is sacred'? Are moral claims a matter of personal view, religious belief or social standard or are they objective in some sense? If they are objective, what make them so? Is there a link between human psychology and the moral claims that humans make?

7.1.2 Normative Ethics:

- Offers theories or accounts of the best way to live. These theories evaluate actions in a systematic way, i.e. they may focus on outcomes or duties or motivation as a means of justifying human conduct.

- Includes ethical theories or approaches such as utilitarianism, deontology, virtue ethics, principlism, narrative ethics and feminist ethics.

Normative ethics poses questions of the following kind: Are there general principles or rules that we could follow which distinguish between right and wrong? Or are there virtues and/or relationships that we can nurture in order to behave well?

7.1.3 Applied Ethics:

- Applies the insights of ethics to social practices.

- For example, environmental ethics considers issues relevant to the relationship between human beings and the natural world, e.g. global warming, animal welfare, limited resources.

- Healthcare ethics is the branch of applied ethics which applies ethical reasoning and standards to the world of healthcare and to the ethical challenges which healthcare professionals, allied professionals, patients and families engage with.

Applied ethics poses questions of the following kind: What should I do in this particular situation? How should we organise society? What do healthcare professionals owe patients in their care? What do humans owe animals and the environment?

While these might be described as three branches of ethics, they often overlap in the course of deliberating about ethical challenges. Anyone with an interest in the issues that arise in end-of-life care – whether they are professionals working in the area or patients or their families – may find themselves doing some work in applied ethics. This is because they are concerned about specific ethically challenging situations in healthcare settings and, perhaps, the specific duties of their profession or family role. However, in addressing these concerns, they may also have worries about how to evaluate their own actions or the actions of others (normative ethics). They may need to explore the meaning and the implications of particular ethical claims, for example they may worry about the extent of their obligation to preserve life if they hold the view that life is sacred (meta-ethics).

8. Module 1 Summary Learning Guides

8.1 A Good Death and Dying

- Death is a fact of life, but beliefs about death and its significance and value are socially constructed.

- Culture and religion are key mediums for understanding the boundary between life and death.

- Recognising cultural diversity implies the need to challenge basic assumptions and to recognise and respect the different values of patients in the illness and dying processes.

- Individuals also differ in the values they hold about dying and death. Research indicates that many people are concerned about family and loved ones being without pain and being able to communicate.

- If there is no universal agreement about what a 'good death' consists of, there is some consensus on the core features of good end-of-life care.

8.2 Defining Features of Utilitarian Moral Theory:

- The moral quality of our decisions is determined entirely by the beneficial consequences following on these decisions.

- Good consequences are understood broadly to mean outcomes such as pleasure, health, well-being, justice, happiness, satisfaction of preferences, etc.

- Moral responsibility is both positive and negative – covering both our actions and our failure to act.

  Motives as morally neutral

- Motives for actions are not relevant for the moral evaluation of that action.

- Motives are simply instrumental means for achieving good ends. Ends justify means. How ought we to live our lives?

- We ought always, in our choices, to work to maximise good consequences and minimise undesirable outcomes.

8.3 Defining Features of Deontological Moral Theory:

- Actions are intrinsically right or wrong depending on whether right principles motivate them.
- Consequences must be considered when making a choice, but they can never be decisive in measuring the moral quality of an action.
- Natural inclinations (positive or negative) might make moral behaviour more or less difficult but they are not part of the moral appraisal of a person.

Motives for acting:

- The motive one has for acting is morally decisive.
- The moral motive for any action is to choose always out of respect for the moral law.

How ought we to live?

- We ought to work conscientiously to become persons of good will.
- A good will observes the rule of universality.

8.4 Principlism claims that:

- Basic commonly shared principles – autonomy, nonmaleficence, beneficence and justice – and the specific action-guiding rules that are derived from them are central to the ethical decision-making process in healthcare situations.
- In any given healthcare situation, any decision or course of action is morally justified if it is consistent with the relevant principles, rules, background theories and judgements in particular situations.
- The success of any chosen course of action, on the part of the health professional, can be measured by the degree to which it achieves an overall cohesion of all of the elements of the decision-making process.

8.5 Narrative Ethics claims that:

- Every moral situation is unique and unrepeatable and its meaning cannot be fully captured by appealing to law-like universal principles.

- In any given healthcare situation, any decision or course of action is justified in terms of its fit with the individual life story or stories of the patient. The credibility of these, in turn, is determined on the basis of narrative reflective equilibrium.

- The objective of narrative reflective equilibrium is not necessarily to unify moral beliefs and commitments but to open up dialogue, challenge received views and explore tensions between individual and shared meanings.

8.6 Feminist Ethics

- is the application of feminist theory to understanding the ethical realm as one in which women are treated as moral equals.

- considers the impact of gender roles and gendered understandings on the moral lives of individual human beings, especially the moral lives of women.

- is sensitive to the power/power differentials and politics inherent in moral relationships.

- highlights the contextual socially embedded nature of moral decision making.

9. Module 1 Activities

9.1 Consider the list of key elements of good end-of-life care:

Are there other elements of a 'good dying' that you think should be included? Explain why.

9.2 Read again the description of what ethics is and ethics is not:

Consider the examples of statements in the table below and categorise them as one (or more) of the following:

- Law

- Hospital policy

- Professional codes

- Public opinion

- Authority

- Religious belief

State also whether you think the statement is

- ethical, i.e. it involves doing the right thing

- unethical, i.e. it involves doing the wrong thing

- non-ethical, i.e. it does not have ethical content; it does not refer to ethical values or reasoning.

You might find it helpful to discuss the examples with a friend or colleague.

Statements	Law?	Policy?	Codes?	Opinion?	Authority?	Religious?	Ethical?	Un-ethical?	Non-ethical?
a. Competent over 16s can consent to medical treatment and care									
b. Cough mixture A is a more effective expectorant than cough mixture B									
c. Healthcare professionals have a duty to intervene in an emergency									
d. The Patients' Charter informs patients about their rights									
e. Patients ought to be informed if they have a serious illness									
f. Consultants' orders should be followed									
g. People have a right to refuse treatment even if it results in their death									
h. Hospital environments should be clean and aesthetically pleasing									
i. 80% of doctors agree that cannabis is therapeutic, therefore it should be legalised									
j. All human life is sacred									

(adapted from Gallagher, 2005)

You may find that many of the statements can be categorised under more than one heading. For example, a) the issue of consent for over 16s is addressed in Irish law but it might also be expressed in hospital policy. You may also consider that it is an ethically good thing to respect the treatment choices of over 16s.

On the other hand, b) the claim that cough mixture A is a more effective expectorant than cough mixture B is a factual (non-ethical) claim. Evidence from clinical trials or practice may prove this claim true or false. It would only become an ethical (or professional and legal) concern if a professional prescribed the least effective expectorant for reasons of personal gain rather than in the best interests of their patient.

The statement relating to professional duties in emergency situations, c), may be a familiar one drawn from your professional code. You may agree or disagree as to whether it is reasonable and ethical to expect professionals to always intervene in emergency situations, even when they are 'off-duty'.

Statement d) concerning the Patients' Charter is likely to be a matter of hospital policy, but it may also reflect Constitutional rights and law and articulate the commitment of a health organisation and its employees to deliver ethically appropriate care.

The obligation to inform most patients if they have a serious condition, e), is usually articulated in professional codes, as well as in hospital policies and laws. It is also considered to be an ethical obligation because truth-telling is generally viewed as a means of affording patients control over information that concerns them, as well as ensuring their participation in decisions affecting their treatment and care.

Statement f) relates to following orders, obeying the directives of others. The important point here is that professionals need to approach such directives critically and ask if they are ethically sound and clinically and technically appropriate.

That a patient has a right to refuse medical treatment even if it leads to their death, g), is a widely held belief of the Irish public (it is a matter of public opinion [Weafer, McCarthy and Loughrey, 2009]) but it is also viewed as an ethically sound claim that has been underpinned by legal decisions, hospital policy documents and professional codes.

The statement h) may appear, at first sight, to be non-ethical, that is, more a matter of aesthetics (concerned with appearance and beauty) than ethics. However, it has been argued on the basis of a recent survey of over 2,000 nurses in the UK that the physical environment contributed to the promotion and diminution of dignity in care (Royal College of Nursing, 2008). The physical environment is, therefore, an ethical issue, as it influences whether people feel valued or not valued.

Statement i) relates to a poll or survey. We do not know exactly which doctors were asked, how many doctors were surveyed, or whether the sample was representative. Moreover, even if this group of professionals holds this view concerning the therapeutic benefits of cannabis, it does not follow that, i, they are correct; ii, that their views should trump the views of other individuals or groups, or, iii, that there might not be other practical/ethical/legal arguments against the legalisation of cannabis.

The final statement j) is a religious claim that links human life with the divine. Some would also argue that the claim can be understood in secular terms to mean that human life is of supreme value, or at least that human life has a deeply significant value. Understood in these terms, the claim is both religious and ethical (modified from Gallagher, 2005).

9.3 Consider the saying that describes utilitarian morality:

'the end justifies the means'. Some commentators think that this policy allows morally reprehensible acts to be committed with the aim of achieving good ends.

a. On the basis of your experience, do you think that this habit of carrying out unjust or dishonest acts as means to achieve good ends is so unusual?

b. What about a doctor's evasion to avoid breaking bad news to a very depressed patient? What about prescribing antibiotics for flu symptoms at the request of a patient?

c. What does the fairly common occurrence of such events tell us? That utilitarianism is well suited to human behaviour?

9.4 Review Kant's rule of universality:

a. Can you give examples where you think this rule should not or could not be observed?

b. Do you agree with Kant that the consequences of our actions are not fully in our control and so should not count in the moral appraisal of our actions?

9.5 The concept of virtue might seem a bit vague,
open to multiple interpretations and unhelpful for giving practical guidance.

a. How do you understand the idea of 'virtue'? Consider someone whom you think is 'virtuous'. How would you describe them? What kinds of behaviour or attitudes of the person would you offer as moral indicators of virtue?

b. Does a 'good' doctor or nurse have certain characteristic 'virtues'? If you had to write a short essay on 'The Caring Professional: A Life of Virtue', what would you have to say? If you believe that virtue is not relevant as a focus in healthcare, try and explain why.

9.6 Consider again the four principles of the PBE approach:
Taking each principle in turn, can you think of examples from practice which illustrate the need for health professionals to respect each principle?

9.7 Read again Brody's account of empathy on page 50:
Do you think it is an accurate representation of the patient/professional relationship? Consider the strengths and weaknesses of his account.

9.8 Feminist theory highlights the significance of power structures and hierarchies
in moral situations. These elements of power seem intractable and yet they are found in educational settings, in healthcare contexts and indeed in families. In the context of healthcare, hierarchies of authority seem resistant to change. But are they?

a. Consider a situation where some moral disagreement occurs in a healthcare setting where power imbalances are at play. These power factors greatly diminish your opportunities to speak, to offer suggestions for resolution of a moral disagreement. What do you do? What would you suggest be done if asked by a colleague or friend of yours?

b. It seems that power structures and healthcare hierarchies are culturally relative. Do healthcare organisations in some countries suffer more from power imbalances than others? If so, how do you explain these cultural differences?

10. Module 1 References and Further Reading

Aristotle, *The Nicomachean Ethics* (trans. J.A.K. Thomson) (Middlesex: Penguin Classics, 1955)

Arras, J. 'Getting Down to Cases: The Revival of Casuistry in Bioethics, *The Journal of Medicine and Philosophy*, 16, 1991, pp.29–51

Beauchamp, T. and Childress, J. *Principles of Biomedical Ethics* (Oxford: Oxford University Press, 1979)

Beauchamp, T. and Childress, J. *Principles of Biomedical Ethics* (4th ed.) (Oxford and New York: Oxford University Press, 1994)

Beauchamp, T. and Childress, J. *Principles of Biomedical Ethics* (5th ed.) (Oxford and New York: Oxford University Press, 2001)

An Bord Altranais, *Code of Professional Conduct for Each Nurse and Midwife* (Dublin: An Bord Altranais, 2000a)

Brody, H. *Stories of Sickness* (New Haven, CT: Yale University Press, 1987)

Carrese, J.A. and Rhodes, L.A. 'Western Bioethics on the Navajo Reservation', *JAMA: Journal of the American Medical Association*, vol. 274, no. 10, 1995, pp.826–30

Cassel, C.K. and Foley, K.M. *Principles for Care of Patients at the End of Life: An Emerging Consensus among the Specialities of Medicine* (New York: Milbank Memorial Fund, 1999)

Chambers, T. *The Fiction of Bioethics: Cases as Literary Texts* (New York: Routledge, 1999). See also *American Journal of Bioethics*, vol. 1, no. 1, 2001 for a range of open peer commentaries, drawn from philosophy, sociology, literature and medicine, on Chambers' book.

Charon, R. 'Narrative Contributions to Medical Ethics: Recognition, Formulation, Interpretation and Validation in the Practice of the Ethicist', in E.R. DuBose, R.P. Hamel and L.J. O'Connell (eds), *A Matter of Principles? Ferment in US Bioethics* (Valley Forge, PA: Trinity Press International, 1994), pp.260–83

College and Association of Registered Nurses of Alberta, 'Position Statement on Hospice Palliative Care', http://www.nurses.ab.ca/Carna-Admin/Uploads/Hospice%20Palliative%20Care.pdf [accessed 1 September 2009]

Cosgrave, T. 'O'Faoláin opens new debate', *Irish Medical Times*, 17 April 2008, http://www.imt.ie/opinion/2008/04/ofaolain_opens_new_debate.html [accessed 21 April 2009]

Council on Ethical and Judicial Affairs, *Surrogate Decision Making* [CEJA Report 4-A-01] (Chicago: American Medical Association, 2001)

Doyle, E. 'A National Conversation about Death', unpublished thesis, University of Edinburgh, 2008

Engelhardt, H.T. *The Foundations of Bioethics* (Oxford and New York: Oxford University Press, 1986)

Frank, A.W. *The Wounded Storyteller: Body, Illness and Ethics* (Chicago: University of Chicago Press, 1995)

Frank, A.W. *The Renewal of Generosity: Illness, Medicine, and How to Live* (Chicago: University of Chicago Press, 2004)

Frankena, W. 'A Critique of Virtue-Based Ethical Systems', in J. Sterba (ed.), *Ethics: The Big Questions* (Oxford: Blackwell, 1998), pp.291–6

Gallagher, A. Block 4. Decision-Making at the End of Life. Course A181: Ethics in Real Life (2005), http://www3.open.ac.uk/courses/bin/p12.dll?C01A181 [accessed 1 November 2009]

General Medical Council, *End-of-Life Treatment and Care. Good Practice in Decision Making: A Draft for Consultation* (London: General Medical Council, 2009)

German National Ethics Council, *Self-determination and Care at the End of Life* (Berlin: German National Ethics Council, 2006)

Gillon, R. 'Medical Ethics: Four Principles Plus Attention to Scope', *British Medical Journal*, vol. 309, no. 6948, 1994, pp.184–8

Holm, S. *Ethical Problems in Clinical Practice* (Manchester: Manchester University Press, 1997)

Hudson Jones, A. 'Narrative in Medical Ethics', in T. Greenhalgh and B. Hurwitz (eds), *Narrative-Based Medicine* (London: British Medical Journal Books, 1998)

Hunter, K.M. *Doctors' Stories: The Narrative Structure of Medical Knowledge* (Princeton, NJ: Princeton University Press, 1992)

Hunter, K.M. 'Narrative', in T.R. Warren (ed.), *Encyclopedia of Bioethics* (New York: Simon & Schuster Macmillan, 1995), pp.1789–94

Irish Council for Bioethics and TNS/MRBI, 'Bioethics Research', http://www.bioethics.ie/uploads/docs/129171–Bioethics%20Research.pdf [accessed 19 August 2009]

Jonsen, A.R. and Toulmin, S. *The Abuse of Casuistry: A History of Moral Reasoning* (Berkeley: University of California Press, 1988)

Kant, I. *Groundwork of the Metaphysics of Morals* (trans. M. Gregor) (Cambridge: Cambridge University Press, 1997)

King, N.M.P. 'Transparency in Neonatal Intensive Care', *The Hastings Center Report*, vol. 22, no. 3, 1992, pp.18–25

Kliever, L.D. 'Death: Western Religious Thought', in S.G. Post (ed.), *Encyclopedia of Bioethics* (3rd ed., vol. 2) (New York: Macmillan, 2004), pp.546–58

Koenig, B.A. and Marshall, P.A. 'Death: Cultural Perspectives', in S.G. Post (ed.), *Encyclopedia of Bioethics* (3rd ed., vol. 2) (New York: Macmillan, 2004)

Kubler-Ross, E. *Death: The Final Stage of Growth* (New Jersey: Prentice-Hall, 1975)

Kuczewski, M.G. 'Commentary: Narrative Views of Personal Identity and Substituted Judgment in Surrogate Decision Making', *Journal of Law, Medicine & Ethics*, vol. 27, no. 1, 1999, pp.32–6

Kukathas, C. and Petit, P. *Rawls: A Theory of Justice and its Critics* (Cambridge: Polity, 1990)

MacIntyre, A. *Whose Justice? Which Rationality?* (London: Duckworth, 1988)

MacIntyre, A. *After Virtue* (2nd ed.) (London: Duckworth, 1999)

McCarthy, J. 'Principlism or Narrative Ethics: Must we Choose Between Them?' *Medical Humanities*, vol. 29, no. 2, 2003, pp.65–71

McCarthy, J., Loughrey, M., Weafer, J. and Dooley, D. 'Conversations with the Irish Public about Death and Dying', *Studies*, vol. 98, no. 392, 2009, pp.457–72

McCarthy, J., Murphy, S. and Loughrey, M. 'Gender and Power: The Irish Hysterectomy Scandal', *Nursing Ethics*, vol. 15, no. 5, 2008, pp.643–55

McCarthy, J., Weafer, J. and Loughrey, M. 'Irish Views on Death and Dying: A National Survey', *Journal of Medical Ethics*, no. 36, 2010, pp.454–8

Medical Council, *A Guide to Ethical Conduct and Behaviour* (6th ed.) (Dublin: Medical Council, 2004)

Medical Council, 'Good Medical Practice in Seeking Informed Consent to Treatment' (2008), http://www.medicalcouncil.ie/_fileupload/news/Informed_Consent.pdf [accessed 1 November 2009]

Medical Council, *Guide to Professional Conduct and Ethics for Registered Medical Practitioners* (7th ed.) (2009), http://www.medicalcouncil.ie [accessed 20 November 2009)]

Mill, J.S. *On Liberty* (Harmondsworth: Penguin, 1981 [1859])

Mill, J.S. in J. Gray (ed.), *On Liberty and Other Essays* (Oxford and New York: Oxford University Press, 1991)

Murphy, S. Personal communication, 2004

Murray, T. and Jennings, B. *The Quest to Reform End-of-Life Care: Rethinking Assumptions and Setting New Directions. A Hastings Center Special Report, 'Improving End-of-Life Care'*, pp.S52–S59

National Commission for the Protection of Human Subjects of Biomedical and Behavioral Research, *Belmont Report: Ethical Principles and Guidelines for the Protection of Human Subjects of Research* (1979), http://ohsr.od.nih.gov/guidelines/belmont.html [accessed 23 April 2009]

National Consensus Project for Quality Palliative Care, *Clinical Practice Guidelines for Quality Palliative Care* (2nd ed.) (2009), http://www.nationalconsensusproject.org/guideline.pdf [accessed 1 November 2009]

NCEPOD (National Confidential Enquiry into Patient Outcome and Death), *Caring to the End?* (London: NCEPOD, 2009), http://www.ncepod.org.uk/2009dah.htm [accessed 1 November 2009]

Nelson, H.L. *Stories and their Limits* (New York: Routledge, 1997)

Nelson, H.L. *Damaged Identities: Narrative Repair* (New York: Cornell University Press, 2001)

New South Wales (NSW) Department of Health, 'Guidelines for End-of-Life Care and Decision Making' (2005) http://www.health.nsw.gov.au/policies/gl/2005/pdf/GL2005_057.pdf [accessed 1 August 2009]

Nussbaum, M. *Love's Knowledge* (Oxford and New York: Oxford University Press, 1992)

Nussbaum, M. *Poetic Justice: The Literary Imagination and Public Life* (Boston: Beacon Press, 1995)

O'Neill, O. *Autonomy and Trust in Bioethics* (Cambridge: Cambridge University Press, 2002)

Our Lady of Lourdes Hospital, 'Care of the Muslim Patient', *Muslim Care* booklet (Drogheda: Our Lady of Lourdes Hospital, 2005), p.11

Pence, G. 'Virtue Theory', in P. Singer (ed.), *A Companion to Ethics* (Oxford, Basil Blackwell, 1991)

Quinlan, C. *Media Messages on Death and Dying* (Dublin: Irish Hospice Foundation, 2009a)

Quinlan, C. *Patient Autonomy at End of Life: Literature Review* (Dublin: Irish Hospice Foundation, 2009b)

Quinlan, C. and O'Neill, C. *Practitioners' Perspectives on Patient Autonomy at End of Life* (Dublin: Irish Hospice Foundation, 2009)

Rawls, J. *A Theory of Justice* (Cambridge, MA: Harvard University Press, 1971)

Ricoeur, P. *Time and Narrative* (vol. 3), (trans. Kathleen Blamey and David Pellauer) (Chicago: University of Chicago Press, 1988)

Royal College of Nursing, *Dignity. Small Changes Make a Big Difference: How You Can Influence to Deliver Dignified Care* (London: Royal College of Nursing, 2008)

Schwartz, L., Preece, P. and Hendry, R.A. *Medical Ethics: A Case-Based Approach* (Edinburgh: Saunders, 2002)

Sherwin, S. *No Longer Patient: Feminist Ethics and Health Care* (Philadelphia: Temple University Press, 1992)

Sisters of Bon Secours, *Care of the Dying Quality Plan* (USA: Sisters of Bon Secours, 2000), pp.11–12

Storch, J.L. 'Nursing Ethics: A Developing Moral Terrain', in J.L. Storch, P. Rodney and R. Starzomski (eds), *Toward a Moral Horizon* (Toronto: Pearson Education, 2004)

Thomas, D. 'Do Not Go Gentle into that Good Night', in D. Jones (ed.), *The Poems of Dylan Thomas* (new revised ed.) (New York: New Directions Publishing Corporation, 2003 [1945])

Thomson, A. *Critical Reasoning in Ethics: A Practical Introduction* (London: Routledge, 1999)

Veatch, R.M. *A Theory of Medical Ethics* (New York: Basic Books, 1981)

Walker, M.U. 'Picking up Pieces, Lives, Stories, and Integrity', in D. Tietzens Meyers (ed.), *Feminists Rethink the Self* (Boulder, CO: Westview Press, 1997)

Walker, M.U. *Moral Understandings: A Feminist Study in Ethics* (London: Routledge, 1998)

Weafer, J. and Associates, *A Nationwide Survey of Public Attitudes and Experiences Regarding Death and Dying* (Dublin: Irish Hospice Foundation, 2004)

Weafer, J., McCarthy, J. and Loughrey M. *Exploring Death and Dying: The Views of the Irish General Public* (Dublin: Irish Hospice Foundation, 2009)

Weafer, J. *A Qualitative Study of Public Perceptions of End-of-Life Issues* (Dublin: Irish Hospice Foundation, 2009)

Woods, S. *Death's Dominion: Ethics at the End of Life* (Berkshire: McGraw-Hill, 2007)

Yeo, M. and Moorhouse, A. *Concepts and Cases in Nursing Ethics* (2nd ed.) (Ontario, Canada: Broadview Press, 1996)

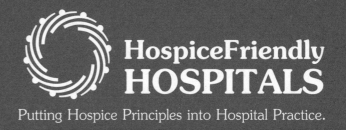

Module 2

The Ethics of Breaking Bad News

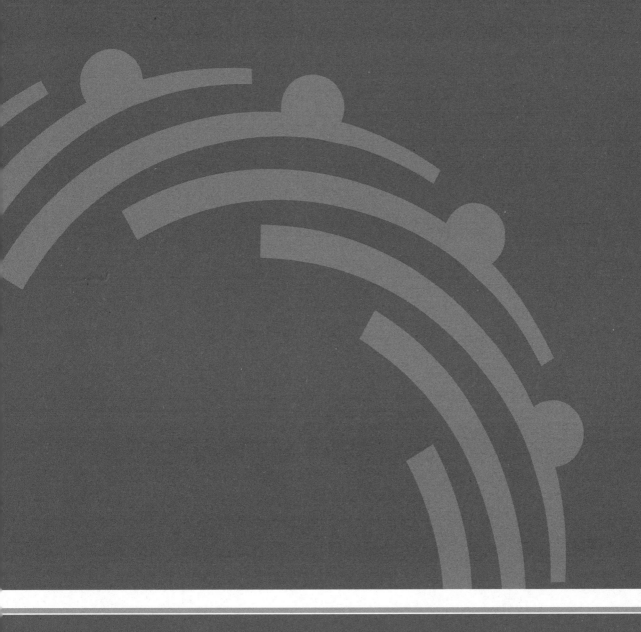

Module 2 Contents   Page

1. Module 2 Key Points

1.1 Most patients want to know:

Research in Ireland and abroad indicates that most patients who are terminally ill want to be told the truth about their condition but health professionals and families tend to withhold (or partially relate) bad news for a variety of reasons.

1.2 The principle of truth-telling:

obliges health professionals to tell patients the truth about their illness in language they can understand, in the presence of those whom the patient has chosen, unless they believe with good reason that telling the truth would cause patients serious harm.

1.3 Arguments for and against breaking bad news:

generally appeal to basic ethical principles such as respect for patient autonomy, doing good and avoiding harm. Objections to disclosure also appeal to serious ethical considerations such as worries about avoiding harm, ensuring patient well-being and maintaining hope.

1.4 Health professionals may exercise caution:

When health professionals believe that telling a patient the truth about their illness risks seriously harming them, they may withhold that information. This action is paternalistic. It is described as the exercise of therapeutic privilege which should be used with care.

1.5 Diverse cultural values need to be respected:

In many cultures, including Irish culture, families may also act paternalistically in withholding information from their loved ones. While there is a need to recognise and respect diverse cultural values regarding disclosure of bad news, it is a matter of debate whether such respect is sufficient reason for a health professional to proceed not to tell a patient about their diagnosis. Health professionals should not ignore the possibility that the patient may wish to have a conversation with them.

1.6 Patients have a right not to know:

A patient's persistent refusal to talk about their illness is an exercise of their autonomy and ought to be respected as far as possible. However, the process of not informing a patient is an ongoing part of the patient/professional relationship and should be subject to review in response to changing circumstances. When a patient is not informed about their condition there may be implications for the requirement of informed consent: without knowledge of diagnosis and prognosis, this consent process would be profoundly impeded.

1.7 Telling the truth is not always appropriate:

The capacity and the circumstances of every patient are unique. There are some situations where it is more important to sensitively communicate with patients in a way that is meaningful to them.

2. Module 2 Definitions

2.1 Autonomy:
is the capacity of self-determination; it is a person's ability to make choices about their own life based on their own beliefs and values.

2.2 Bad News:
information that seriously and negatively alters an individual's expectations of his or her future.

2.3 Paternalism:
involves an action that overrides a person's decision or controls their actions in the interests of what is considered to be their own good. Paternalism is described as strong paternalism when the person whose decisions and actions are being controlled is autonomous (capable of making their own decisions). It is described as weak paternalism when the person whose decisions and actions are being controlled is not autonomous.

2.4 Principle of Autonomy:
requires that, in a healthcare context, health professionals recognise and support the unique values, priorities and preferences of patients.

2.5 Principle of Beneficence:
requires that health professionals 'do good' for patients – that they are actively concerned for patient well-being.

2.6 Principle of Nonmaleficence:
requires that health professionals 'do no harm' – that they avoid or minimise harm to patients.

2.7 Therapeutic Privilege:
entitles health professionals to withhold information if they think the information given to the patient would run the risk of seriously harming the patient.

3. Module 2 Background

3.1 Right to Information

As a mark of respect for patient autonomy, Irish healthcare providers – organisations, hospitals, clinics, professionals – are increasingly committed to including patients in the decisions made about their medical treatment and care. Knowledge of one's health or information about illness seems, in general, a condition for choices about the future. So one way of enhancing patients' roles in decision making is to provide them with diagnostic and prognostic information about their health status. Access to such information is now conceived of as a right enshrined in the Irish Patients' Charter (Irish Patients' Association, 2008). These rights are also affirmed in professional codes and laws (An Bord Altranais, 2000; Medical Council, 2009; Irish Constitution, 1937). However, while all patients might be considered to have a right to be reasonably informed about their medical condition, the obligations of health professionals in relation to the information needs of patients who are terminally ill are particularly challenging.

Breaking bad news to individuals who are seriously ill and have a poor prognosis is a complex and contentious issue. Arguments for disclosure of bad news generally appeal to basic ethical principles such as respect for patient autonomy, doing good (beneficence) and avoiding harm (nonmaleficence). Objections to disclosure also appeal to serious ethical considerations such as worries about avoiding harm, ensuring patient well-being and maintaining hope (see Arguments For and Against Breaking Bad News). In addition, the situation is made more complex because of the number of people who may be involved. These include patients, families and health professionals and, while these individuals and groups may be equally concerned for the interests of the patient, they may differ as to how those interests might best be protected and/or promoted. These concerns deepen for those patients who lack the capacity to understand their situation or who are unable to express their own views.

3.2 International Research

International research on health professionals', patients' and families' experiences and attitudes in relation to the breaking of bad news is beginning to throw some light on current trends (Fujimori and Uchitomi, 2009). A systematic review on the subject of breaking bad news broadly found that while clinicians believed that patients should be told the truth about their illness, many hold back information (Hancock, Clayton and Parker et al., 2007). Reasons for not engaging in truthful disclosure included worries about patient well being, the stress incurred by having such conversations, a general discomfort in discussing death, a belief that doctors were not well trained in how to conduct such conversations and worries that there was no time to engage patients in what might become a lengthy conversation (Hancock et al., 2007).

Despite clinicians' concerns, however, research also indicates that most patients are, at least in Western countries such as the United States (US) and the United Kingdom (UK), not seriously harmed by such disclosures (Hancock et al., 2007). To take one example: a recent major study conducted in the US demonstrated that patients with advanced cancer who were able to have open discussions about their condition with health professionals had better outcomes than patients who had no such discussion (Wright et al., 2008). The latter were subjected to more aggressive medical care in their final week of life and were reported as having a poorer quality of life near their death. In addition, the caregivers of these patients were found to be at an increased risk of developing a depressive illness in the wake of their loved one's death.

On the other hand, research also suggests that there is a marked reluctance to disclose information directly to patients in many countries where there is much emphasis on the role of the family and religious beliefs in the lives of terminally ill patients. Traditionally, in these countries, the family, not the patient, takes centre stage. Also central is the deference to the decision-making authority of the doctor. This deference combines with a respect for family and a belief that family knowledge is essential regarding diagnosis and prognosis in order to protect a loved one from emotional suffering. Some southern European countries – Italy and Greece – and many Eastern and African cultures share this view of clinician and family participation taking precedence over patient knowledge and autonomy (Johnstone, 2004). According to Candib (2002), in cultures such as these, the family, not the individual, is the unit of identity and responsibility: 'The patient knows that family is protecting her and that this is what families should do […] non-disclosure is not a matter of lying. Ambiguity may be seen as the most suitable strategy to allow the patient to maintain tranquillity.'
(Candib, 2002, p.214).

It seems very important then that discussions concerning end-of-life are contextualised. This is because the experience and understanding of the death and dying process are clearly influenced by social, religious and cultural norms.

4. Irish Research

The question arises, is the culture in relation to breaking bad news in Ireland closer to the US/UK experience or to the experience of countries such as Italy, Greece or Pakistan? To answer this, it is important to ascertain and critically consider the extant Irish data pertaining to truth-telling/disclosure at end of life.

In Ireland, a concern for patient well-being as well as a cultural dis-ease around dying and death and lack of time also motivates health professionals in their decisions whether to communicate bad news or not. Two excerpts from research undertaken in 2009 points to a sharp distinction between the communicative practices in many general hospitals and those in some long-term care facilities. Consider the following account of practices in general hospitals:

The practice in general in hospitals in terms of communication around dying and death is to follow the patient's lead, to answer any direct questions. This means that clinicians seldom volunteer information, the patient must ask for the information. Frequently communication practice among clinicians communicating with patients around dying and death involves clinicians responding to patient probes or questions with another question. For instance the patient might say something like, 'I'm not a well as I was'. To this a clinician would respond 'why do you say that?' A patient might ask 'how am I doing?' to this a clinician would typically respond, 'how do you think you're doing?' In this way, slowing and indirectly, a conversation will unfold between a clinician and a patient.

Given that this research has already established that patients in hospital lose their identities, their sense of self, and much of their personal power, given too that the clinicians who participated in the research acknowledged the deference that patients pay to clinicians, and the propensity of patients in hospital to acquiesce to physician power and inevitability of hospitalised patients rapidly becoming part of hospital workflows, and the time needed for such conversations, it seems likely that it would be perhaps an exceptional patient who would lead and direct such a conversation.

Even in terms of the model of the twelve aspects of daily living that all patients are interviewed and assessed on admission to hospital, the one question within the model which is never asked is the question on dying. It is never asked.

The participants in the research also highlighted the euphemisms that are used by clinicians when talking to patients about dying and death. Patients might be told that 'they are going downhill', that 'they are not that well', that 'it's taking them a bit longer now to pull back this time', or that' 'it's going to be a little more difficult than was originally thought'. Consultants were said to be very cautious and deliberately oblique with the language they use with patients. Information given to patients around end-of-life issues tends to be very guarded, with the information giver constantly trying to second-guess how the information is being received. Consultants would typically talk to patients about 'inflammations' and 'shadows' when describing a tumour, even a malignant tumour. They would talk to patients about 'lumps' and 'bumps' and about whether the 'lump' or 'bump' was a malignancy or a non-malignancy.

There is the difficulty too of patients and families simply not understanding the clinicians. There was one case reported in the research of the wife of a man who was dying being told that her husband was 'deteriorating', when the woman did not know what the word 'deteriorating' meant. Patients and their relatives often don't know what the consultants are talking about, and frequently they do not have the courage or capacity to question them.

Nurses have a substantial role in communication in hospitals, not least in terms of interpreting the communications of consultants for patients. Patients seeking information were said to be often passed from pillar to post around the hospital as practitioner after practitioner evaded the question. In practice, direct questions about dying and death from patients at end-of-life in hospital are very rare, direct replies from clinicians even rarer.
(Quinlan and O'Neill, 2009, pp.90–2)

While Quinlan and O'Neill paint a bleak picture of current practices in relation to professional–patient communication in many Irish hospitals, the news is more positive in at least some long-term care facilities:

The emphasis in the long-term care facility for adults with intellectual disabilities was on quality of life. Patient autonomy was respected and was constantly the focus of the carers and clinicians within the hospital. The willingness of the senior management of the hospital to take risks with individual patients in order to enhance their autonomy and support their wishes shaped the experience of the facility for those living there.

One of the clinicians in that facility reported the case of one of the patients who was terminally ill. This patient knew her prognosis, she had been given that by the doctor and she decided herself that she did not want to go to an acute hospital, she did not want to have surgery. The doctor advised the patient and the patient's family, but respected the patient's wishes. The woman, who had an intellectual disability, stayed in the long-term care facility in which she had lived her life and she died there. That was her choice.

Another participant said of another patient in this long-term care facility:
"In my recent experience, while spending some time with a service user who was actually diagnosed with a terminal illness I sat with her and asked her if she had any wishes she would like us to look after and her wish was to visit Lourdes. She actually had been to Lourdes before but she felt herself that she just had the need to go to Lourdes again and she just felt that her condition was deteriorating. So while I was talking to her I documented what she was saying and her wish was granted. Another concern that this same person actually had was that she would visit her parents' grave and this was a huge wish for her because she herself felt 'well I want to know where I'm going to be buried' and that was looked after. So they were just two very simple [wishes] simple to us, we were well able to fulfil that duty – and to her it was a huge issue.'"
(Quinlan and O'Neill, 2009, pp.53–4)

The emphasis in the long-term care facility described by Quinlan and O'Neill is on individual people, their unique stories and circumstances. No doubt, the fact that this is a long-term stay facility means that attention to individual needs and, significantly, communication about what is meaningful to individual patients is prioritised. This focus is missing from the picture drawn of general hospitals where the relationships are often impersonal and breaking bad news is generally carried out reluctantly, avoided or shrouded in mystery.

From the patient perspective, several recent Irish studies indicate that most patients (over 80%) who are terminally ill want to be told the truth about their diagnosis and prognosis (Keating, Nayeem, Gilmartin et al., 2005; O'Keeffe et al. 2000; Weafer 2009a, 2009b, Weafer, McCarthy and Loughrey, 2009). However, even though patients may want to be informed, Irish research suggests that, in general, relatives are more likely to be informed about patients' illnesses than patients themselves (Keegan, McGee, Hogan et al., 1999; O'Keeffe et al, 2000). The research also suggests that there is a gap between what relatives think patients want to know and what patients actually want to know: patients want to be informed even though their relatives believe that they do not (O'Keeffe et al., 2000). Finally, the research indicates that a mutual concern for each others' well-being characterises the relationship between patients and their next of kin: both groups want to protect each other from the painful news (O'Keeffe et al., 2000; Quinlan and O'Neill, 2009).

To return to the question posed at the outset of this section – as to whether the culture in relation to breaking bad news in Ireland is closer to the US and the UK experience or to the experience of countries such as Italy, Greece or Pakistan – the answer seems fairly clear.

Many Irish patients want information as do their counterparts in the US and UK. However, the Irish patient also shares something in common with patients in Italy and Greece – an embeddedness in family relationships. In this context, the family may play a more central role in the communicative process and the patient's voice may be harder for health professionals to hear. For some patients and families, this may be welcomed. For others, patients and their family members may be confused about the role that family should play.

Following on this research, it would seem that a major challenge for health professionals working in an Irish context is to understand that no single approach to breaking bad news will suffice; they must be prepared to respond to the individual and unique set of circumstances of each patient and his or her family. A related challenge for healthcare organisations is to ensure that patients, families and professionals have a clearer understanding of their respective roles in information provision. Some reflection on the ethical concerns that arise in relation to truth-telling in healthcare practice in general may be a useful start. This is addressed in the following section.

5. Ethical Concerns

The value of truth-telling as a contributor to patient well-being that is respectful of personal autonomy has long been considered by ethicists in all traditions of philosophy.

5.1 Principle of Truth-telling

The following formulation of the general principle of truth-telling incorporates several elements for practice:

The health professional should tell the patient:

1. the truth about their illness,

2. in a measured manner,

3. in language the patient can understand,

4. in the presence of those whom the patient has chosen,

5. unless there are good reasons to believe that a degree of harm, more serious than a temporary emotional depression, would follow as a result of telling the truth.

This general principle can be viewed as respecting several patients' rights:

- The right to information which is accurate and true

- The right to decide how much information they feel they need and a right not to receive information

- The right to decide who should be present during the consultation, i.e. family member including children and/or significant others.

- The right to decide who should be informed about their condition and what information that person(s) should receive. (adapted from Irish Hospice Foundation, 2008)

5.2 Arguments For and Against Breaking Bad News

The arguments for and against breaking bad news concern basic ethical principles or guidelines for practice: respect autonomy, do good (beneficence) and avoid harm (nonmaleficence) and can be clustered under four separate headings: autonomy, clinical benefit, psychological benefit and practical reality (Higgs, 1999, pp.507–12).

5.2.1 Patient Autonomy

For breaking bad news: The patient as a human being has an entitlement to know what is discovered about their health and what options are available for treatment and care. Respecting autonomy implies respect for a person's own choices with regard to their own lives and precludes anyone else manipulating them in order to achieve ends that are not their own. Being kept in ignorance by concealing the reality of illness shows a lack of respect for a person's desire to have some control in the direction of their treatment, care and plans for life.

Against breaking bad news: The patient does not wish to know and has made this clear. In some situations and circumstances, competent individuals choose not to be informed about their condition.

A second argument against breaking bad news is that the patient is not capable of understanding the truth. This argument addresses concerns in relation to patients who may be cognitively impaired, confused or emotionally distressed. Care must be taken that the standard for understanding one's illness is not set so high that no patient except clinicians themselves would qualify for hearing of their diagnosis, etc.

The obligation of the general principle of truth-telling is to explain an illness to the patient in language they can understand. This obliges professionals to pay close and creative attention to the process of information giving but the circumstances of some patients may not always make this possible.

5.2.2 Clinical Benefit (Beneficence and Nonmaleficence)

For breaking bad news: Treatment is considerably facilitated if the patient knows what they are being treated for, what therapeutic options they could choose and why doctors or nurses might recommend certain treatments over others. This collaborative approach encourages patients to adhere to treatment and care procedures and to provide more information about the effects of these on them. It encourages patients to communicate their needs and to provide a more complete picture of the whole of their concerns in relation to proposed treatments.

Against breaking bad news: If the patient is informed about their diagnosis, the concern is that they will refuse to adhere to treatment and care that would benefit them. In order to ensure that professionals are not deceiving competent patients, simply because they disagree with what the professional deems is in their best interests, this requires sound judgement that to divulge the information would be potentially, and seriously, harmful.

5.2.3 Psychological Benefit (Beneficence and Nonmaleficence)

For breaking bad news: Disclosure builds trust between patients and health professionals. Knowing and understanding diagnoses and prognoses that are communicated with hope helps to provide psychological support against isolation in illness. Such conversation with hope that everything will be done to help the patient can minimise the worst imaginings and fears about the disease process. Knowing that therapies and pain control are available for an illness enables the patient to seek help from medical staff, nurses and family members. Deception and concealment hinder such positive benefits. Moreover, sustained deception can create a climate of secrecy and lies which staff, relatives and friends must endorse and which will surround the patient, further isolating them from the support that they might need in order to prepare for their dying and death.

Against breaking bad news: The truth would harm the patient by causing serious distress and taking away hope. Deception is perceived to maintain hope. As with the clinical benefit argument; this requires sound medical judgement that to divulge the information would be potentially harmful to a depressed, emotionally drained or unstable person.

5.2.4 Practical Reality

For breaking bad news: The patient will find out about their condition whether they are told by a health professional or not. The patient finds out by intelligent guessing. A charade of pretence is usually unsuccessful in protecting the patient from the truth. Guessing about one's illness rather than being treated with respect as a competent adult affects trust and openness with the health professionals and families involved in the deception.

Against breaking bad news: The patient is not in a position (practically or cognitively) to find out the truth.

6. Cases: Breaking Bad News in Practice

6.1 Case 1: Strong Paternalism – Talking to the Doctors

Consider the following case, recounted by a nurse working in the west of Ireland, which represents some of the attitudes and practices in relation to breaking bad news that currently prevail in Irish hospitals:

Talking to the Doctors

And the whole culture lends itself to dealing with the family as opposed to dealing with the patient because if somebody's relative comes and says they want the progress up to date and the patient is dying then the consultant will say 'let the family come and talk to me or when the family comes in I'll talk with the family' and they may not have discussed the resuscitation status with the patient directly but it will be discussed with the families.

When you talk about prognosis with families, the one thing is they're very protective of what you tell the patient or what you have discussed with the patient. Protecting them in the sense that 'oh I hope you didn't tell them that their disease has progressed or that they're not able to swallow? It's almost like keeping the person in the dark. I think it's a real protective thing: 'don't be telling'.

Where I work, the layout of the ward makes it difficult so that if you have families coming down the ward they'll almost sort of nearly shield their faces after speaking to the doctor to make sure that their mother or father doesn't see them going out because if they see them going out it is always an indication that they are after being told bad news.

Just the other day we had a gentleman, Patrick, who came in because the doctors wanted to speak to him because his wife, Mary, was quite ill and death was, you know, soon. So we rang the husband to come in and he wanted to know over the phone, 'was she that ill?', 'Had she deteriorated that much?' So we found it very hard to say 'well actually your wife is dying, you need to come quickly'. So when he came in he didn't want to go in to see Mary because he said, 'I know she'll know I'm going to talk to the doctors and I don't want her to know that'. So he spoke to the doctors and when he went in to see his wife, she said, 'I know you've been talking to the doctors'. Mary just knew by the reaction on his face and she goes 'I know you've been talking to the doctors, tell me what they told you'. And Patrick didn't tell her at all, it was like they all denied what was going on and yet the tears were streaming down their faces.

(adapted from Quinlan and O'Neill, 2008)

6.1.1 Discussion

Case 1 involves the collusion of health professionals and a relative in deceiving a patient. Taking the arguments for and against breaking bad news and applying them to Case 1 brings a number of ethical concerns to the fore.

All four arguments in favour of breaking the truth apply in Mary's case. In relation to 5.2.1 Patient Autonomy, Mary is a competent person and there seems to be no doubt about her ability to understand the reality of her situation. Yet both her husband and her doctor do not respect her autonomy by withholding information that she may need to make choices about her treatment and care and life plans in general. In addition, Mary's right to control over that information is also disrespected; her husband is told about her condition before she is and he is told by a health professional in the absence of permission from Mary. In effect, Mary's entitlement both to honesty and confidentiality is breached and the deception effectively treats her as a means to others' ends (See Module 7 for a more detailed discussion of confidentiality).

Arguably, Patrick does not actively consciously deceive his wife. He does collude with the health professionals in that he asks them to give him information before Mary is told. On the other hand, his query is understandable because of the fact that he was telephoned by staff, an extraordinary action, that implies that Mary's situation is bad. In effect, Patrick does not tell Mary because he can't – not because he exercised a choice not to tell her.

The contrary autonomy argument which favours deception when a patient asks not to be told bad news does not apply in this case as Mary has directly asked her husband what the doctors have told him about her condition. There is no question of this patient waiving her right to know.

Concern for 5.2.2 Clinical Benefit also applies to Case 1 as it seems that Mary's treatment and care is ongoing. In this case, Mary may benefit therapeutically if she has information about her diagnosis, prognosis and the options available to her.

The contrary argument in favour of appeal to therapeutic privilege does not seem persuasive as there is no indication that Mary will refuse treatment that might benefit her.

The 5.2.3 Psychological Benefit that derives from keeping a patient in the information loop clearly applies to Mary's situation; she seems to want to talk openly about her illness. Mary is suffering because information directly related to her is being withheld from her. Moreover, she is denied emotional support and the opportunity to discuss her fears in relation to her deteriorating condition.

As Lyckholm (2005) argues:

[I]f we are to take the charge of caring for very ill and vulnerable patients, then truth telling must be one on our most precious duties. It is important for patients to know what lies ahead of them so they may make final life choices. It is out of respect for their autonomy that we must be honest about their prognoses. Patients need to plan financially, psychologically, and emotionally. They need the chance to make peace, to say I love you, to say goodbye. (p.3037)

The argument justifying deception because it is perceived to maintain hope does not apply to Mary; without relevant information about the disease process and pain management, Mary is distressed and her situation may well seem hopeless to her. In addition, Patrick also struggles in isolation with the news, he wants to avoid Mary because he knows that she will know implicitly by the look on his face and the fact that the doctors had spoken to him that the news was bad.

The 5.2.4 Practical Reality favouring truth-telling also applies to Case 1: Mary knows that Patrick has received bad news about her condition. The lack of openness between Mary and Patrick and between Mary and the nurses and doctors caring for her seems to be distressing to all concerned. There is no doubt that Mary is capable of understanding what is going on; the deception, rather than avoiding confusion and emotional upset, adds to it.

In Case 1, both the doctor and, to a lesser degree, the husband adopt the stance of strong paternalism. Strong paternalism refers to actions that obstruct the exercise of choice by an autonomous person. The motive for strong paternalism here may well be to benefit the patient, Mary, (the obligation of beneficence) but a pertinent question is always: Is this decision truly being taken for the well-being of the patient or are other motives dominant such as self-interest or self-protection? Thomas Hill links the ideas of a 'right of autonomy' and the idea of a 'rational decision-maker', offering some insight into the case at hand:

The right of autonomy is only a right to make one's choices free from certain interferences by others. Among these interferences are illegitimate threats, manipulations, and blocking or distorting the perception of options. A rational decision maker wants not only to have a clear head and ability to respond wisely to the problems present to him; he wants also to see the problems and the important facts that bear on them realistically and in perspective. Thus one can also manipulate a person by feeding him information selectively, by covering up pertinent evidence, and by planting false clues in order to give a distorted picture of the problem situation. (Hill, 1991, pp.32–3)

Hill's worries in relation to the role that others might play in interfering with or limiting the autonomy of individuals seem to be at the heart of many experiences that Irish health professionals have with terminally ill patients and their families.

Therapeutic Privilege

The exercise of paternalism by the doctor in Case 1 can also be described as therapeutic privilege. Therapeutic privilege assumes that the health professional knows best what is in the interests of the patient. If one grants this, then we see a subtle move from medical expertise to moral expertise. The 'privilege' idea in therapeutic privilege is an entitlement for the healthcare professional to withhold information if they think the information given to the patient would run the risk of seriously harming the patient. Notice how this privilege was incorporated in the general principle of truth-telling outlined above.

Beauchamp and Childress think that use of the therapeutic privilege is very controversial because it can be over-used in order to avoid difficult challenges in communication with patients. What is required is a sound medical judgement that to divulge the information would be potentially harmful to a depressed, emotionally drained or unstable person (Beauchamp and Childress, 2008).

Is an appeal to therapeutic privilege in Case 1 a beneficent decision? Mary is not unstable or depressed, though she is indeed worried. Information about the seriousness of her illness is likely to cause considerable distress, tears and fear. But fear and distress is the state that Mary is in while not knowing. The application of the therapeutic privilege in this case seems totally unjustified. Non-disclosure prevents Mary from beginning the human process of internalising the very difficult news of her illness and making plans for her care and her future. One could argue that the practice of medicine and nursing precisely involves clinicians in learning the art of compassion, listening and creativity in helping patients and families in distress during and after receiving bad news. If this process is considered tangential to healthcare practice, a reassessment of the goals of healthcare provision might be warranted.

The medical doctor and ethics writer Jay Katz proposes a new model of trust in the healthcare context, a model that endorses the fundamental importance of communication to achievement of good medical practice and respectful patient care.

Both parties need to relate to one another as equals and unequals. Their equalities and inequalities complement one another. [Health professionals] know more about the disease. Patients know more about their own needs. Neither knows at the outset what each can do for the other. This trust cannot be earned through deeds alone. It requires words as well. It relies not only on [health professionals'] technical competence but also on their willingness to share the burden of decision making with patients and on their verbal competence to do so. It is a trust that requires professionals to trust themselves in order to trust their patients, for to trust patients, [they] first must learn to trust themselves to face up to and acknowledge the tragic limitations of their own professional knowledge (Katz, 2002, p.102).

6.1.2 Suggested Professional Responsibilities

- Mary is a competent person and there seems to be no doubt about her ability to understand the reality of her situation. Efforts should be made to determine if the patient wants to know the truth about her situation. If it is clear that she does, she should be informed of her prognosis along the lines of the principle of truth-telling and best practice in relation to breaking bad news (See Irish Hospice Foundation 2006; Buckman 2005).

- The fears and concerns of Mary's husband, Patrick, need to be addressed in order to enable both him and her to come to terms with the fact that Mary is dying.

- The practice of disclosing information about a (competent) patient's illness to family members without the patient's permission breaches patient confidentiality. It is a mark of respect for patient autonomy that they control who, and who may not, have access to information about them.

- The fact that Mary does not know about the seriousness of her situation has implications for her capacity to provide informed consent for treatment decisions and care. It also means that she is unable to make plans about her dying and death including how she might spend her final days. Truth-telling in this case might be described as a 'precious duty' (Lyckholm, 2002).

6.2 Case 2: Paternalism of Families – Backwards Autonomy

The following case, recounted by a palliative care consultant working in a general hospital outside Dublin, tells of his attempts to advocate to protect the autonomy of a vulnerable patient. These attempts are thwarted by the paternalism of the patient's family. As the research indicates, this is, unfortunately, fairly typical of what can happen when families are deeply involved in the care of older and dying relatives. Asked how he might explore with patients about how much they understood about their condition, the doctor told the following story of 'backwards autonomy'.

Backwards Autonomy

So I say to the patient 'you've been in hospital a long time, you've had a lot of scans and blood tests done, do you feel you know what's going on? Do you feel you know enough or would you like to know more?' and eight or nine times out of ten the patient will say, 'I want to know'. And in a situation where the family are uncomfortable with that we would invite them to be present for that conversation, but I would never, ever undertake with the family not to tell the patient. Sometimes, the Palliative Care Team become involved when a family will say 'we'd love you to see ...' it's typically an older person, so it's typically a parent rather than a child, they'll say 'It's great that you're coming to see dad but don't tell him you're Palliative Care and don't tell him he's cancer and don't tell him he's sick'. We would sort of understand that but again we would explain that we will go at the patient's speed and the patient doesn't need to know but the patient also has the right to know if they choose. And we would always work with that. Very occasionally, but still probably once a month, we would have patients who we end up not seeing because that's not acceptable to the family. There's been backwards autonomy in the first place: it's been given to the family to decide whether or not the patient is seen by Palliative Care. I mean that should never arise as the issue in the first place but that happens and typically it's somebody who is frail, they can't come into the clinic to see us without the support of their family and the family say 'well you've got to guarantee me you won't tell them that they have cancer otherwise I'm not bringing them in'. It's very, very rare but we do have it, we had a case last week and the family just said 'well sorry, we're not bringing Sean in then if that's what you're going to do'.

In that case, the patient, Sean, is at home and I know from the referring physician, and even from talking to the family, that this patient is very unwell, needs the type of support that we can offer and our community teams can offer but this patient went home and the doctor whose care they were under agreed not to tell them their diagnosis. They are now at home, the family aren't telling the diagnosis and the patient isn't being allowed access Palliative Care because we will not agree to not telling them the diagnosis. We're also not saying that we have to tell them, but we're saying that if the patient asks us why this has happened over the last two months that we will explain that to them in their own speed and in a gentle way. So I think that's somebody whose autonomy isn't being recognised and it's someone who is cognitively intact.

(adapted from Quinlan and O'Neill, 2009. pp.68–9)

6.2.1 Discussion

Case 2 is ethically similar to Case 1 in that both cases involve families who act paternalistically towards their relatives. However, there are differences also from an ethical perspective. In Case 1, both the family and the health professionals involved collude to keep the patient, Mary, in the dark about her condition. In Case 2, however, while Sean's family adopt the stance of strong paternalism, this is being resisted by the palliative care consultant whose approach is orientated towards involving Sean in decisions around his treatment and care to whatever level that is possible. The family's motivation may well be to protect Sean but they are obstructing his choice to know about his health status and his capacity to make decisions in relation to it. Their threat to prevent Sean from seeing the palliative care team because of their fears that the team will communicate bad news to Sean directly impacts on the kind and quality of treatment he can receive (clinical benefit).

Both cases are also ethically similar in that both Mary's and Sean's families are informed first about their health status: in effect, they did not seem to have control over who had access to information about them and when they would be informed. In both cases, their entitlement to confidentiality was not respected. In Case 1, Patrick was informed first by the doctor involved; in Case 2, the paternalism of the family was facilitated by the local general practitioner who seems to have informed the family first, a gesture the palliative care consultant describes as 'backwards autonomy'.

No patient likes the tragic news of serious illness. Sadness is painfully normal. Anticipating that another will be saddened or distressed at bad news should not be confused with evidence that they do not wish to know of their illness. Should health professionals second-guess a patient's sincerity in asking the questions to understand? The consultant, in Sean's case, is happy to wait and see, after meeting with and talking with Sean, what kind of information he might want to have. The consultant states that he will also respect Sean's right not to know. On the contrary, the family are not allowing Sean to exercise either a right to know or not to know: they are deciding for him.

Claiming that the truth will bring harm to a patient requires that one reflects honestly on the evidence for anticipated harm. On reflection, evidence may be more difficult than realised. Is concern about Mary's and Sean's well-being central to the decision made by their families? The consciences of the authors of both of these cases are very uneasy. This is, perhaps, because they see no evidence for deception.

The palliative care consultant in Sean's case offers strong evidence that the 5.2.4 Practical Reality argument in favour of breaking bad news should be taken seriously, especially in relation to older people. He observes:

People tend to underestimate [the understanding that older people have]. If you have someone who is 70 or 80 or 90 their peers, their friends, their family have died, they are more familiar with death and that process than the 40 year old son or daughter and we don't allow for that. And we don't allow for the fact that patients at 70 or 80, even if they have some mild cognitive impairment, generally they have a very good awareness of what's going on and they're aware that they're a completely different person to who they were 3 or 6 months ago and they know there's something going on. They may well have been sitting in a hospital, a six bedded ward here, where the three patients opposite them were all young people with no hair on chemotherapy and everyone is assuming that the 82 year old won't have guessed that cancer could be an issue here.
(adapted from Quinlan and O'Neill, 2008)

Sean has had a long and serious illness and he is, most likely, aware that his situation is very serious and/or terminal. However, his health status makes him profoundly vulnerable to the will of other people. This kind of vulnerability is captured by the philosopher Sisela Bok:

It has always been especially easy to keep knowledge from terminally ill patients. They are most vulnerable, least able to take action to learn what they need to know, or to protect their autonomy. The very fact of being so ill greatly increases the likelihood of control by others. And the fear of being helpless in the face of such control is growing. The sense of possible prolonged pain, the uncertainty, increasing weakness, loss of powers, chance of senility, sense of being a burden.
(edited from Bok, 1978, pp.231–3)

6.2.2 Suggested Professional Responsibilities

- Sean's family's threat to prevent Sean from seeing the palliative care team is obstructing his ability to make a choice to know about his health status and to control who else may know about his condition. Efforts should be made to understand the family's concerns in this regard. They also need to be made aware of the health professional's duty to tell the truth (where appropriate) and to protect patient confidentiality.

- Preventing Sean from seeing the palliative care team also impacts on the kind and quality of treatment he can receive. Efforts need to be made to understand the family members' reluctance to involve Sean, to address their concerns and to explain to them the implications of their refusal and the professional's duty of care to Sean.

- Sean's ability to participate in decision making around his treatment and care is hindered by his lack of knowledge. The family, not the patient, are making the decisions in this case. It needs to be established if this is what the patient himself wants to happen.

6.3 Case 3: Familial, Religious and Medical Authority – Family at the Centre

If we look at a Pakistani perspective on medical decision making we see the way in which family and religion play a significant role in the treatment and care of loved ones who are terminally ill. This is markedly different from secular Western societies, such as the US and the UK, where patient autonomy is generally accepted as the cornerstone of healthcare ethics when it comes to choices in medical care and end-of-life decisions. However, the following case is very similar to the earlier cases and indicates that Irish culture is, often, closely aligned with cultures that place much emphasis on the role of the family and religious beliefs in the lives of terminally ill loved ones.

Family at the Centre

After training as a doctor in the United States for many years, I accepted an academic position at a medical university in Pakistan. One of my first experiences there was to tell two brothers sitting across the desk from me that all investigations indicated their elderly father had widespread metastatic cancer, and therefore not long to live. The patient, who lived with the oldest son and his family, was not present during this conversation, although an adult daughter, a daughter-in-law, and an adult grandson were. After listening attentively to what I had to say, and obviously upset at this news, one of the sons said, 'We do not want him to know that he has cancer. How long he lives is in the hands of God in any case, and it is not right to make my father lose hope while he is so ill.' He then added, 'Doctor Sahib, tell us what we should do next. You know best. You are not just our doctor, you are like our mother.' **(Moazam, 2000, p.28)**

6.3.1 Discussion

In Case 3, like Case 2, the family, not the patient, takes centre stage. Also central to this case is the deference to the decision-making authority of the doctor. This deference combines with a respect for family and a belief that family knowledge is essential regarding diagnosis and prognosis in order to protect a loved one from emotional suffering. This attitude is not unique to Pakistan. Many Eastern and African cultures also share this view of clinician and family participation taking precedence over patient knowledge and autonomy. According to Candib (2002), in cultures such as these, the family, not the individual, is the unit of identity and responsibility: 'The patient knows that family is protecting her and that this is what families should do […] non-disclosure is not a matter of lying. Ambiguity may be seen as the most suitable strategy to allow the patient to maintain tranquillity' (Candib, 2002, p.214).

As illustrated by the narratives from health professionals (Quinlan and O'Neill, 2008, 2009), Irish family members are also protective of their loved ones when they insist that they, and not the patient, are to receive medical information. In coping with this diversion of autonomy from patient to family, health professionals working in Ireland have explained that it is most challenging and stressful especially when families are insistent.

Interviews with health professionals from both rural and urban hospitals around Ireland, illustrated in Cases 1 and 2, reflect the difficulties for some health professionals in trying to keep the patient's right to honest information primary in the face of family requests to the contrary. The motive for doing this, from the family's point of view, may be paternalistic – wishing to protect the loved one from distress and anxiety associated with knowledge of their near death. Alternatively and/or in addition, the family may not be able to communicate directly/at all with the patient in the face of current, immediate frightening news and so can cope better by talking about and making decisions from a distance. In sum, it may be a question of limited ability rather than, simply, protection.

Medical Authority

For the most part, within the cultural setting of Case 3, the doctor remains the authority in matters relating to diagnoses and prognoses, treatment interventions and life-prolonging decisions. The family wishes the doctor to direct rather than just facilitate medical decision making. The important religious perspective of trust in a deity is also firmly part of the religious and cultural context of this case. As in Ireland, religious customs may be very important at the time of death and provide identity and comfort for families of the deceased. The case from Pakistan suggests also that for persons embedded in the faith tradition shown in this case, end of life may ultimately be perceived to be in the hands of God and issues of faith may be integral to overall healing at the end of life.

Drawing on the empirical research undertaken by the HfH (Quinlan and O'Neill, 2008, 2009; Weafer, 2009a, 2009b) as well as other relevant existing Irish studies, there is a body of evidence suggesting that in Ireland too, many family members tend to respect divine and also medical authority over individual autonomy.

Both Cases 2 and 3 involve a conflict between family wishes and health professionals' convictions about giving information to the patient. The families of the elderly gentlemen in both cases tell the doctors, with conviction, that their fathers should not be told any bad news about their condition. These cases highlight the question as to whether the practice of telling family members bad news before (or instead of) a competent and conscious patient is ever morally justifiable. When healthcare professionals gather at meetings and are asked who should be given information about a patient's diagnoses or prognoses, virtually all will reply that the operative principle is that the competent patient should be offered the information first. Yet, in spite of this verbal nod towards patient entitlements, in practice, even in many countries in the Western world, and certainly in Ireland, this still does not happen.

Reasons given for this discrepancy are that it is simply easier to tell relatives first (or only). Facing relatives' distress is simply not as difficult as facing the likely greater distress of the patient hearing of a serious condition. But is this a valid moral justification for over-riding the entitlement of the patient to know?

The first point to make is that the health professional's difficulty or ease in the communication process does not amount to a moral justification. Intimidation by insistent relatives can be stressful but similarly such intimidation is not tantamount to a moral justification. Emotional discomfort is a psychological report, not an ethical explanation. The communication process in clinical settings is one of the obligations or duties of health professionals. Many obligations and duties are difficult and that is clearly part of the challenge and sometimes anxiety associated with a chosen career.

In most cases, it is the health professional's responsibility to judge how much information to give to a patient, how to communicate this and over what kind of time-frame. Randall and Downie comment on this type of situation: 'The carer's feelings in this regard are not morally relevant. This may seem a hard thing to say, but it needs to be said if the patients' right to the truth is to be upheld' (1996, p.84).

If the good of the patient is paramount, and if we assume that respect for the patient requires allowing them self-determination or voice of some kind in decisions, then it is at least important that the doctor tries to get some evidence that the patient in Case 3 wishes his voice to be heard through his family. One way of achieving this might be to offer the patient the 'option of truth' when breaking bad news regardless of where the patient comes from. Candib (2002) suggests using questions like: 'Will you want to be making the decisions about your care with the doctors, or do you want your family to be making those decisions?' And 'When we understand what is causing your illness, will you want us to tell you about it or to talk with your family about it?'

In addition, the health professionals in both Cases 2 and 3 can do more to try and understand the relatives' request not to inform their father. Health professionals do not need to second guess the family's reasons, precarious speculation at best. However, doctors and nurses can initiate a conversation in private with relatives (and separately with different family members) about why they think their father should not be told. Note that consensus may not be reached within families that the patient should/should not be told bad news and so disagreements emerge from within the 'family'. One way of addressing this might be to request that a nominated person be identified from within the family with whom the team can deal directly regarding care decisions about the patient. This can provide valuable information for health professionals about the patient's personality and whether there are previous situations where their father coped badly with distressful news and crises (Randall and Downie, 1996).

6.3.2 Suggested Professional Responsibilities

- The question is: should health professionals simply agree with the request and proceed to treatments or provide only comfort care without informing patients about their diagnoses and prognoses? Respecting the cultural values of many families in Ireland or in Pakistan may not justify a generalisation of all Irish or Pakistani individuals. The doctor, in brief, should not ignore the possibility that the patient may wish to have a conversation with the doctor. He or she might offer the patient the 'option of truth'.

- One of the questions that diverse cultural values raise is whether or not the respect owed to the family's cultural practices about information giving is sufficient moral reason for health professionals to proceed not to tell the patient about his condition. Respecting diverse cultural values does not mean that the doctor automatically takes the word of the family. Does the doctor, for example in Case 3, know that the father does not wish to be informed of his grave situation? He should try to confirm the word of the family that their father wishes communication to be with them. Doctors and nurses can and perhaps must try to test the validity of this request from family.

6.4 Case 4: The Right Not to Know – Must She Know?

Case 4 is drawn from research funded by the Irish Hospice Foundation that investigates the grief experiences of same-sex couples in an Irish context. According to the authors of the research, the 'belief by health professionals that patients should be informed of their diagnosis resulted in one of the participants being what she perceived as "forced" to inform her partner of her diagnosis [of terminal illness]. This was despite the fact that her partner had previously told her she did not want to know her diagnosis' (Higgins and Glacken 2009, p.172). The authors report on Brid's distress at having to share 'the devastating news of her impending death with her partner':

Must She Know?

I said [to the doctor], 'Surely her right to not know should be adhered to'. And he said, 'No' … and the following morning I went in [hospital]. I was in with her at 4 o'clock in the morning. And she was sitting in the chair beside the bed. And she said to me, 'What are you doing here at this time?' And I closed the door and I pulled the curtains … I said to the nurses, 'I've got to go in. If anyone's to tell her, I'd have to tell her'. And I had to tell her … and it was the most difficult thing I had to do. [Very upset and tearful.] She looked at me and I said, 'Will you forgive me for telling you?' 'But' she said, 'I didn't want to know'. **(Higgins and Glacken 2009, p.172)**

6.4.1 Discussion

The reader is not aware of all of the circumstances surrounding Case 4, but what is clear is that the doctor in this case has an expression of the patient's personal preference but is unwilling to respect it. Moreover, this case is similar to cases 1, 2 and 3: the family member of a competent patient is informed about the patient's condition before and/or instead of the patient themselves.

A patient's choice not to know is an exercise of their autonomy and ought to be respected as far as possible. However, as breaking bad news is best understood as part of an ongoing relationship where the news is shared and reviewed in an ongoing way, so too the process of not informing a patient is an ongoing part of the patient/professional relationship and should also be subject to review in response to changing circumstances. In Case 4, the doctor's brief and (seemingly curt) response, 'No', indicates that he has no interest in engaging with the patient or her partner in relation to the reasons why the patient does not want to be informed. It might be, for example, that some patients cope better with less information, while others wish to exercise control over the flow of information and resent being sidelined in this respect. Whatever her reasons, an opportunity is lost here to address the patient's concerns about knowing/not knowing and the patient's partner, Brid, is left to cope with sharing the news alone. The task of doing so may well add additional stress to the women's relationship at a time when time is precious and in circumstances that are already deeply traumatic.

It might be that the doctor in this case is concerned that if the patient is not informed about the seriousness of her condition there may be implications for the requirement of informed consent. In general, competent patients are both morally and legally entitled to information from professionals about their illness. The important caveat here is the expressed request from a competent patient that she does not wish to be informed or consulted. The difficulty might be that there may be need for ongoing consent or refusal for therapies. Without knowing of diagnosis and prognosis, this consent process would be profoundly impeded. It follows that foregoing the possibility of consent conversations with a competent patient should be done only for very good reasons. However, it is not clear that the insistence on disclosure on the part of the doctor in Case 4 is based on concern about the informed consent process. If this were the case, it seems strange that he is happy to derogate the responsibility for sharing medical information to the patient's family.

This leads us to a further question that this case prompts: what kind of information is at stake here? Higgins and Glacken use the term 'diagnosis' and the phrase 'news of her impending death' in their description of the case. Few might dispute that 'diagnosis' is a medical term and, as such, it could be argued that communication about a poor diagnosis is something that health professionals should undertake with (willing and competent) patients and family (where appropriate).

The phrase 'news of her impending death', however, highlights the profound human drama that underlies the medical terminology. This phrase could be viewed as medical information but it can also be understood as news that is profoundly personal, spiritual and existential. In short, news about dying and death is not a simple matter of fact and sharing it demands more of health professionals than, perhaps, health professionals, patients and society as a whole are willing or ready to acknowledge.

6.4.2 Professional Responsibilities

- If, in spite of being told that her condition really needs discussion and is quite serious, the patient persists in declining conversations, it is difficult to justify imposing the truth about her condition on the patient.

- It is essential to view the patient's refusal of information as part of an ongoing conversation that demands a willingness on the doctor to try to understand the patient's reasons for not wanting to know.

- If the patient requires further therapeutic and/or palliative treatment for her condition, it is important to engage the patient as fully as is reasonably possible in planning her care. At the same time, health professionals should respect the patient's resistance to knowing what undergoing these treatments implies about her medical prognosis.

- The patient's family should not be abandoned by the doctor, and perhaps, in turn, by the nurses. Sensitive communication with the patient and with Brid may address fears and worries and prevent conflict and confrontation from developing.

- Health professionals should be aware of best practice in relation to patients who identify as lesbian or gay. See Health Service Executive (2009) for *Good practice guidelines for health service providers working with lesbian, gay, bisexual and transgender people.*

6.5 Case 5: Communicating with Patients who Lack Capacity – The Forgetful Mourner

So far, this module has focused on the insights that can be gained from considering cases involving the breaking of bad news to competent patients in the light of the obligations that basic principles such as respecting patient autonomy and acting for the good of patients confer. The next case involves a patient who is not autonomous and it raises additional challenges and demands additional skills on the part of health professionals in order to ensure respectful and good patient care. The case involves the breaking of bad news to a patient who is suffering from Alzheimer's disease. The bad news, in this case, relates not to the patient's own condition but to the death of her son.

The Forgetful Mourner

An eighty six year old Italian American woman with moderate dementia, Joanna, is admitted to a nursing home when her son Tony, with whom she has been living, falls ill. When, after two years, Tony dies suddenly the staff in the nursing home are especially concerned for Joanna. In the days and weeks that follow the funeral, she continues to ask how Tony is doing as if he is still alive. After consulting with staff, the director of the Alzheimer unit decides that Joanna's questions should be answered truthfully: she should be told that Tony has died. Each time this is done, however, Joanna becomes distraught, enduring the pain of her son's death over and over again. While everyone finds this very hard, the Director hopes that their patience and persistence will enable Joanna to remember what really happened. The only alternative seems to be a grave and sustained deception on the part of everyone who has a relationship with her.

As it turns out, Joanna is told of her son's death at least fifteen times, and each time she experiences the grief of her loss anew. Then, one of the nurses suggests that Joanna put on the black dress she had been wearing on the day she attended Tony's funeral. This she does and it seems to help her to remember. Even though Joanna continues to talk about Tony, she no longer asks how he is doing. **(Adapted from Yang-Lewis and Moody, 1995)**

6.5.1 Discussion

One response to the actions of the director might endorse the view that, however painful it is, in this case, telling the truth to Joanna, in whatever fashion, is the right and respectful thing to do because it conforms with the principle of truth-telling, avoids the sustained deception of Joanna and acknowledges the importance of her relationship with her son (Yang-Lewis, 1995). It is, after all, Joanna's memory that is eroded, but not, necessarily, her sense of self and her relationships with others, especially her son.

An alternative approach, however, might argue that the director's commitment to truth-telling is misguided as it ignores the pointless anguish and pain that truth-telling visits on Joanna (Moody, 1995). The experimental and imaginative approach of the nurse, on this view, is the more ethically acceptable because she focuses on the communication rather than the truth element of the principle of truth-telling. The nurse's suggestion that Joanna wear the black dress is motivated by the desire to communicate with the patient in a way that is meaningful to her. The immediate effect of wearing the black dress somehow meets Joanna's sense of loss and validates her feeling of grief around her son. Ultimately, it may or may not succeed in getting Joanna to intellectually understand and accept the truth about her son's death. On this view, it is communication with the aim of meeting the patient in a way that is meaningful to them, not truth-telling, which is ethically important.

6.5.2 Professional Responsibilities

- The ethical challenge in this case is that health professionals have a duty to consider both Joanna's autonomy interests as well as her well-being.

- Even though Joanna might not be considered competent or capable of understanding the news about her son in the usual way she nevertheless has autonomy interests in the sense that she still has a sense of her own life, her relationships and concerns. The patient's autonomy, thus broadly construed, needs to be respected.

- Respect for Joanna's autonomy needs to be balanced by concern for her well-being. Health professionals might consider the breaking of bad news as a task of communication in the widest sense where communication is understood as more than the provision of cognitive information. The goal of communication could be to enable Joanna to understand what has happened to her son in a way which is meaningful for her.

6.6 Case 6: The Need for Sensitivity – Why Tell the Truth?

The final case in this module also raises a question about the appropriateness of always telling the truth. It involves a general practitioner (GP) whose breaking of bad news to a patient worries one of her colleagues and prompts him to reflect on the context within which the truth gets told.

Why Tell the Truth?

We all commiserated as our colleague told us about her awful consultation the previous day. She had had to tell a man in his fifties that his ultrasound scan had shown a mass in the head of his pancreas, almost certainly a carcinoma. The man clearly hadn't been expecting bad news, and had turned up at the surgery on his own, with a rather jaunty manner. To make matters worse, she had never met the man previously – she was covering for someone else that day. We squirmed and offered our sympathy as she described the encounter unfolding from moment to moment. She was honest enough to admit that she hadn't actually liked the man, who had been a bit smelly. At the end of the consultation she had wanted to hug him, or at the very least to touch him on the arm, but found herself unable to. We were all experienced educators as well as clinicians, and we tried to cover every angle in our discussion: the painfully inappropriate circumstances in which we often have to break bad news; the way in which negative impressions can disable our compassion; and how we aspire to the impossible task of spelling out a death sentence nicely, and feel like failures when it never quite happens that way. Yet afterwards I pondered on her story and I couldn't get another, heretical thought out of my mind: why did the doctor have to tell the truth?

(Launer, 2005, p.385)

6.6.1 Discussion

The author of this story is somewhat taken aback at the frankness of his colleague and he contemplates the variety of ways in which the GP might have postponed telling the patient of his full scan results, at least until a relative or friend could arrive or until the man's regular doctor could be there. Launer imagines some prevaricating language that the GP might have used: 'The result isn't back yet', 'It's back but it's not entirely clear', 'I'm a bit puzzled about its significance and I need to discuss it with a colleague'. Even if such subterfuge had made the patient more anxious, it was still preferable, for Launer, to the shock he received without anyone to support him in it.

Module 2 The Ethics of Breaking Bad News

At the heart of Launer's concern is that an excessive bias towards patient autonomy might prompt health professionals to assume that there is only one right action: to tell the truth. He advises caution and sensitivity towards the unique circumstances of each patient so that decisions and actions are focussed on the individual and sought through conversation rather than fixed prior notions of what should be done.

Case 6 illustrates the tension that can exist for stressed and busy health professionals who, anxious to respect patient autonomy and to avoid acting paternalistically, are insensitive to the import of their conversations on unsuspecting and ill-prepared patients. In such cases, Launer advises not simple subterfuge but deception, even lying ('The results aren't back yet'). While it could be argued that lying is more ethically unacceptable than prevarification (see Further Discussion), what this case underlines is the need for health professionals to consider the unique circumstances of each patient and to exercise caution and sensitivity in relating bad news to them.

6.6.2 Suggested Professional Responsibilities

- Health professionals need to remember that the communication of bad news is more than the communication of matters of fact.

- The views of patients in relation to when, and with whom, they might be provided with information about their condition should, where possible, be invited.

- Sensitivity to the unique circumstances of the patient is important. The need and availability of support from family members and/or others should be assessed and identified.

- The emotional labour of breaking bad news should be recognised by healthcare organisations. Every ward/unit/centre should have a disclosure policy and training in relation to communicating bad news and the documentation of disclosures. Psychosocial support for the professionals involved in communicating bad news and/or other members of the healthcare team should be considered.

- Clinical practice guidelines should be put in place in hospital units and healthcare settings to support health professionals in the communication of bad news. For an example of such guidelines, see Clayton, Hancock, Butow, Tattersall and Currow (2007).

7. Module 2 Further Discussion

The arguments for and against breaking bad news might also be framed in terms of two traditional moral theories where truth-telling and respect for individual autonomy are seen as central to human relationships.

7.1 Deontology: Focus on Duty

According to deontology, some actions are simply wrong (See Module 1). They are 'intrinsically wrong'. In claiming that some actions are intrinsically wrong, the eighteenth-century German philosopher Immanuel Kant means that no anticipated good outcome can give moral warrant or justification for carrying out these actions. To use an example, let us say that torturing innocent human beings is intrinsically wrong. This means that no amount of anticipated positive results or good outcomes from torture (such as getting valuable information) can make such torture 'right'. Likewise, to say that lying cannot be morally defended means that no amount of seemingly good outcomes, for the liar or the one lied to, justifies lying.

Staying with these examples, why is it that good consequences would never warrant torture of the innocent or the act of lying? In the *Metaphysical Principles of Virtue* [1797] (1968), Kant explains the relationship between truthfulness and the dignity of humanity in a person. Right actions promote or foster human dignity and respect for human beings. Wrong actions undermine dignity and respect, of the one lying and the person lied to.

> *The greatest violation of man's duty to himself considered only as a moral being is the opposite of veracity: lying. Dishonour, which goes with lying, accompanies the liar, like his shadow. Lying is the throwing away and, as it were, the obliteration of one's dignity as a human being. Lying, as intentional untruth in general, does not need to be harmful to others in order to be blameworthy. Even a really good end may be intended by lying. Yet to lie even for these reasons is through its mere form a crime of man against his own person and a baseness which must make a man contemptible in his own eyes* (Kant. [1797], 1968, pp.90–1).

Notice that from this rigorous deontological perspective, lying, even for reasons of supposed kindness or benevolence, is still wrong because it debases the one lying. Secondly, Kant thinks that lying also treats the person we lie to with disrespect for their autonomy: we are using the other person as a means for our own ends – perhaps to make the job easier or because we cannot bring ourselves to share bad news. Kant puts it this way: 'Lying is a crime of man [woman] against his [her] own person.' He asks: 'Should I lie to extricate myself from a difficult situation?' No, is the categorical response. No matter the motivation, in Kant's philosophy, expected good consequences do not make the lying right. Consequences are irrelevant to the moral evaluation of actions.

7.2 Utilitarianism: Focus on Consequences

The deontological theory is strikingly different from other ethical theories such as utilitarianism. Whereas deontology argues that some actions are simply wrong regardless of the good consequences, utilitarianism is a consequentialist theory (See Module 1). This indicates the centrality of consequences of actions when we are morally evaluating an action. Acts are not right or wrong in themselves. Utilitarians stress that the rightness or wrongness of an act is determined by looking to what follows from the choices of individuals. If we maximise human well-being or happiness it is a moral action. If human suffering and degradation occur then the action is immoral. The challenges of utilitarianism become clear: human beings take great responsibility for anticipating the outcomes of choices.

Rather than argue, as Kant did, that consequences are irrelevant to the moral quality of actions, the nineteenth-century utilitarian philosopher John Stuart Mill took the maxim of utilitarianism to be: 'Do what has the best effects over-all'. Unlike Kantian ethics, Mill argues that it might be necessary to lie if doing so would likely, and in a particular situation, protect individuals from harm. Mill asks: 'What if lying would serve to achieve the greater happiness and welfare of individuals and society?' Utilitarians see their great strength in emphasising what is good or bad for people based on the preferences of people. What matters in terms of the goal of morality are specific consequences for happiness and human well-being affecting persons' lives. This is in contrast with deontologists who stress the importance of abstract rules, divine commands or intuitions that are supposed to define what is moral.

7.3 Moral Principles and Exceptions

7.3.1 Justification

In many situations of healthcare you may be asked to explain how you would justify or defend your views about, for example, truth-telling, confidentiality, or constraints on autonomy. Being prepared to give reasons means that we are willing to continue to grow as moral agents. Justification involves giving reasons for adherence to truth-telling in general. But justification is also about giving reasons why an exception to truthfulness is necessary in a particular situation. For example, the doctor in Mary's case (Case 1) may generally agree with the practice of truth-telling but judge now in the concrete circumstances that it is not (immediately) appropriate. If this is so, then the doctor is clearly choosing to make an exception to the general principle of truth-telling. This path requires justification.

The nature of the general ethical principle of truth-telling is precisely that: it expresses a basic value or set of values that we wish to protect. We can, with consistency, strongly affirm the general principle and yet recognise that there might be circumstances where we must set aside the general presumption because other competing values are deemed more important at this point in time. So the rule in the general principle operates 'most of the time' and functions as a 'rule of thumb' for most situations.

7.3.2 Exceptions

If we find ourselves appealing to the exceptions much more than the general principle, then we are probably beginning to seriously doubt the value contained in the general rule or principle. Alternatively, we might verbally endorse the value of being truthful but through repeated exceptions reveal a lack of sincerity or 'weakness of will' in our conviction about the value of truthfulness.

Accepting general principles is one way of endorsing the cumulative experience of human valuing. When we endorse the moral importance of certain values we are agreeing to the general acceptability of what is called an 'ethical norm'. The norm of 'telling the truth as a general rule' is defended by appeal to the moral value of respect for the autonomy of individuals whose condition of health is primarily their business, their concern and an area of profound meaning in their life.

Like all exceptions to ethical principles, if we put aside the general rule in a particular case, reflection is required regarding the concrete patient and specific clinical realities that are known. Taking the full range of human, patient, personal and health realities into account, we must then consider the reasons for thinking that a particular case is an exception and that withholding information, partial deception or total deception is called for.

8. Module 2 Summary Learning Guides

8.1 Truth-Telling

- is defended as a fundamental moral value in healthcare practice
- is founded on respect for personal autonomy
- can be expressed in the form of a general principle
- requires skilful communication and listening to foster hope for coping with one's illness.

The principle of truth-telling is not absolute but it:

- allows for exceptions in certain specific situations
- requires that any exceptions be justified or defended by evidence from the concrete realities of a case
- considers therapeutic privilege as one such exception but one that requires caution in its use.

8.2 Arguments For and Against Breaking Bad News

1. Patient Autonomy

- For: The patient as a human being has an entitlement to know what is discovered about their health and what options are available for treatment and care.
- Against: The patient does not wish to know and has made this clear. The patient is not capable of understanding the truth.

2. Clinical Benefit

- For: Treatment is considerably facilitated if the patient knows what they are being treated for, what therapeutic options they could choose and why doctors or nurses might recommend certain treatments over others.
- Against: If the patient is informed about their diagnosis, the concern is that they will refuse to adhere to treatment and care that would benefit them.

3. Psychological Benefit

- For: Knowing and understanding diagnoses that are communicated with hope helps to provide psychological support against isolation in illness.
- Against: The truth would harm the patient by causing serious distress and taking away hope.

4. Practical Reality

- For: The patient will find out their diagnosis whether they are told by a health professional or not.

- Against: The patient is not in a position to find out the truth.

8.3 Traditional Ethical Approaches to Truth-Telling

If you approach truth-telling as a Kantian deontologist you would believe:

- that lying is intrinsically wrong

- that lying is against the moral law

- that, by lying to others, we treat both them and ourselves with disrespect

- that no anticipated good consequences from lying will make it right.

If you approach truth-telling as a consequentialist or utilitarian, you would believe:

- that no actions are intrinsically and always wrong

- that the rightness or wrongness of lying depends on the consequences of lying

- that the consequences must foster well-being and minimise suffering

- that the judgement of likely consequences is rigorously demanding and requires that you know the patient and context thoroughly.

9. Module 2 Activities

9.1 Recall the principle of truth-telling:

a. Would you add anything further to these points on truth-telling?

b. Would you challenge anything in this statement?

c. Use the following web link: http://www.hospicefriendlyhospitals.net/resources-and-courses/itemlist/category/20-resources-communications.html (accessed 1 December 2009) to download the document, How Do I Break Bad News? (Irish Hospice Foundation, 2009). Read the Guidelines and identify three of the ethical values that inform these guidelines. Source Buckman (2005) and critically consider the SPIKES strategy for communicating bad news.

9.2 Reflect back on the particulars of Case 1:

a. In reading Case 1, jot down your first, unanalysed response to the decisions taken.

b. If Mary does not understand her illness because she has not been taken seriously as a questioning patient, the possibility of achieving consent to treatment is undermined. What if the doctor decides to administer steroids in an effort to control Mary's pain? Mary may well ask, What is the medication? Will it help? What would you tell her?

c. Are the consequences of not informing Mary in Case 1 more conducive to maximising the good (for who?) than the results of informing her?

d. How would you gauge the likely consequences of telling or not telling Mary the truth of her condition?

9.3 Reflect back on the particulars of Case 2:

a. What do you think the doctor in this case means by 'backwards autonomy'? What other ethical values besides truth-telling have been set aside here?

b. The strong paternalism practised by the family in Sean's case involves more than limiting his access to information; it also has repercussions for his care. What are the ethical dilemmas for the health professionals involved?

c. Gauging consequences is difficult but very important if one is reasoning as a utilitarian. A good utilitarian has to ask: Were there good reasons for obstructions to Sean's liberty? How would you gauge the likely consequences of telling or not telling Sean the truth of his condition?

d. If you were the consultant involved, how might you respond to the conditions that the family place on you, the palliative care team, and the GP?

9.4 Reflect back on the particulars of Case 3:

a. Notice how different the focus is if one approaches the family as a group of people bound together by relationships and stories that tie them: the focus turns on the family as an integral whole needing help and listening. Consider how a health professional might help this family absorb and negotiate their father's illness.

b. Identify the ethical values that are at risk in Cases 2 and 3. Compare and contrast Cases 2 and 3 from an ethical perspective.

9.5 Reflect back on the particulars of Case 4:

a. It might be suggested that the couple in this case were treated insensitively because the doctor was uncomfortable with the fact that the patient was in a lesbian relationship. Consider this possibility. Consider in what ways homophobia might impact on the care and treatment offered to lesbian and gay patients. Jot down your first unanalysed response.

b. Download the Health Service Executive Guidelines on good practice with LGBT patients at the following link: http://www.hse.ie/eng/newsmedia/Archive/LGBT_HEALTH_Towards_ meeting_the_Health_care_Needs_of_Lesbian,_Gay,_Bisexual_and_Transgender_People. html

c. Are there any guidelines that you might have difficulty in applying? Have you any to add?

9.6 Reflect back on the particulars of Case 5:

a. What are the values at risk in this case? What are the values that need to be nurtured?

b. Critically consider the motivation of the director and the nurse in this case. What values might underpin their different responses to Joanna's situation?

c. Read Case 5 and consider the principle of truth-telling in the light of Joanna's situation. Note that the principle includes emphasis on the role of communication in the process of truth-telling. What, in your view, is the difference between 'truth-telling' and 'communication'?

9.7 Reflect back on the particulars of Case 6:

a. Take each of the four arguments for and against disclosing bad news and apply them to this case.

b. In your view, was the GP right to tell the truth? Or are concerns about the consequences of telling the truth more persuasive?

c. It could be argued that if health professionals are obliged to provide information, patients also have a responsibility to face the truth and to participate in a meaningful way in decisions about their treatment and care. This is all the more compelling when a patient's resistance to being told the truth may have implications for the well-being of others. See Module 4 for discussion of the harm principle and Module 7 for application of the harm principle to confidentiality. Consider whether or not the harm principle is applicable to the circumstances of Cases 5 and 6.

d. Practically speaking, some claim that it is difficult, if not futile, to impose the truth on someone who really does not want to hear it (Biggar, 2009). Can you recall any cases from practice which would lend support to this claim?

10. Module 2 References and Further Reading

Back, A., Arnold, R., & Tulsky, J. (2009) Mastering communication with seriously ill patients. Cambridge: Cambridge University Press

Beauchamp, T., & Childress, J. (2008). Principles of biomedical ethics (6th ed.). Oxford, New York: Oxford University Press

Beauchamp, T. and Childress, J. *Principles of Biomedical Ethics* (5th ed.) (Oxford and New York: Oxford University Press, 2001)

Biggar, N. Personal communication, 2009

Bok, S. *Lying: Moral Choice in Public and Private Life* (Sussex: Harvester Press, 1978)

Bok, S. *Secrets: On the Ethics of Concealment and Revelation* (New York: Vintage, 1983)

An Bord Altranais, *Code of Professional Conduct for Each Nurse and Midwife* (Dublin: An Bord Altranais, 2000a)

Brazier, M. and Cave, E. *Medicine, Patients and the Law* (4th ed.) (London: Penguin Books, 2007)

Buckman, R.A. Breaking Bad News: The S-P-I-K-E-S Strategy, *Community Oncology*, vol. 2, no. 2, 2005, pp.138–42

Candib, L.M. 'Truth Telling and Advance Planning at the End of Life: Problems with Autonomy in a Multicultural World', *Families, Systems & Health: The Journal of Collaborative Family HealthCare*, vol. 20, no. 3, 2002, pp.213–29

Clayton, J.M., Hancock, K.M., Butow, P.N., Tattersall, M.H.N., & Currow, D.C. (2007) Clinical practice guidelines for communicating prognosis and end-of-life issues with adults in the advanced stages of a life-limiting illness, and their caregivers. *MJA 186* (12) S77-S108 (Supplement)

Constitution of Ireland (Bunreacht na hÉireann), 1937

Council of Europe, Article 8. 'Right to Respect for Private and Family Life', The European Convention on Human Rights and Fundamental Freedoms as Amended by Protocol No. 11 (ETS No. 155) (Strasbourg: Council of Europe, 1998)

Department of Justice Equality and Law Reform, Scheme of Mental Capacity Bill 2008, http://www.justice.ie/en/JELR/Pages/Scheme_of_Mental_Capacity_Bill_2008 [accessed 18 August 2009]

Elger, B.S. and Harding, T.W. 'Should Cancer Patients Be Informed about their Diagnosis and Prognosis? Future Doctors and Lawyers Differ', *Journal of Medical Ethics*, vol. 28, no. 4,

2002, pp.258–65

Fujimori, M. and Uchitomi, Y. 'Preferences of Cancer Patients Regarding Communication of Bad News: A Systematic Literature Review', *Japanese Journal of Clinical Oncology*, vol. 39, no. 4, 2009, pp.201–16

Hancock, K., Clayton, J.M., Parker, S.M., Walder, S., Butow, P.N., Carrick, S., Currow, D., Ghersi, D., Glare, P., Hagerty, R. and Tattersall, M. 'Truth-Telling in Discussing Prognosis in Advanced Life-Limiting Illnesses: A Systematic Review', *Palliative Medicine*, vol. 21, no. 6, 2007, pp.507–17

Health Service Executive (HSE) *Good Practice Guidelines for Health Service Providers Working with Lesbian, Gay, Bisexual and Transgender People* (Dublin: HSE, 2009b), http://www. hse.ie/eng/newsmedia/Archive/LGBT_HEALTH_Towards_meeting_the_Health_care_Needs_of_Lesbian,_Gay,_Bisexual_and_Transgender_People.html [accessed 1 June 2009]

Higgins, A. and Glacken, M. 'Sculpting the Distress: Easing or Exacerbating the Grief Experience of Same-Sex Couples', *International Journal of Palliative Nursing*, vol. 15, no. 4, 2009, pp.170–6

Higgs, R. 'On Telling Patients the Truth', in H. Kuhse and P. Singer (eds), *Bioethics: An Anthology* (Oxford: Blackwell Publishers, 1999), pp.507–12

Hill, T.E. (ed.), *Autonomy and Self Respect* (Cambridge: Cambridge University Press, 1991)

Hunter v. Mann [1974] 2 All ER 414 QBD England

Irish Council for Bioethics and TNS/MRBI, 'Bioethics Research', http://www.bioethics.ie/uploads/docs/129171–Bioethics%20Research.pdf [accessed 19 August 2009]

Irish Hospice Foundation, *How Do I Break Bad News?* (2009), http://www.hospicefriendlyhospitals.net/resources-and-courses/itemlist/category/20-resources-communications.html [accessed 1 December 2009]

Irish Patients' Association, 'Your Rights and Responsibilities: The Irish Patients Charter' (2008), http://www.nrh.ie/LIVE_Docs/Patient%20Rights%20&%20Responsibilities.pdf [accessed 19 August 2009]

Johnstone, M. *Bioethics: A Nursing Perspective* (4th ed.) (Sydney: Churchill Livingstone, 2004)

Kant, I. *The Metaphysical Principles of Virtue* (trans. J. Ellington and W. Wick) (Indianapolis: Bobbs-Merrill Co., 1968)

Katz, J. *The Silent World of Doctor and Patient* (Baltimore: Johns Hopkins University Press, 2002)

Keating, D.T., Nayeem, K., Gilmartin, J.J. and O'Keeffe, S.T. 'Advance Directives for Truth Disclosure', *Chest*, vol. 128, no. 2, 2005, pp.1037–9

Keegan, O., McGee, H., Hogan, M., Kunin, H., O'Brien, S. and O'Siorain, L. 'Relatives' Views of Health Care in the Last Year of Life, *International Journal of Palliative Nursing*, vol. 7, no. 9, 2001, pp.449–56

Launer, J. 'Breaking the News', *QJM*, vol. 98, no. 5, 2005, pp.385–6

Lyckholm, L. 'Let's Be Honest', *Journal of Clinical Oncology*, vol. 20, no. 13, 2005, p.3037

McCartan, P., Fanning, M. and Conlon, M. *Breaking Bad News: A Literature Review and Guidelines for Breaking Bad News to Patients and Relatives* (Dublin: Beaumont Hospital, 1999)

McCarthy, J. 'Principlism or Narrative Ethics: Must we Choose Between Them?' *Medical Humanities*, vol. 29, no. 2, 2003, pp.65–71

Medical Council, *A Guide to Ethical Conduct and Behaviour* (6th ed.) (Dublin: Medical Council, 2004)

Medical Council, *Guide to Professional Conduct and Ethics for Registered Medical Practitioners* (7th ed.) (2009), http://www.medicalcouncil.ie [accessed 20 November 2009)]

Mill, J.S. *On Liberty* (Harmondsworth: Penguin, 1981 [1859])

Moazam, F. 'Families, Patients and Physicians in Medical Decisionmaking: A Pakistani Perspective', *Hastings Center Report*, vol. 30, no. 6, 2000, pp.28–37

Moody, H.R. 'Commentary', *Hastings Center Report*, vol. 25, no. 1, 1995, p.33

National Institute of Health (NIH), 'National Institutes of Mental Health. Suicide in the US: Statistics and Prevention' (2009), http://www.nimh.nih.gov/health/publications/suicide-in-the-us-statistics-and-prevention/index.shtml#children [accessed 19 August 2009]

Neff, P. 'Truth or Consequences: What to Do When the Patient Doesn't Want to Know', *Journal of Clinical Oncology*, vol. 20, no. 13, 2002, pp.3035–7

O'Keeffe, S.T. 'Development and Implementation of Resuscitation Guidelines: A Personal Experience', *Age & Ageing*, vol. 30, no. 1, 2001, pp.19–25

O'Keeffe, S.T., Noone, I. and Pillay, I. 'Telling the Truth about Cancer: Views of Elderly Patients and their Relatives', *Irish Medical Journal*, vol. 93, no. 4, 2000, pp.104–5

Quinlan, C. and O'Neill, C. 'Practitioners' Narrative Submissions, Interviews and Focus Groups' (Unpublished) (Dublin: Irish Hospice Foundation, 2008)

Quinlan, C. and O'Neill, C. *Practitioners' Perspectives on Patient Autonomy at End of Life* (Dublin: Irish Hospice Foundation, 2009)

Randall, F. and Downie, R.S. *Palliative Care Ethics: A Good Companion* (Oxford and New York: Oxford University Press, 1996)

Rayson, D. 'Sweet Time Unafflicted', *Journal of Clinical Oncology* (Supplement), vol. 21, no. 9, 2003, pp.46–8

Torrance, I. 'Confidentiality and its Limits: Some Contributions from Christianity', *Journal of Medical Ethics*, vol. 29, 2003, pp.8–9

Veatch, R.M. 'Abandoning Informed Consent', *Hastings Center Report*, vol. 25, no. 2, 1995, pp.5–12

Weafer, J. *A Qualitative Study of Public Perceptions of End-of-Life Issues* (Dublin: Irish Hospice Foundation, 2009a)

Weafer, J. *The Views of Political Representatives* (Dublin: Irish Hospice Foundation, 2009b)

Weafer, J. and Associates, *A Nationwide Survey of Public Attitudes and Experiences Regarding Death and Dying* (Dublin: Irish Hospice Foundation, 2004)

Weafer, J., McCarthy, J. and Loughrey M. *Exploring Death and Dying: The Views of the Irish General Public* (Dublin: Irish Hospice Foundation, 2009)

Yang-Lewis, T. 'Commentary', *Hastings Center Report*, vol. 25, no. 1, 1995, pp.32–3

Yang-Lewis, T. and Moody H.R. 'The Forgetful Mourner', *Hastings Center Report*, vol. 25, no. 1, 1995, p.32

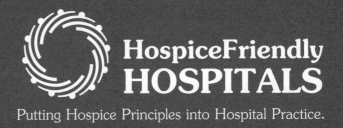

HospiceFriendly HOSPITALS

Putting Hospice Principles into Hospital Practice.

Module 3

Healthcare Decision-making and the Role of Rights

Module 3 Contents   Page

1. Module 3 Key Points

1.1 Patients have rights and these must be respected in healthcare decision making:

Patients have both moral rights and legal rights which must be respected in healthcare decision making. This includes decisions about the end of life.

1.2 Moral rights and legal rights are different:

A person may have a moral right to something but this moral right may not be enforceable in a court of law. This does not mean that the moral right is less important than a legal right. However, it can mean that a moral right is more difficult to enforce.

1.3 Rights are both positive and negative:

Rights can be seen as a right to something – a positive right – and a right that someone does not do something to you – a negative right. Most legal rights tend to be negative rights. This does not mean that negative rights are more important than positive rights. However, the enforcement of positive rights can be more difficult to achieve. In particular, positive rights may require the allocation of resources.

1.4 All patients have rights:

Rights are not restricted to certain patients only. All patients have rights. Patients who are children, patients who have disabilities, patients who lack the capacity to make decisions for themselves all have rights and these must be respected in healthcare decision making in respect of these patients.

1.5 Rights can sometimes be viewed in too limited a way:

Rights should not be thought of as negative rights or as legal rights only. This is too limited a view. It is essential to remember that people have positive rights and moral rights.

1.6 Rights are not absolute:

Rights may be restricted for a number of reasons, including the protection of the rights of others or the protection of societal interests. The extent to which a person's rights may legitimately be restricted varies depending on the circumstances.

1.7 A rights-based approach offers important possibilities in respect of patient care:

A rights-based approach to decision making can have important advantages for patient care. It places the patient at the centre of the decision-making process. In an end-of-life context, it recognises that all decisions must centre on the patient and his or her needs.

1.8 An exclusive focus on rights can be problematic:

A focus on rights without reference to the social situation in which people live (and die) can provide too narrow a focus.

1.9 Good care requires more than just respecting people's rights:

It is not enough simply to respect patients' rights. Good care requires more than this. Yet, while respect for rights does not provide the whole basis for care, it is an important aspect of appropriate patient care.

2. Module 3 Definitions

2.1 Positive Rights:

an individual's right to some social or personal or institutional benefit or provision.

2.2 Negative Rights:

the right to demand that a person or persons desist from doing something to you.

2.3 Moral Rights:

a justified claim that entitles us to demand that other persons act or desist from acting in certain ways.

2.4 Legal Rights:

rights enforceable in a Court of Law.

2.5 Constitution of Ireland:

a legal instrument which provides the foundation for all laws in Ireland. The Constitution was adopted in 1937 and sets out certain fundamental rights. All laws must comply with the Constitution and if a law is found to be unconstitutional, it is invalid, to the extent of the unconstitutionality. The Constitution may be amended only by a referendum of the people.

2.6 European Convention on Human Rights:

a human rights instrument adopted by the Council of Europe in 1950 to protect human rights and fundamental freedoms in Europe. Until 2003, Ireland was a signatory to the European Convention on Human Rights but judgements of the European Court of Human Rights in Strasbourg were of persuasive effect only. The European Convention on Human Rights Act 2003 made the Convention part of domestic Irish law. This means the Convention can be argued in an Irish court.

2.7 Charter of Patient Rights:

the European Charter of Patient Rights agreed in Rome in 2002 sets out 14 rights of the patient. The Charter is not legally enforceable but is an important indicator of best practice.

2.8 The United Nations Convention on the Rights of the Child:

an international human rights instrument adopted by the United Nations in 1989 which sets out the human rights of children. Ireland has signed and ratified the Convention. This means that Ireland is bound by the Convention.

2.9 The United Nations Convention on the Rights of Persons with Disabilities:

an international human rights instrument adopted by the United Nations in 2006 which sets out the human rights of persons with disabilities. Ireland has signed the Convention but has not ratified it. This means that the Convention is not legally binding on the state at this point but that the state has committed to be bound by the Convention at a later date.

2.10 Council of Europe Recommendation Concerning the Legal Protection of Incapable Adults:

a recommendation adopted by the Council of Europe in 1999 covering the protection of adults lacking decision-making capacity. This Recommendation is not legally binding but is an example of best practice in this area.

3. Module 3 Background

3.1 Medical Ethics and the Rise of Rights

For much of the history of medicine, the most important imperatives were doing good for the patient, frequently referred to as beneficence, and the protection of life, often referred to as the sanctity of life principle. This ethical view derives from the Judaeo-Christian tradition whereby life was seen as having an intrinsic value unrelated to the individual's views regarding his own life. The principle is based, in Paul Ramsey's words, on the fact that '[every human being is a unique, unrepeatable opportunity to praise God. His life is entirely an ordination, a loan and a stewardship' (Ramsey, 1971, p.11). The matter of patient rights was largely irrelevant. However, in the late 1960s, attitudes began to change. Medical ethicists, especially in the United States, began to emphasise the importance of patient rights and in particular to draw attention to the role of patient autonomy. The right of autonomy is of such significance in the context of healthcare decision making that it is considered in more detail in Module 4.

It has now become commonplace to speak about patient rights in the context of healthcare decision making. As the philosopher Onora O'Neill writes, since the mid-1970s 'no themes have become more central in large parts of bioethics, and especially in medical ethics, than the importance of respecting individual rights and individual autonomy' (2002, p.2). However, as O'Neill has also argued, this focus on rights is not unproblematic. She points to the cost to other values, including trust, which derives from a fixation with rights. Others (Callahan, 2003) have argued that the individualistic focus on rights fails to recognise the social context within which individuals operate.

In this module, we look at the issues which arise in respect of a rights-based approach to healthcare decision making in decisions made towards the end of life. The goal is to understand the possibilities and limits of a rights-based approach to decision making at the end of life and to appreciate how a rights-based approach operates in practice.

3.2 Different Kinds of Rights

In order to appreciate the role of rights in decision making at the end of life, it is important to distinguish between different kinds of rights. The first distinction is between positive rights and negative rights. The second distinction is between moral rights and legal rights.

3.2.1 Positive Rights and Negative Rights

Rights impose either negative or positive duties or obligations on others. We develop this distinction in the context of what we mean by 'a right to die'.

Negative rights: the right to demand that a person or persons desist from doing something to you. Applied to the 'right to die', this means, for example, that we have a negative right to refuse treatments or life-prolonging therapies.

Positive rights: the right to some social or personal or institutional benefit or provision. Applied to the 'right to a good dying', this means that we can claim or expect some state or healthcare institutional provisions that would facilitate a 'good dying', for example adequate pain relief, appropriate information, a caring and private environment.

A positive right to die might also be interpreted to mean a right to have active steps taken to end a person's life or to assist a person in ending his or her own life. The term 'euthanasia' is often used to refer to these situations. Additionally, the term 'assisted suicide' is sometimes used (where a person seeks assistance in ending his or her own life). The legal and ethical challenges to which these issues give rise are discussed in more detail in other modules. For present purposes, the important point is that neither is permissible under Irish law.

Under Irish law, any person who deliberately ends the life of another person is potentially guilty of murder. It makes no difference that the person consented to the action or even that he or she requested that this should happen. The law does not permit a person to consent to his or her own death. A person who assists another person in ending his or her own life is also criminally liable. Under Irish law, suicide ceased to be a criminal offence under the Criminal Law (Suicide) Act 1993. However, the act states that anyone who 'aids, abets, counsels or procures' the suicide of another person commits a criminal offence which is punishable with a possible maximum sentence of 14 years.

Therefore, a positive right to die in the sense of a right to have active steps taken to end one's life or to assistance in ending one's life would run contrary to the law. This is not the meaning of positive rights adopted in this module. However, other aspects of positive rights, such as a right to a 'good dying', are lawful and are very significant if we are to develop the best way to ensure that people have the most appropriate care and treatment at the end of their lives.

3.2.2 Moral Rights and Legal Rights

When thinking about the role of rights in healthcare decision making, it is important to distinguish between moral rights and legal rights.

A moral right, if accepted within a community, is a justified claim that entitles us to demand that other persons act or desist from acting in certain ways.

For example, we have a moral right to be treated with dignity and that people do not act in a way which is degrading or inconsistent with our dignity. Moral rights are politically important. The existence of a moral right is empowering for the individual whose right is recognised and the recognition of the right can have powerful rhetorical force. However, the existence of a moral right does not create a legal obligation in others to respect that right.

A legal right is a right which is legally enforceable in a court of law. Legal rights create legal obligations in another person or the state. Some legal rights are also moral rights but not all moral rights are legal rights.

To date, most legal interventions in respect of rights in an end-of-life context have involved the cessation of unwanted interventions rather than the delivery of appropriate care. This means that most legal rights have tended to be seen as negative rights rather than positive rights.

The fact that legal rights tend to be negative rather than positive means that the contribution of the law in this area is inevitably limited. This means that, while law is important in decisions about treatment at the end of life, the law provides only a small part of the picture in developing an appropriate framework for end-of-life care.

4. The Scope of Rights

Both legal and moral rights are important in thinking about decisions at the end of life. As will be seen below, there are advantages in a rights-based approach to patient care. However, it is also important to recognise the limited scope of a rights-based approach. Rights are not absolute and may justifiably be subject to limitations. Nor can it be expected that a simple reference to rights will resolve difficult ethical questions. Rights may also be in conflict. There may be a conflict between the rights of the dying person and those of other people or a conflict between different rights of the dying person. There may also be a conflict between individual rights and broader societal interests. A classic example of this conflict in action has been the debate surrounding assisted suicide. There may also be a conflict between respect for individual rights and a societal commitment to the principle of sanctity of life.

An exclusive focus on rights as the basis for a framework for a good dying is overly limited and does not, of itself, provide an appropriate approach to patient care. Other matters, including beneficence and care, are also essential components of an appropriate framework.

4.1 Rights and Absolutes

Few, if any, rights are absolute. Even rights which we think of as fundamental, such as the right to life, may be restricted in certain circumstances. The most common basis upon which rights are restricted is that respect for one person's right will have a negative impact on another person's right. In some circumstances, societal interests may also justify interfering with a person's right. For example, as discussed in Module 4, in various legal cases in respect of a right to assisted suicide the courts have held that the person's right to autonomy (in choosing when to end his or her life) could be overridden on the basis of a societal interest in protecting vulnerable people from possible pressure to end their lives. The difficult question is when such justifications will arise and how an appropriate balance may be struck between competing rights and interests. With legal rights, these questions are decided by courts. Increasingly commonly, courts adopt a proportional approach to the resolution of these kinds of questions. If a right is found to exist, the court asks whether interference with the right can be justified and whether the degree of interference is proportional in light of the justification. With moral rights, resolution of the appropriate balance depends on informed debate and discussion.

4.2 Rights and Responsibilities

Patients have rights but they also have responsibilities. Brazier (2006, p.401) identifies the direct link between increased recognition of patient rights and an increased recognition of patient responsibilities: 'In a relationship where the recipients of medical care were infantilised, patients' responsibilities seem to me to be of a much lesser order.' Thus, she argues that 'it is the empowerment of patients that brings responsibilities'.

Freedom of choice (which is central to a rights-based approach centred on the right of autonomy) brings with it a moral responsibility to consider the impact of one's choice on others. For example, a person's decision to decline life-saving treatment places an ethical obligation on the person to consider the impact of his or her decision on family members or others. Again, a distinction must be made between moral obligations and legal obligations. As Brazier (2006, p.422) reminds us, 'identifying when and how these moral obligations become legally enforceable remains difficult'. We may argue that a person has a moral obligation to take account of the impact of his or her decisions on others but imposing a legal obligation to do this is a different matter.

4.3 The Contribution of a Rights-Based Approach

A rights-based approach to decisions taken at the end of life has important advantages for patient care. It places the patient at the centre of the decision-making process and allows a patient to exert a degree of control over how and when she dies.

The value of this approach can be seen in one of the narratives outlined by Quinlan and O'Neill (2008, p.19):

> *Rita had a very peaceful happy death. She refused some treatment and her wishes were granted. She never discussed death with any staff, but in the end had a very peaceful pain-free death in the company of her family.*

Here, Rita's rights, in particular her right not to have treatment which she did not feel appropriate, was respected and Rita's death was peaceful and pain free.
Arguments based on positive rights can also make a very significant contribution to delivering appropriate care and in particular in respect of the important matter of access to necessary resources. In end-of-life care, there are repeated concerns about the lack of resources necessary to make a 'good dying' a more likely outcome.

As Quinlan and O'Neill's (2009, pp.29–30) interviews show, the pressure on resources, even when people are dying, was evident. There is pressure for beds. A hospital may need the bed for the next patient and practitioners recount how, even when a patient is still dying, staff may come to the ward and ask if the patient has gone to the mortuary yet. There is resource pressure in providing access to appropriate treatment and diagnostic processes at an appropriate time. There is resource pressure in facilitating dying people, both adults and children, in spending their last days at home. One incident recounted by Quinlan and O'Neill (2009, p.30) reminds us that, when someone has a short time to live, even relatively short delays can have a huge impact on the patient's quality of life and death. The practitioner describes a young man who had to spend over five weeks in hospital in order to have routine procedures because resource pressures led to delays. For a young man with a limited life expectancy, this was time which he would have been happier to spend elsewhere.

The impact of limited resources is also felt in respect of communication. Communication is fundamental if a patient's right to a dignified dying is to be a reality. Yet, based on practitioner interviews, one of the most consistent frustrations experienced is in respect of communication. This frustration stems in large part from shortage of staff and lack of time on busy wards.

Resources have to be pleaded for in social and political arenas. While positive rights may not necessarily be legally enforceable, the rhetoric of rights ensures that the issue of resources is recognised as an ethical issue as well as a political one. As Munro (2001, p. 463) notes, 'the rhetorical value of rights discourse must not be underestimated.' It is essential that rights are understood as encompassing both positive and negative rights and that it is recognised that people have positive rights to a 'good dying'.

4.4 The Limits of a Rights-Based Approach

While a rights-based approach makes an important contribution to an appropriate framework (and in respect of legal rights is a legal obligation), an exclusive focus on rights is limited in several respects. First, rights are formulated in an abstract way and sometimes the rhetoric of rights may seem far removed from the reality of treatment decisions in practice. It is one thing to say that a patient has rights, it is quite another to understand what respect for a patient's rights requires in any particular situation.

Secondly, while rights can be both positive and negative, very often a rights-based approach will be seen to extend only to negative rights. This is in part because the law has tended to recognise negative rights rather than positive rights. This approach to rights can lead to a rights-based approach which protects a patient's right to refuse unwanted treatment but does little in furthering the provision of appropriate treatment (in the broadest sense including medical treatment but also an appropriate environment, communication, etc).

Thirdly, an exclusive focus on rights omits important aspects of the ethical picture. Beauchamp and Childress' influential four principles approach to ethics identifies beneficence, nonmaleficence and justice alongside autonomy. An appropriate framework for decisions at the end of life requires more than simply respecting patients' rights. If we look at the example of Rita's situation discussed earlier, her right to refuse treatment was an important aspect of her peaceful death but so too was the fact that her family were present and the care of the professionals involved. Focussing on rights alone fails to accord sufficient recognition to these broader but equally essential aspects of patient care at the end of life.

5. Rights in Practice

Rights must have a basis or source. It is not enough simply to assert that a person has a right to something. There must be a means whereby the existence of the right may be asserted.

5.1 Sources of Moral Rights

Moral rights derive from our membership of the moral community. In this sense, moral rights may sometimes be contested. For example, some people may argue for a moral right to choose to die even if this requires active steps, such as euthanasia, while others may equally vigorously contest the existence of such a moral right.

5.2 Sources of Legal Rights

In relation to legal rights, the rights derive from a more tangible source. For a right to be legally enforceable, it must for the main part derive from some form of legal instrument. Like moral rights, legal rights can be contested. However, with legal rights, the final determination of whether or not a legal right exists, what the right means and whether interference with the right may be justified is made by a court. Legal rights tend to be more limited in scope and will often tend to be negative rather than positive rights. For this reason, it is important to remember that legal rights should not be thought of as providing the whole basis for patient rights in respect of healthcare decision making (and that rights alone do not provide a full basis for care).

Nonetheless, legal rights provide the foundation for healthcare decisions and therefore it is necessary to discuss the sources of patients' legal rights in more detail.

5.3 Legal Rights as Citizens

Patients at the end of life have the same rights as any other members of society. Therefore the human rights frameworks which apply to all citizens in general also apply to these patients. In Ireland, these rights derive first, from the Irish Constitution (Bunreacht na hÉireann) and secondly, from the European Convention on Human Rights. Both of these human rights instruments impose obligations on others to respect rights and a patient may assert his or her rights in a court. These rights are practically important because a patient can take steps to enforce them and because health professionals are legally obliged to respect them.

5.3.1 Rights and the Irish Constitution

The Irish Constitution was introduced in 1937. It provides the basis for protection of individual rights. All legislation must comply with the provisions of the Constitution. The 'fundamental rights' part of the Constitution is found in Articles 40–45. Of these Articles,

the most important source for patient rights is Article 40.3.1.
This Article states as follows:

The State guarantees in its laws to respect, and, as far as practicable, by its laws to defend and vindicate the personal rights of the citizen.

From this general statement, the Irish courts have identified a range of rights (often referred to as 'unenumerated' or unstated rights). The rights identified by the courts have included a right to autonomy or self-determination; a right to privacy; a right to dignity; a right to bodily integrity; a right to freedom from inhuman and degrading treatment. The Irish Constitution also expressly protects the right to life. Article 40.3.2 states that the state shall protect, as best it may, the life of every citizen from unjust attack and, in the case of injustice done, vindicate that life.

Two other articles of the Constitution are relevant in respect of children. Article 41 protects the authority of the family (based on marriage) while Article 42 protects parents' rights in respect of their children. Article 42.5 can be especially important in relation to healthcare decision making involving children. This article states that, in exceptional cases, where parents for physical or moral reasons fail in their duty to their children, the state may endeavour to supply the place of the parents but always with due regard to the rights of the child. Other than this, there is currently no express statement of the rights of the child in the Constitution.

The Irish Constitution is much less strong in its endorsement of positive rights. Article 45 sets out 'directive principles of social policy'. This states that justice and charity must inform national institutions and that the vulnerable must be protected. However, these principles cannot be enforced in a court of law. Therefore, as with the other positive rights discussed above, these are matters for political and ethical engagement rather than legal enforcement.

5.3.2   Rights under the European Convention on Human Rights

Since 2003, the European Convention on Human Rights (ECHR) has been incorporated into Irish law. This means that the ECHR is directly enforceable in the Irish courts. However, if there is a conflict between the Irish Constitution and the ECHR, constitutional rights take priority. The ECHR was adopted in 1950 to protect human rights and fundamental freedoms in Europe. A number of the rights protected by the ECHR are important in the context of end-of-life decisions. These include: the right to life which is protected by Article 2; the right to freedom from inhuman and degrading treatment which is protected by Article 3; the right to respect for private and family life which is protected by Article 8; and the right to freedom of thought, conscience and religion which is protected by Article 9.

5.4   Other Sources of Rights

5.4.1   Charter of Patients' Rights

In addition to general rights under the Irish Constitution and the ECHR, there is a specific Charter of Patients' Rights. Unlike rights protected under the Irish Constitution and the ECHR, these rights are not directly enforceable in a court. They are also stated in general terms and many are aspirational in nature. However, they are important indicators of best practice. The European Charter of Patients' Rights agreed in Rome in 2002 sets out 14 rights of the patient. The following rights are most important in the context of healthcare decisions, including decisions at the end of life.

Right to Information: Every individual has a right of access to all kinds of information regarding their state of health.

Right to Consent: Every individual has a right of access to all information that might enable him or her to actively participate in the decisions regarding his or her health; this information is a prerequisite for any procedure and treatment.

Right of Free Choice: Each individual has the right to freely choose from different treatment procedures and providers on the basis of adequate information.

Right to Privacy and Confidentiality: Each individual has the right to the confidentiality of personal information, including information regarding his or her state of health and potential diagnostic or therapeutic procedures.

Right to Avoid Unnecessary Suffering and Pain: Each individual has the right to avoid as much suffering and pain as possible, in each phase of his or her illness.

5.4.2   International Human Rights Instruments

There are also a number of international human rights instruments which have a broader remit than application to patients but which are relevant to certain kinds of patients. Among the most important of these instruments are:

The United Nations Convention on the Rights of the Child:
This Convention was adopted by the United Nations General Assembly on 20 November 1989 and entered into force on 20 September 1990. Ireland signed the Convention on 30 September 1990 and ratified it without reservation on 21 September 1992. This means that Ireland is bound by the Convention. The Convention sets out the human rights of children

which must be observed by states. The Article of the Convention which is most relevant to healthcare decision making is Article 12. This says that:

States parties shall assure to the child who is capable of forming his or her own views the right to express those views freely in all matters affecting the child, the views of the child being given due weight in accordance with the age and maturity of the child.

This requires that, in healthcare decisions, including decisions about dying, the child has a right to participate in the decision-making process and his or her views must be taken into account increasingly as he or she becomes older and/or more mature (Kilkelly and Donnelly, 2006; 2011).

United Nations Convention on the Rights of Persons with Disabilities:
This Convention was adopted by the United Nations General Assembly in December 2006 and entered into force on 3 May 2008. The Convention was signed by Ireland on 30 March 2007. However, it has not yet been ratified by Ireland. This means that the state has not yet formally agreed to be bound by the Convention. It is likely that, when legislation relating to adults lacking capacity is introduced (expected to happen in 2012), the state will ratify the Convention and it will then be bound to observe the rights set out in the Convention.

The Convention sets out a framework to protect the human rights of people with disabilities – both physical and mental/intellectual disabilities. Among the Articles of most relevance to healthcare decision making, and in particular to decisions at the end of life are:
Article 3 sets out general principles underpinning the Convention. These include respect for inherent dignity and individual autonomy, including the freedom to make one's own choices, and independence of persons.
Article 10 reaffirms the inherent right to life of all persons with disabilities.
Article 17 states that every person with disabilities has a right to respect for his or her physical and mental integrity on an equal basis with others.

Council of Europe Recommendation Concerning the Legal Protection of Incapable Adults:
This Recommendation was adopted by the Council of Europe in 1999. The Recommendation adopts as its fundamental principle 'respect for the dignity of each person as a human being'. It requires that the laws, procedures and practices relating to the protection of adults lacking capacity should be based on respect for their 'human rights and fundamental freedoms'. The Recommendation is an indicator of best practice and is not legally binding.

6. Cases: Exploring Rights in Action

It is a relatively straightforward matter to list the rights relevant to end-of-life decisions. The most obvious of these are the right to life, the right to autonomy or self-determination, the right to bodily integrity, the right to dignity, the right to freedom from inhuman and degrading treatment. However, it is a much more complex and difficult matter to determine how rights apply in practice and how a rights-based approach to end of life decisions should work. This section will explore some of the issues through four case studies. These show the contribution which a rights-based approach can make but they also show the limits of a rights-based approach and remind us that good care requires more than simply respect for rights.

6.1 Case 1: The Limits of Negative Rights – refusing pain relief

Consider the following case which is based on a narrative from a practitioner recounted by Quinlan and O'Neill (2008, p.18) and which shows some of the limits of the rights-based approach to care. As is clear from the narrative, the incident described did not occur in Ireland. Nonetheless, the issues to which it gives rise are applicable here:

> *Refusing pain relief*
>
> *In Australia, a young mother in early 30's had an inoperable tumour at back of her nose and throat. In the end stages, this girl refused pain relief or sedatives. She did not want much medical intervention. It was the most distressing death I ever witnessed as she could not breathe and depended on a nasal tube as her only airway. This frequently blocked and needed regular suctioning. It was very distressing for her, her family and staff. She was from a very poor social background and had little or no education. Staff tried to assist her as much as possible but it was an awful death for her.* (Quinlan and O'Neill, 2008, p.18)

6.1.1   Discussion

This case shows the limits of an approach to rights which is based simply on negative rights. Here, the patient refused pain relief or sedatives. In this, she was exercising her right to autonomy by refusing medical intervention/treatment. This right is recognised under the Irish Constitution (In re a Ward of Court, 1995; Fitzpatrick v K, 2008) and under the European Convention on Human Rights (Pretty v UK, 2004). The right is undoubtedly very important and is discussed in more detail in Module 4.

However, the striking thing about this narrative is how very limited the right of autonomy can be. The young woman's right to refuse treatment was respected but, on the basis of this narrative, very little was done in a positive way to improve the dying process for her. Respect for the patient's autonomy here raised conflicts with the healthcare staff's concern about the well-being of the patient and yet they believed that the value of autonomy as expressed by the patient should have priority.

Arguing that something positive should have been done to improve the dying process for this patient does not mean that the woman's autonomous wishes should not be respected. However, if one thinks about the circumstances, there may have been positive ways in which the woman's right to make her own choices and decisions could have been respected while at the same time helping to ensure that her death was made as bearable for her as was possible in light of her circumstances.

For example, the narrative states that the woman was from a very poor social background and had little or no education. Presumably, also, she was very frightened and distressed. In addition to her physical pain, it is highly likely that she suffered 'soul pain' (discussed in detail in Module 5). It may be that, if it had been possible to talk with her, to explain and discuss her situation and to provide her with the support she needed, she might have been able to choose a way of dying which was less difficult for her (and less traumatic for her carers and family members). The choice should not be between respecting her right to refuse treatment and imposing treatment she does not wish. Rather it should be possible to find ways to provide positive help suitable for her situation.

Contrast the very different approach evident in the following example, also drawn from Quinlan and O'Neill (2009, p.32):

A couple of years ago now when I was in Palliative Medicine in another centre, adult Palliative Medicine, we came across a gentleman who was referred to us after he had attempted to commit suicide and he had thrown himself into the local river, was referred to us then. The reason that he had tried to commit suicide was that he had a diagnosis of cancer which he'd lived with well for about eight years at this stage but was developing increasing pain and he was worried that if his pain was so bad at this stage and not controlled, how bad was it going to be when he was closer to death and it was really his fear about symptoms, you know, not being controlled. So he was able to relay all this to us, we then got his pain under control, relatively easily I suppose, it's what we do every day, and we were able to reassure him that his pain would never have to be out of control as it had been and thereby his suicidal ideation completely resolved.

Because the health professionals were able to reassure this man, he was able to live out his life in the best way possible in the circumstances. Rather than ending his life by suicide, he felt content to live out his life to the end because he knew that his pain could be controlled.

If one contrasts this example with Case 1, this example shows the contribution to be made by positive rights to a 'good dying.' This approach to rights is much broader in scope and much more significant for many patients than simply respecting patients' decisions.

Of course, respect for patients' decisions is very important but so too is respect for the positive rights needed to ensure that patients' decisions are made in a way which maximises patient control. Empirical research shows unanimity on the significance of adequate pain relief. As one hospice worker commented, 'the main thing is that it's just pain relief. Our big thing in the unit is pain relief, that person is never in pain.' (Quinlan and O'Neill, 2008). Without adequate pain relief, it is very difficult for patients to have and to retain control of their situation. It is just as important to remember that patients have a positive right to appropriate pain relief and to appropriate explanations and communications from professionals as it is to remember that patients have a negative right to refuse treatment.

6.1.2   Suggested Professional Responsibilities

- Where a person refuses treatment, especially pain relief, efforts should be made to engage with the person and to understand the basis for the decision. Patients' decisions may be based on fear or lack of understanding and communication may help to alleviate these factors. The person may still wish to refuse the treatment and if he or she does so and he or she has the necessary degree of decision-making capacity, his or her wish to do so should be respected.

- Where possible, where a person refuses a particular treatment, alternative options should be made available to the person. Reasonable choice requires the availability of more than one option.

- Efforts should be made to engage with the patient in a way which is accessible to him or her in light of education level, background, etc. Different people require different kinds of communication and in many instances, a blanket approach based on simple provision of information will not suffice.

- Every effort should be made to ensure both that adequate pain relief is made available and that patients are reassured in this regard. Even if patients have not actively sought reassurance, they may have fears about pain which they find difficult to articulate. Sometimes it may be necessary to repeatedly provide reassurance about pain relief for patients.

6.2 Case 2: Constitutional Rights - In Re a Ward of Court 1995

One of the reasons why rights tend sometimes to be thought of as negative rather than positive – with the limits which this involves – is that the law's approach to rights usually focuses on negative rights rather than positive rights. This is evident in the following case study which is based on the facts of an important Irish Supreme Court decision on end of life. In the case study, we can see legal reasoning at work and we also see the possibilities and the limits of a law-focussed approach to rights.

In re a Ward of Court 1995

This case came before the Supreme Court in 1995. It concerned a woman who had been in a near- Persistent Vegetative State (PVS) for twenty-three years. She was unable to communicate although she may have had minimal ability to recognise and track people with her eyes. She was unable to move or swallow and was fed by gastrostomy (PEG) tube.

The Ward's family asked the court to have the PEG tube removed which removal would, inevitably, lead to the woman's death. In reaching its decision in favour of removing the tube, the Supreme Court regarded as relevant a number of rights protected under the Irish Constitution. These included the right to autonomy or self-determination, the right to privacy, the right to dignity, the right to bodily integrity, the right to life and the right to die and the right to equality. The court stated that the fact that the woman lacked decision-making capacity did not diminish her rights. To distinguish between people with capacity and people without capacity would be 'invidious'.

Bearing in mind the significance of the woman's rights, the Supreme Court decided that decisions such as this should be made on the basis of the best interests of the person taken from the point of view of a 'prudent and loving' parent. In the circumstances, the PEG tube should be removed.

6.2.1   Discussion

The decision in In re a Ward of Court is important for many reasons. The fact that the case came before the court at all is striking. There was clearly a strong disagreement between the health professionals and family members. There is a suggestion that the ward's family had attempted to communicate about the possibility of discontinuing life supports including re-insertions of the PEG tube and use of antibiotics and resuscitation when their loved one arrested and that these efforts at communication were resisted. The institution where the Ward was cared for had ethical objections to discontinuing life supports, especially discontinuing the PEG tube, because they understood this as aiding the progression towards dying.

Sometimes disagreements between health professionals and family members will be inevitable; there may be very good reasons why family members and health professionals do not agree. If this is the case, it may well be that a situation such as this may only be resolved through recourse to courts. However, there may be situations where better communication between health professionals, family members and patients would resolve some of the difficulties and avoid the need for the engagement of the legal system. In particular, knee-jerk reactions by professionals to family requests must be avoided. Resolution is much more likely in a context of engagement, communication and explanation rather than dogmatic assertions by professionals. And even if resolution is not possible in the particular circumstances, a process of communication and engagement enhances the experience for all concerned: the patient, the family and the health professionals.

In re a Ward of Court is also important because it involves the Supreme Court setting out in the clearest terms that patients have rights in respect of dying and that these rights do not stop simply because a person lacks or loses capacity. The fact that the woman was in a near PVS did not diminish her rights. She still had rights to autonomy, bodily integrity, dignity and privacy. These rights arise under the Constitution and all people and institutions who deal with her (and with other patients) have a legal obligation to respect these rights. Failure to do so would leave the healthcare professional/institution liable for failing to respect individual rights.

While the recognition that people have rights, regardless of capacity, was a very important contribution, the Supreme Court was less clear in setting out what exactly the rights actually meant in the circumstances of the case before them. In fact, the court did little more than list the rights implicated and provided no analysis of how they operated and interacted with each other and with the principle of sanctity of life. The decision has been criticised for its lack of conceptual coherence (Keown, 1996; Hogan and Whyte 2004, pp.1397–1401).

The Supreme Court left many questions unanswered. For example, what does it mean to respect the right of autonomy of a woman who clearly lacks the ability to make decisions and who has not left any clear indication of what she would have wanted to happen in the situation which arises? This means that health professionals trying to provide rights-based end-of-life care are left with limited legal guidance regarding what exactly is required. Patients' rights have to be respected but the detail of what respect for patient rights requires is more difficult. This is why a focus on legal rights alone provides too limited a basis for a rights-based approach to a good dying. This case reminds us that a meaningful rights-based approach to healthcare decision making must encompass positive as well as negative rights and moral as well as legal rights.

In In re a Ward of Court, the Supreme Court did not differentiate between withdrawal of artificial nutrition and hydration (ANH) and other forms of treatment withdrawal. However, following the decision, both the Medical Council and An Bord Altranais issued statements making a clear differentiation on these grounds. This special status of nutrition and hydration is reflected in the current Medical Council *Guide to Professional Conduct and Ethics for Registered Medical Practitioners* (2009) which states that 'Nutrition and hydration are basic needs of human beings. All patients are entitled to be provided with nutrition and hydration in a way that meets their needs' (par.19.1). However, the Code has moved away from the more absolute position of previous Codes, which had required that 'all reasonable and practical efforts should be made to maintain' nutrition and hydration. Rather, it now states that '[i]f a patient is unable to take sufficient nutrition and hydration orally, you should assess what alternative forms are possible and appropriate in the circumstances.' Medical professionals are reminded that they should 'bear in mind the burden or risks to the patient, the patient's wishes if known, and the overall benefit to be achieved.' The ethical issues to which withdrawal of ANH give rise are discussed in detail in Module 6.

The decision of the Supreme Court in In re a Ward of Court shows both the potential and the limitations of legal rights. Recognising that patients have legally enforceable rights places patients in a stronger position in asserting their rights. However, legal rights are just the first part of the picture. Good care requires more than just respecting people's legal rights.

6.2.2 Suggested Professional Responsibilities

- It is essential to maintain good communication with family members. This does not mean that family members' views should take precedence over the legal and ethical obligation of the healthcare professional to provide care to the patient. However, appropriate communication can alleviate family concerns and can sometimes prevent confrontational situations developing.

- If in doubt about the legal rights implicated in a particular decision, professionals should seek advice as to how to proceed. This is especially important in the event of disputes between family members or between professionals and family members.

6.3 Case 3: Children, Rights and Healthcare Decision-making – Glass v UK 2004

Good care requires more than just respecting people's legal rights. This is shown in the next case study which is also based on a legal case but which shows a range of factors relevant to good decision making which go beyond simply respecting legal rights.

Decisions involving children, especially decisions where children are dying, are very traumatic and difficult for all parties involved. As Quinlan and O'Neill (2009, p.56) remind us:

> A sick child in a family is as much at the mercy of the family dynamics as any sick person within a family. Sometimes the dynamics are good and sometimes they are not so good. Where the not so good family dynamics interfere with the care of the child the clinicians may need to intervene, and facilitate a resolution, as they intervene in any such family. Such interventions are often unwelcome and as such they can be difficult and challenging for the clinicians as well as the families. All of this goes to further the complexity of the situation of the patient in hospital and expressions and experiences of patient autonomy and practices around patient autonomy in hospital care settings.

The challenges involved in making decisions where children or young people are very ill or dying are very clear in the case discussed below. This case came before the European Court of Human Rights in 2004. The case had first been brought before the courts in the United Kingdom and these courts had held that there had been no breach of rights in the circumstances (which are outlined in more detail below). The family were unhappy with the conclusion and brought the case to the European Court of Human Rights. As in Ireland, the European Convention on Human Rights is part of domestic law in the United Kingdom and decisions of the European Court of Human Rights are binding on citizens and the state.

Glass v UK 2004

David Glass was a teenager with severe intellectual and physical disabilities and with a very poor life expectancy. He had been admitted to hospital many times in the past with respiratory failure and this was a pattern which was likely to continue.

David was admitted to hospital following respiratory failure. The health professionals responsible for his care considered that his condition had reached the point where any further resuscitation was futile. They put a DNR (do not resuscitate) order on his file without consulting with his family.

The health professionals also believed that David was in pain and they provided him with palliative care in the form of morphine, again without consulting his family. David's family objected to the placing of the DNR on this file and to the administration of morphine which they feared would speed up his death. They attempted to remove the DNR from the file and to disconnect the morphine feed. A fracas ensued between family members and the health professionals and family members were physically ejected from David's room by security staff. David's mother (acting as representative for the family) first brought the case before the English courts, arguing that the placing of the DNR and the administration of morphine without the consent of David's family was a breach of the family's rights and also of David's rights. The action was unsuccessful before the English courts. Mrs Glass brought the matter to the European Court of Human Rights. She argued that the hospital had failed to respect both her own right and David's right to private and family life as protected by Article 8 of the European Convention on Human Rights.

The European Court held that the hospital authorities had breached David's right to private and family life. The professionals involved should have consulted with David's family before reaching the decisions on his care. The court did not consider that the family's views should have decided the matter. Ultimately, the important question was whether the decision made was in David's best interests. This could be decided by the professionals involved or, in the event of a dispute, by a court. However, David was entitled to have his family consulted before a decision regarding his best interests was reached. The court did not offer any view on whether Mrs Glass's rights were breached.

6.3.1 Discussion

This case is important for a number of reasons. First, even if one does not consider the matter from a perspective of legal rights, it is very obvious that the hospital's way of dealing with the Glass family was inappropriate. Cases like this can come to litigation precisely because of failures on the part of health care staff to communicate in an ongoing way and assure families that they are being heard. This case also arose in part because the resuscitation process was neither clarified nor documented on the ward and the family's wishes or family expectations were not documented. Once again, a failure of communication by staff with family intensified the family's frustration.

Some of the practitioner perspectives recounted by Quinlan and O'Neill (2009, p.81) remind us of how important it is that resuscitation status is clear and that patients and family members are aware of the position. Failure to clarify can result in the patient, family and staff being insecure and anxious about a DNR (do not resuscitate) order.

This can be made more difficult because some consultants may be reluctant to document the existence of a DNR order. The position may also raise difficulties when, as happened in Case 3, families may insist on resuscitation and a conflict arises on the ward.

More than anything, Case 3 serves as a reminder of the need for good communication. This does not mean that families and professionals will always agree. But it does maximise the chances of agreement and an appropriate resolution and it ensures that, even if the participants fail to reach agreement, the discussion takes place in the best possible way for the patient, the family and the health professionals.

The second reason that Case 3 is important is that it recognises that patients are members of families. It was David's right that his family be consulted. Respect for patient rights requires family involvement. In Ireland, family rights are further enhanced by Articles 41 and 42 of the Irish Constitution. Here, the rights recognised are the rights of the family and of parents. In North Western Health Board v HW and CW (2001), the Irish Supreme Court held that parents had a constitutional right to make healthcare decisions for their children (in this case, the parents sought to refuse the routine PKU test aimed at detecting certain genetic abnormalities). The right is not absolute. The state can intervene where parents fail in their moral duty but this may arise only in an 'exceptional case' (as set out in Article 42(5) of the Constitution of Ireland) where, for example, the child's life is at risk: see Temple Street v D and Anor [2011] IEHC 1.

A great deal has been written about the way in which families have been treated in healthcare decision making in respect of children (for example, Bristol Royal Infirmary Inquiry, 2001; Kilkelly and Donnelly, 2006). In the inquiry into practices surrounding children's heart surgery at the Bristol Royal Infirmary, it became clear that some professionals dealing with parents were not giving clear indications to parents about their children's situations. Sometimes this was a deliberate practice, aimed at ensuring that parents maintained hope or did not communicate distress to children. However, as the Bristol parents recognised (2001, p.282): 'I think you need to know. It hurts … It hurts to hear it, but you need to know the truth. I do not want to be told that everything is going to be jolly and fine. It is a fact of life … You do not want people to be cruel to you but you need honesty in a situation like that.'

Case 3 reminds us that children and their families have a right to full information and appropriate communication. Families have to be consulted in decisions at the end of life of their children and their views must be taken into account in reaching decisions. This does not mean that family views will or should always prevail but consultation, communication and engagement are essential.

Case 3 is also important because, while it recognises that patients are members of families, it also reminds us that patients are individuals too. David had a right to have his family consulted as regards what was in his best interests. But the decision was not wholly that of David's family. Rather the decision had to be what was best for David. His family were an important part of this decision but ultimately it was David's best interests which were at stake. These were to be determined by the health professionals in consultation with his family and, if a dispute continued, by the court.

Family involvement is, of course, not just an issue in respect of children. It can equally arise in the context of elderly people as the following example from Quinlan and O'Neill (2009, p.37) makes clear:

> *I have a very recent experience that upset me greatly and that I'm still trying to have conversations with the individuals concerned and it was for a patient who had, whom I happened to come across on their admission to the hospital four days previously. So I knew their history very well. They had had palliative radiotherapy for CA of the lung, a gentleman in his early 80s, and he had a chest infection on admission to hospital. I met up with the family about three days later when I took a report from a colleague at 5 pm in the evening, to hear that the patient's condition had deteriorated. His oxygen saturations had dropped. He was on the medical unit and had been transferred to the high care unit and he was disimproving. I asked what the plan of care was for him and I was told that the family wanted him to have every possible chance. The consultant was not on duty that day. There was someone acting for him until 5 pm in the evening and as far as they were aware, the gentleman was to be resuscitated. I asked had the fact that he had a chest infection as well as CA of the lung (he knew what was wrong with him) been discussed with the patient and I was told no, because the family wanted him to have every chance. Before I got to the end of that report the emergency bleep went off and it was for this patient. When I got to the unit the patient was intubated. I asked the nurses about it. They said yes the family wanted – the doctor had discussed it with the family and they did want resuscitation measures taken if anything happened. They knew that their father was getting worse. The father himself had expressed that he didn't want tubes or anything like that, so I was very annoyed really. I couldn't understand how it had gotten to this stage.* (2009, p.34)

Here it would seem that the family's views took precedence over those of the patient (who died an hour later). Quinlan and O'Neill's study of practitioner perspectives suggest that this is not unusual. One practitioner quoted states:

Sometimes their wishes may not be respected. You might like have a patient and you might know the patient quite well and know that they probably want conservative treatment or palliative care. The families might want this done or want them transferred to [named acute hospital]. The next thing they're getting bloods and x-rays and the whole lot done and know in your heart and soul, this is not what this patient wants. **(2009, p.37)**

It is easy to understand why families respond in these kinds of ways. Families may find it difficult to 'let go' of a loved one; they may be suspicious of medical professionals, perhaps doubting that the professionals have their loved one's best interests at heart; they will often be frightened and traumatised by the impending death. With these difficult challenges around life-support decisions, one contributor suggests that perhaps a Palliative Care Team would be of great benefit to sound decision making. This team would deal specifically with end-of-life families. The contributor suggested:

…if there was a system there or there was services there, that we actually had a team that were able to approach a family and say: 'Listen, this is what we'll do over the next few hours' or 'listen, this is what you have in the weeks ahead.

Once again, communication does not solve all the difficulties which may arise but good communication provides the basis for the best experience possible.

As discussed above, the challenges for a rights-based approach to decision making are significant when family members are involved. Patients who are children have a right to have their families involved in decisions about their dying. But ultimately, the patient must be central. His or her views must provide the basis for decisions about care. Of course, it will not always be possible for a patient to express his or her views. In Case 3, David had very serious intellectual and physical disabilities and very limited abilities to communicate. Very young children may also have difficulty communicating what they want although most children are able to express preferences from a relatively young age (Alderson and Montgomery, 1996; Kilkelly and Donnelly, 2006; Bridgeman, 2007). The issue of children's autonomy and respect for children's choices will be discussed in more detail in Module 4.

6.3.2 Suggested Professional Responsibilities

- Professionals should maintain communication with family members. This is especially important in respect of highly charged situations such as the recording of a DNR on a patient's file.

- Where possible, health professionals should inform families about what to expect in the dying process. Many families will not know what to expect and informing them of what is likely will make the process easier and reduce the possibilities of conflict between families and health professionals. This may also involve reassurance about pain relief and distress.

- Professionals should think about the time at which they talk to family members and the environment in which discussions take place. Rushed conversations in public places cannot provide the kind of reassurance needed and may lead to feelings of resentment and anger among family members which may create further difficulties for the patient, the family and the health professionals involved.

- Resuscitation status should be made clear to family members and, if a DNR is recorded on a patient's file, the reason why a DNR is considered appropriate should be made clear. The meaning and limits of a DNR should be explained in full to family members.

- While families should be informed and involved and their views should be sought and weight should be accorded to these, the duty to act in the best interests of the patient must always remain central.

- When dealing with children and young people, professionals should make efforts to explain what is going on in a way that is accessible and should involve children and young people in decisions about their care insofar as this is possible in light of the child's age and maturity.

6.4 Case 4: Rights, Incapacity and Decision making – why resuscitation?

This case study explores the rights issues which arise where patients have difficulty formulating their views or communicating their preferences, perhaps because they have dementia, Alzheimer's disease, intellectual disabilities or other conditions which limit their decision-making abilities. The role of advance healthcare directives in such circumstances will be discussed in more detail in Module 4. However, even if these measures are legally provided for, they will not apply in all situations. The question which then arises is how are patient rights to be respected when there is no indication of what the patient would have wanted and he or she is not in a position to communicate. The final case examined in this module on the role of rights in healthcare decision making looks at rights, incapacity and decision making.

This case study is based on a case adapted from Quinlan and O'Neill. It is based on a real experience as recounted by a practitioner – however, as recounted it is not clear whether the patient had given any indication of preference or, indeed, whether or not he had the capacity to do so. The facts have therefore been adapted in order to allow discussion of the situation where a patient clearly lacks capacity and is nearing the end of life.

Why Resuscitation?

I'm on the resuscitation team, when we arrived at the scene, you know, the first thing I could see, God, this is such an unethical resuscitation, if it was my relative in the bed I'd be so upset. It was an 86 year old gentleman with Alzheimer's disease that was admitted that night by a medical registrar that had not consulted with his consultant, and had not consulted with the anaesthetic consultant, to review this patient. He had end stage chronic obstructive airway disease that was on maximum medical treatment and home oxygen. So, I mean, the sort of thing we're talking about – resuscitation, that's why often patients and relatives are not explained to properly, or talking about will they benefit from their heart being shocked or will they benefit from being put on a life support machine? Now, this gentleman would not have benefited from that because he would never come off of the life support machine, research would have shown with end stage Chronic Obstructive Pulmonary Disease (COPD). The poor little gentleman was very skeletal and he had a pigeon chest as well. You know, and the first thing I could say – I arrived at the scene the same time as the anaesthetist and the medical registrar that called the rest of us there – and I said,

> *'This gentleman is for resuscitation, is he'? And yes – and we were going through with it, and all his ribs were cracking as we were doing the procedure. And I said, God, this is very unethical, has this been discussed with the gentleman or relatives? And the registrar said, 'No' and the anaesthetist just chimed in as well, he said, 'This is quite unethical.' And he just was continuing leading on, and he just said, 'Oh well, we won't compress as much on the chest compressions, we'll do it gentler.' But the thing with resuscitation, you either do it properly or you don't do it at all. There are no half measures; we don't act out the role. He died; once the resuscitation was called off he died. He wasn't going to survive resuscitation.'* (Adapted from Quinlan and O'Neill, 2009, p.31)

6.4.1   Discussion

This case raises the issue of rights outside of the situation where a patient has given a clear indication of his or her treatment preferences. It raises a number of ethical issues regarding futility, the use of life-prolonging methods and moral distress which are explored in more detail in Module 6. The present discussion is concerned with the issue of rights and whether intervention in a situation such as this is respectful of the patient's rights.

A number of rights are relevant to a discussion of Case 4. First, the patient had a right to life. As discussed above, the right to life is protected by the Irish Constitution, the European Convention on Human Rights as well as under United Nations human rights instruments. The right to life is one of the most fundamental rights. It derives from the ethical principle of the sanctity of life and it is a right which is universal. A person cannot be deprived of his or her right to life because he or she is disabled or because he or she lacks capacity. It would be both unlawful and unethical to deny treatment to a patient on this basis. Yet the right to life is not absolute. It is generally accepted that treatment is not required where treatment would be futile or, in Keown's words, 'not worthwhile' (Keown, 1997, p.485). Keown, (1997, p.485) describes a treatment as not worthwhile in this sense 'either because it offers no reasonable hope of benefit or because, even though it does, the expected benefit would be outweighed by burdens which the treatment would impose, such as excessive pain.'

Other rights are also at stake. A person has a right to dignity, a right to freedom from inhuman and degrading treatment and a right to bodily integrity. The patient in Case 4 had his ribs cracked during the administration of resuscitation. By any standards, this is an invasion of his right to bodily integrity and by many standards, it constitutes inhuman treatment. His right to dignity was also compromised. His last moments of life were spent having his ribs broken during a highly invasive process.

Of course, in many cases, if a person had his or her ribs cracked during the administration of cardiopulmonary resuscitation (CPR), we would accept that, while this was an invasion of his or her right to dignity or bodily integrity, it was justified because it saves his life. Imagine if the man in Case 4 had been 30 years younger and had been admitted following a heart attack. Nobody would argue that CPR should not be administered even if there was a risk of broken ribs and of loss of dignity during the process. However, in a case such as Case 4, a real question arises as to whether the administration of the CPR was worthwhile and whether the violation of the patient's right to dignity, bodily integrity and freedom from inhuman and degrading treatment could be justified on the basis of the patient's right to life.

The interplay of rights in these kinds of situations was explored in an English case of R (Burke) v the General Medical Council and Others (2004). Although the Irish courts might act differently, this case is helpful in showing how complex the interplay of rights can be and how difficult it is to reach appropriate conclusions. The case concerned a 44-year-old man named Leslie Burke who had motor neurone disease – a progressive condition which would ultimately lead to his death. The likely progression of the disease was that a time would come when Mr Burke would be completely unable to move or to communicate with his carers but he would still be sentient. Mr Burke was concerned that, under the General Medical Council (GMC) Guidelines: *Withholding and Withdrawing Life-Prolonging Treatment: Good Practice in Decision-Making* (2002), at this stage of his illness, the medical professionals caring for him would be able to decide that it was in his best interests to have artificial hydration and nutrition removed. He would not be able to object to the decision. Mr Burke considered that death from deprivation of ANH would be undignified and he was very concerned that he should not die in this way. He wanted an express confirmation that this would not occur.

In the English High Court, Judge Munby found that the GMC Guidelines failed to protect the patient's right to autonomy in determining when ANH should be withdrawn. In his view, where a patient has made his or her views known (in a case like this, by means of an advance instruction), this should determine when ANH should be withdrawn. Where a patient has not made his or her views known, Judge Munby held that the relevant factor in deciding when life-sustaining treatment should be withdrawn was 'intolerability'. It was only if life was intolerable for the patient that the withdrawal of treatment leading to the patient's death should take place. Judge Munby's decision was overruled by the English Court of Appeal, which approved the GMC Guidelines. The Court of Appeal considered that it was for the medical professionals acting in a patient's best interests and not for the patient to decide when ANH should be withdrawn. The court also rejected the use of a standard based on intolerability where the patient's views are not known and said instead that a simple best interests test should apply.

The decision in Burke is a reminder that, in end-of-life situations, while the right to life is very important, it does not 'trump' other rights in all circumstances and sometimes treatment should be withheld or withdrawn depending on the circumstances. Following Burke, and taking account of other developments, including the introduction of the Mental Capacity Act 2005, government strategies on end-of-life care in England and Scotland, new GMC guidance on Consent: Patients and Doctors Making Decisions together (2008), and new research, the GMC has issued new guidance on withholding and withdrawing treatment (GMC, 2010). This guidance lays down a framework in respect of decisions on life-prolonging treatment for patients with and without capacity. The guidance advises doctors to encourage patients to plan for end-of-life care in respect of both advance requests for treatment and advance refusals of treatment. The role of advance planning is discussed in more detail in Module 4. In a substantial change from the former GMC guidance (which was at issue in the Burke case), doctors are advised that ANH may be withdrawn from a patient who lacks capacity, where death is not imminent, if 'it is considered that providing clinically assisted nutrition or hydration would not be in [the patient's] best interests.' (Dyer 2009, p.875).

6.4.2 Suggested Professional Responsibilities

- Professionals have an ongoing duty to respect the right to life of a person who lacks decision-making capacity. However, this duty must be balanced with the duty to protect the patient from inhuman or degrading treatment and the duty to respect the patient's right to dignity and bodily integrity.

- Patients should be encouraged to plan for end-of-life care while they have the capacity to do so. In this respect, communication and (appropriate) reassurance is essential to ensuring that patients can make decisions which are informed and which represent their considered views.

7. Module 3 Further Discussion

Rights are important tools in the provision of appropriate care for patients at the end of their lives. The rights to autonomy, to dignity, to bodily integrity, to freedom from inhuman and degrading treatment as well as the rights to information, to consent and to free choice are powerful ideals and, in some cases, legal obligations. To state the rights applicable in decisions at the end of life is easy enough but, as the practitioner interviews show, giving practical effect to rights is much more difficult. Patients may get little information about their condition and so are unable to form realistic expectations or they may get no information or, indeed, misinformation. Decisions may be made in emergency situations by professionals who have not had the opportunity to reflect on the rights involved or indeed who may not have a full picture of the circumstances at issue.

There is a recognisable gap between these rights and their application in end-of-life care. This is not meant to be pessimistic but rather to signal the need to take account of the practical operation of patient rights in developing a framework for end-of-life care. It is essential that resources are allocated to allow for patient-focussed communication and for education and training to ensure that professionals who are involved in these important decisions are aware that patients have rights and to ensure that these rights are respected in one of the most important decision-making situations that any of us will encounter – that is, decisions about care at the end of life.

8. Module 3 Summary Learning Guides

8.1 The Nature of Rights

- There are different kinds of rights. The rights discussed in this module have been:
  Positive Rights: Right to something
  Negative Rights: Rights that someone should desist from something
  Moral Rights: Rights justified on the basis of membership of the moral community
  Legal Rights: Rights enforceable in a court of law
- Each aspect of rights is important. An appropriate framework for rights in respect of decisions at the end of life must recognise positive as well as negative rights and moral rights as well as legal rights. It is especially important that, in discussing rights, the discussion is not limited to (largely negative) legal rights.

8.2 The Contribution of Rights

- Rights make an important contribution to patient care because respect for patient rights makes the patient central to the decision-making process.

- Arguments based on positive rights provides a basis for essential resources.

- There is a legal obligation to respect patients' legal rights
  But good patient care requires more than just respect for rights.

8.3 Sources of Legal Rights

- Irish Constitution
- European Convention on Human Rights
- European Charter of Patients' Rights (not legally enforceable)
- United Nations Conventions

8.4 Positive Rights Implicated in End-of-Life Care

- Right to information
- Right to pain relief
- Right to communication
- Right to a 'good dying'

These rights have a basis in legal rights, including the right to dignity, to protection from inhuman and degrading treatment and the right to bodily integrity. They are also moral rights. An appropriate framework for end-of-life care requires that these rights be recognised.

8.5 All Patients Have Rights

Rights are not restricted to adult patients with decision-making capacity. All patients have rights.

Children's rights include:

- The right to participate in decisions about their care – including end-of-life care – in accordance with their age and maturity
- The right to have their family consulted and involved in the decision-making process
- The right to have treatment decisions made in their best interests
- The right to life, to dignity, to protection from inhuman and degrading treatment

Adults who lack decision-making capacity have rights. These include:

- The right to participate in decisions made insofar as this is possible
- The right to life
- The right to dignity
- The right to protection from inhuman and degrading treatment

The right to life is not absolute but must be balanced with other rights.

9. Module 3 Activities

9.1 Recall the distinction between positive and negative rights:

a. Would you add anything further to these points on the distinction?

b. Which kind of rights seem to you to contribute best to appropriate decision making at the end of life?

c. Which negative rights do you think are most relevant to treatment decisions at the end of life?

d. Which positive rights do you think are most relevant to treatment decisions at the end of life?

9.2 Reflect back on the particulars of Case 1:

a. In reading Case 1, jot down your first, unanalysed response to the facts set out.

b. Do you think that the health professionals should have done more for the woman in this case?

c. What kind of structures would facilitate health professionals in doing more in a case along the lines of Case 1?

d. Compare Case 1 with the contrasting example given. Is the approach taken in the contrasting example a better way of protecting patient rights than the approach outlined in Case 1? If so, why?

9.3 Reflect back on the particulars of Case 2:

a. In your view, is it a good or a bad thing for cases like this to come before the courts?

b. In your view, what should the Supreme Court have done when faced with this case?

c. The Supreme Court listed a set of rights, including the right of autonomy, dignity, bodily integrity and dignity. How do you think that these rights were relevant to the circumstances which arose in Case 2?

d. Can you think of any other rights (both positive and negative) which may have been relevant in the facts arising in Case 2?

e. If you were the health professionals involved, would you have taken a similar position to that taken by the health professionals? If so, why; if not, why not?

f. Was the Supreme Court correct in the approach taken to ANH? Would you take a similar approach? Is the approach taken by the Medical Council Guide consistent with the approach of the Supreme Court?

9.4 Reflect back on the particulars of Case 3:

a. Were the health professionals wrong in placing a DNR order on the patient's file without consulting his family? Were they wrong in administering morphine without consulting his family? Is there any difference between the two decisions?

b. How involved should parents be in end-of-life decisions about their children?

c. Is it justified to retain information about a child's situation from parents in order to preserve hope/prevent the parents from distressing the child?

d. How would you resolve a conflict where you believe that parents are making inappropriate decisions about their dying child? What factors would influence you in resolving the conflict?

9.5 Reflect back on the particulars of Case 4:

a. What are the rights at risk in this case?

b. How should the right to life be balanced against other rights where a patient lacks the capacity to make his or her own views or preferences known?

c. Do you agree with a standard for withdrawing or withholding treatment based on whether the treatment is 'worthwhile' or based on whether the patient's life would be 'intolerable'? Can you think of other possible standards which might be used in resolving the conflict between rights in making decisions about end-of-life care for patients lacking capacity?

10. Module 3 References and Further Reading

Active Citizenship Network, European Charter of Patients' Rights (Brussels: Active Citizenship Network, 2002)

Airedale NHS Trust v Bland [1993] AC 789

Alderson, P. and Montgomery, J. *Health Care Choices: Making Decisions with Children* (London: Institute for Public Policy Research (IPPR), 1996)

Beauchamp, T. and Childress, J. *Principles of Biomedical Ethics* (5th ed.) (Oxford and New York: Oxford University Press, 2001)

Brazier, M. 'Do No Harm: Do Patients Have Responsibilities Too?
The Cambridge Law Journal, vol. 65, no. 2, 2006, pp.397–422

Bridgeman, J. *Parental Responsibility, Young Children and Healthcare Law* (Cambridge: Cambridge University Press, 2007)

Bristol Royal Infirmary Inquiry, *Learning from Bristol: The Report of the Public Inquiry into Children's Heart Surgery at the Bristol Royal Infirmary 1984–1995* (2001), Cm 5297(1)

Buchanan, A. and Brock, D. *Deciding for Others: The Ethics of Surrogate Decision Making* (Cambridge: Cambridge University Press, 1989)

Callahan, D. 'Individual Good and Common Good: A Communitarian Approach to Bioethics', *Perspectives in Biology and Medicine*, vol. 46, no. 4, 2003, pp.496–611

Constitution of Ireland (Bunreacht na hÉireann), 1937

Council of Europe, The European Convention for the Protection of Human Rights and Fundamental Freedoms as Amended by Protocol No. 11 (ETS No. 155) (Rome: Council of Europe, 1950)

Council of Europe Committee of Ministers, Recommendation no. R (99) 4 of the Committee of Ministers to Member States on Principles Concerning the Legal Protection of Incapable Adults (Strasbourg: Council of Europe, 1999)

Criminal Law (Suicide) Act No. 11 (1993)

Donnelly, M. Consent: Bridging the Gap between Doctor and Patient (Cork: Cork University Press, 2002)

Donnelly, M. 'The Right of Autonomy in Irish Law', *Medico-Legal Journal of Ireland*, vol. 14, 2008, pp.34–40

Donnelly, M. and Kilkelly, U. 'Child-Friendly Healthcare: Delivering on the Right to be Heard', *Medical Law Review*, vol. 19, 2011, pp.27–54

Draper, H. and Sorell, T. 'Patients' Responsibilities in Medical Ethics', *Bioethics*, vol. 16, no. 4, 2002, pp.335–52

Dyer, C. 'GMC is to Reconsider Guidance on End-of-Life Care', *British Medical Journal*, vol. 338, no. b875, 2009, p.561

European Convention on Human Rights Act 2003, No. 20 of 2003

Fitzpatrick v K [2008] IEHC 104

General Medical Council, *Withholding and Withdrawing Life-Prolonging Treatments: Good Practice in Decision Making* (London: General Medical Council, 2002)

General Medical Council, *Consent: Patients and Doctors Making Decisions Together*, GMC/CMDT/0408 (London: General Medical Council, 2008)

General Medical Council, *Treatment and Care Towards the End of Life: Good Practice in Decision Making* (London: General Medical Council, 2010)

Gillon, R. 'Ethics Needs Principles – Four Can Encompass the Rest – And Respect for Autonomy Should be "First Among Equals"', *Journal of Medical Ethics*, vol. 29, no. 5, 2003, pp.307–12

Glass v United Kingdom [2004] ECHR 102, Application No. 61827/00

Hogan, G. and Whyte, G. *J.M. Kelly: The Irish Constitution* (4th ed.) (Dublin: Lexis Nexis Butterworths, 1994)

Huxtable, R. and Forbes, K. 'Glass v United Kingdom: Maternal Instinct v Medical Opinion', *Child and Family Law Quarterly*, vol. 16, no. 3, 2004, pp.339–54

In re a Ward of Court [1996] 2 IR 79

Keown, J. 'Life and Death in Dublin', *The Cambridge Law Journal*, vol. 55, no. 1, 1996, pp.6–8

Keown, J. 'Restoring Moral and Intellectual Shape to the Law after Bland', *Law Quarterly Review*, vol. 113, 1997, pp.481–503

Kilkelly, U. and Donnelly, M. *The Child's Right to be Heard in the Healthcare Setting: Perspectives of Children, Parents and Health Professionals* (Dublin: Office of the Minister for Children, 2006)

Law Reform Commission, *Bioethics: Advance Care Directives [LRC 94 – 2009]* (Dublin: Law Reform Commission, 2009)

Medical Council, *A Guide to Ethical Conduct and Behaviour* (6th ed.) (Dublin: Medical Council, 2004)

Medical Council, *Guide to Professional Conduct and Ethics for Registered Medical Practitioners* (7th ed.) (2009), http://www.medicalcouncil.ie [accessed 20 November 2009)]

Mental Capacity Act 2005 (England and Wales)

Munro, V.E. 'Square Pegs in Round Holes: The Dilemma of Conjoined Twins and Individual Rights', *Social & Legal Studies*, vol. 10, no. 4, 2001, p.459

North Western Health Board v HW and CW [2001] 2 IR 622

O'Neill, O. 'The Dark Side of Human Rights', *International Affairs*, vol. 81, no. 2, 2005, pp.427–39

O'Neill, O. *Autonomy and Trust in Bioethics* (Cambridge: Cambridge University Press, 2002)

Pellegrino, E.D. and Thomasma, D.C. *For the Patient's Good: The Restoration of Beneficence in Health Care* (Oxford and New York: Oxford University Press, 1988)

Pretty v UK [2002] ECHR 2346/02

Quinlan, C. *Media Messages on Death and Dying* (Dublin: Irish Hospice Foundation, 2009a)

Quinlan, C. and O'Neill, C. 'Practitioners' Narrative Submissions' (Unpublished) (Dublin: Irish Hospice Foundation, 2008)

Quinlan, C. and O'Neill, C. *Practitioners' Perspectives on Patient Autonomy at End of Life* (Dublin: Irish Hospice Foundation, 2009)

R (Burke) v the General Medical Council and Others [2004] EWHC 1879 (Admin); [2005] EWCA Civ 1003 (CA)

Ramsey, P. 'The Morality of Abortion', in J. Rachels (ed.), *Moral Problems: A Collection of Philosophical Essays* (New York: Harper Row, 1971)

Re C [1989] 1 WLR 240

Temple Street v D and Anor [2011] IEHC 1

United Nations General Assembly, United Nations Convention on the Rights of the Child, General Assembly Resolution 44/25 of 20 November 1989, http://www.un.org/documents/ga/res/44/a44r025.htm [accessed 2 August 2009]

United Nations General Assembly, Convention on the Rights of Persons with Disabilities, General Assembly Resolution A/RES/61/106 of 13 December 2006, http://www.un.org/disabilities/convention/conventionfull.shtml [accessed 2 August 2009]

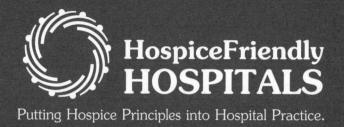

HospiceFriendly
HOSPITALS

Putting Hospice Principles into Hospital Practice.

Module 4

Patient Autonomy in Law
and Practice

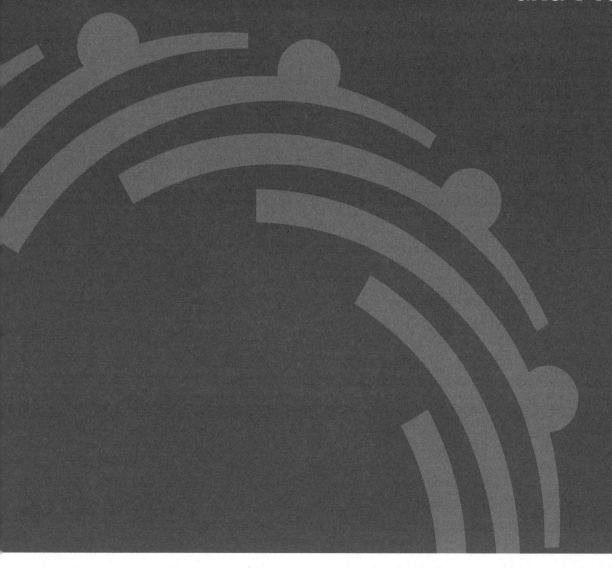

Module 4 Contents   Page

1. Module 4 Key Points

1.1 Autonomy is not just about the right to say no:

The right of autonomy is not just about refusing treatment or procedures; it is also about the positive right to be involved in decisions about treatment.

1.2 Respect for autonomy is especially important in a hospital setting:

A patient in a hospital setting is in an inherently vulnerable position; he or she is part of a big and sometimes impersonal institution and is inherently restricted in many of the choices which he or she can make.

1.3 Autonomy is a contested notion:

There is ongoing debate among healthcare ethicists and others regarding the proper status for autonomy. For some, autonomy provides the basis for patient rights and is the most important of all the ethical standards. However, this claim is disputed by others who place importance on values such as trust and maintaining personal and social relationships.

1.4 A capable/competent patient has the right to refuse treatment:

This is a legal right which is protected under the Irish Constitution and the European Convention on Human Rights.

1.5 There are three requirements for autonomous decisions:

Information, Capacity and Freedom: Not all decisions are autonomous: an autonomous decision is one which is made with adequate information; where the patient has decision-making capacity and where the patient is not unduly influenced or pressured by others.

1.6 The legal right of autonomy does not extend to allow patients assert a 'right to die':

Courts in a number of countries have rejected the argument that the right of autonomy gives people a 'right to die' in the sense of a right to have active steps taken to end a person's life or to assist a person in ending his or her own life.

1.7 Information is key to autonomous decision making:

Without adequate information, a patient cannot make autonomous decisions. Protection of patient autonomy imposes a positive duty to provide information in an appropriate way. However, simply providing information does not ensure autonomous decision making.

1.8 Legal capacity is a threshold and not a comparison:

A person's legal capacity is decided according to whether or not he or she meets a designated standard.

1.9 Every adult is presumed to have capacity to make decisions:

Regardless of age, intellectual disability or mental illness, all adults are presumed to have the capacity to make decisions.

1.10 The legal test for capacity asks three questions:

Can the patient understand the information relevant to the decision? Can he or she believe this information? Can he or she make a decision based on the information?

1.11 Capacity assessment:

Respect for the principle of autonomy requires that capacity be assessed in a way which is fair and appropriate and which is free from prejudices based on external factors such as old age, mental illness or intellectual disability.

1.12 Respect for the principle of autonomy:

This requires efforts to be made to develop and enhance patients' capacity and to facilitate them in making decisions where this is possible

1.13 Autonomous decisions are decisions which are freely made:

The positive right of autonomy requires that efforts be made to ensure that patients are free to make their own decisions and that patients have the maximum control possible over the manner of their dying.

1.14 Advance Directives provide vital control for patients over their dying:

An Advance Directive can prolong life as well as decide when life should end.

1.15 Autonomy and incapable adults:

It should not be presumed that simply because a person lacks the capacity to make an autonomous decision, his or her views should simply be disregarded. An autonomy-centred approach to end-of-life decisions requires that efforts must be made to facilitate the participation of patients lacking capacity in making decisions.

2. Module 4 Definitions

2.1 Autonomy:

the capacity of self-determination; it is a person's ability to make choices about their own life based on their own beliefs and values.

2.2 Absolute Right:

a right which cannot be interfered with in any circumstances. Autonomy is not an absolute right.

2.3 Advance Directive:

a decision made by a person while he or she has decision-making capacity regarding the medical treatment which he or she would wish to receive (and more frequently not to receive) if he or she subsequently loses capacity.

2.4 Capacity/Competence:

the ability to make decisions based on designated standards.

2.5 Duty to Disclose:

the duty of a medical professional to disclose material risks to a patient in advance of treatment.

2.6 Enduring Power of Attorney:

power which a person grants while he or she has capacity giving another person the power to make certain designated decisions if the person granting the power of attorney subsequently loses capacity.

2.7 'Living Will':

another term for an Advance Directive.

2.8 Paternalism:

involves an action that overrides a person's decision or controls their actions in the interests of what is considered to be their own good.

2.9 Principle of Autonomy:

requires that, in a healthcare context, health professionals recognise and support the unique values, priorities and preferences of patients.

2.10 Principle of Beneficence:

doing good for the patient.

2.11 Right to Refuse Treatment:

a legal and ethical right of a patient.

2.12 Sanctity of Life:

a principle whereby life is seen as having an intrinsic value unrelated to the individual's views regarding his or her own life.

2.13 Self-determination:

another way of saying 'autonomy' – sometimes used in legal discussions.

3. Module 4 Background

3.1 A Matter of Policy

One of the goals of the Irish Health Service Executive Strategic Plan for 2008–13 is 'to develop the role of the "expert patient", especially those with long-term illnesses, in developing their own care plan and in looking after their own condition' (p.14).

Two of the related actions to achieve this goal are the promotion of patients as 'partners with health professionals' and the education of staff on the 'importance of patient involvement in their care' (*National Strategy for Service User Involvement in the Irish Health Service 2008-2013*). The document defines 'involvement' as:

> *A process by which people are enabled to become actively and genuinely involved in defining the issues of concern to them, in making decisions about factors that affect their lives, in formulating and implementing polices, in planning, developing and delivering services and in taking action to achieve change.* (2008, p.6)

In emphasising the idea of individual patient participation in care planning and self-care, this HSE strategic plan brings Ireland into line with international efforts to change the way in which illness is managed in the twenty-first century by health professionals and, increasingly, by patients themselves. This focus on patient-directed and patient-centred care is construed as giving expression to patient autonomy and it is articulated in the 7th edition of the Irish Guide to Professional Conduct and Ethics for Registered Medical Practitioners (2009) in relation to the requirement of the informed consent of patients to medical treatment:

> *You should ensure that informed consent has been given by a patient before any medical treatment is carried out. The ethical and legal rationale behind this is to respect the patient's autonomy and their right to control their own life. The basic idea of personal autonomy is that everyone's actions and decisions are their own. Therefore, the patient has the right to decide what happens to their own body.* (Section 33.1, p.34)

The notion of patient autonomy is especially relevant to one particularly vulnerable group of individuals: patients who are dying.

3.2 Defining Patient Autonomy

The term 'autonomy' derives from the Greek words autos ('self') and nomos ('rule', 'law', 'governance'), and originally referred to the self-rule of Greek independent city-states. Today, however, autonomy is associated not just with nations but also with persons, decisions and actions and it is linked with other meanings such as self-governance, liberty, self-authorship, free will and self-determination.

The moral principle of autonomy requires that, in a healthcare context, health professionals recognise and support the unique values, priorities and preferences of patients. In end-of-life care, they can do this by enabling patients to direct their own journeys from living to dying and death. This requires that patients be encouraged to participate in decisions relating to their treatment and care.

Respecting patient autonomy does not mean that health professionals only respect the choices of persons who are deemed autonomous. It requires that they respect whatever level of autonomy the person is capable of. Where the dying person is incompetent or impaired or suffers from some psychological, emotional, physiological or social disability, the principle of autonomy obliges health professionals and organisations to create the conditions that foster capacity. They do this through, for example, the early provision of treatment or care plans and consulting with family members and friends about what the person would have wished in the circumstances.

3.3 The Nature of the Right of Autonomy

The right of autonomy or self-determination protects the individual's 'interest in making significant decisions about his or her own life' (Buchanan and Brock, 1989, p.36). This right is often seen as being encapsulated by John Stuart Mill's ([1859], 1991, p.4) words, 'Over himself, over his own body and mind, the individual is sovereign'.

Respect for autonomy requires that autonomous decisions must be respected even if we do not agree with them. In the words of Ronald Dworkin, '[w]e allow someone to choose death over radical amputation or a blood transfusion, if that is his informed wish, because we acknowledge his right to a life structured by his own values' (1993, p.27).

The right of autonomy is both a moral right and a legal one. As members of the moral community, we have a moral obligation to respect our fellow citizens' right of autonomy. We also have a legal obligation to respect the right. In this sense, autonomy may be seen as a negative right (see discussion on positive and negative rights in Module 3). It is a right not to be interfered with. This has often been the legal response to the right and in the healthcare context, the legal right of autonomy is often viewed as simply the right to refuse treatment.

3.4 Autonomy is Not an Absolute Right

Autonomy is not an absolute right. The most commonly recognised justification for interference with autonomy is that respect for the right will cause harm to another person (often described as the 'harm' principle; see Further Discussion). For example, where a person has a contagious and dangerous disease, say tuberculosis, a degree of interference with his or her autonomous rights (to refuse treatment, to freely interact with others) may be justified on the basis of the harm which would be caused to others who might well become infected with the disease if the person's right of autonomy were respected.

Respect for autonomy is also premised on 'all the persons concerned being of full age, and the ordinary amount of understanding' (Mill, [1859], 1991 p.84). Children and people without decision-making capacity do not have the same right of autonomy as capable adults. However, this does not mean that their views are irrelevant. Insofar as is possible, account should be taken of the views of people lacking capacity in healthcare decisions, including decisions at the end of life.

3.5 Autonomy as a Positive Right

The right of autonomy should also be viewed as a positive right. Respect for the right is as much about empowering patients as about patients refusing treatment. Many in the healthcare profession would argue that the right of patient autonomy should be accompanied by more positive help to enable patients to die in a context that protects their dignity and privacy. This is clear in the range of practitioner responses to Quinlan and O'Neill's request to define patient autonomy (2009, pp.44–5). Practitioners responded:

'I suppose it's the right and the ability of the patient to make a choice'.

'It's the choice of what kind of treatment the patient is going to receive and the degree of treatment, if it's going to be just like minimal or more aggressive'.

'I suppose it's more the patients' right to make choices around that and, you know, that we would be respectful to the patients' wishes [...]'.

'[...] that we would take their wishes into consideration and act on them at all times [...]'.

'It's to do with, maybe not just the treatment, but things like patients' family involvement and special particular requests that the patient might have as to whether we can, you know, the balance between whether we can have whatever the patient wants from a practical point of view'.

This means that autonomy is not just about the right to say no; it is also about the right to be involved in decisions about how one's treatment proceeds and the environment in which one dies.

This is the view of autonomy developed in this module – a view of autonomy as a positive right to be involved in decisions at the end of life and to have the steps taken to ensure that this happens.

4. Ethical Debates Regarding the Status of Autonomy

As discussed in Module 3, the principle of autonomy has traditionally played a very limited role in medical ethics. Historically, healthcare decisions were based on the principles of beneficence (doing good for the patient) and sanctity of life (recognising an intrinsic value in life) with little or no reference to the patient's own views of their interests or of the value of their lives. However, from this position of insignificance in traditional medical ethics, in recent decades, the principle of respect for patient autonomy has come to be widely recognised in healthcare decision making.

Autonomy is now regarded as a fundamental ethical principle (Beauchamp and Childress, 2008) governing healthcare decisions. However, it is a contested notion. For some, it is the most fundamental ethical principle governing the relationship between medical professional and patient (Gillon, 2003). For others (O'Neill, 2002; Callahan, 1984, 2003), autonomy provides, 'a thin gruel for the future of bioethics' (Callahan, 2003, p.499).

4.1 Critiques of Autonomy

The elevated role of autonomy has been criticised for a number of reasons. Critics argue that the autonomy principle is too individualistic and that it fails to take account of the essential interconnectedness of people or the complexity of the ways in which people make healthcare decisions (Schneider, 1998; Callahan, 1984, 2003; O'Neill, 2002; Donnelly, 2010). Many argue that a broad and more concrete understanding of autonomy is required.

One significant deficiency in the way that autonomy is usually understood is that it supports an abstract view of persons as independent, self-sufficient centres of decision-making. When associated with free market economies such as ours, this view of autonomy conjures up an image of an independent individual who chooses from amongst an array of commodities; in the healthcare arena, the patient is a consumer and the commodity is a medicine or treatment. It could be argued that this distorts the relationship between the patient and the professional, and between the citizen and the state which has responsibility for healthcare provision.

Daniel Callahan puts his criticism as follows:

> *[Autonomy] buys our freedom to be ourselves, and to be free of undue influence by others, at too high a price. It establishes contractual relationships as the principal and highest form of relationships. It elevates isolation and separation as the necessary starting point of human commitments.* (1984, p.41)

Onora O'Neill (2002) identifies the cost to other values and in particular the important value of trust, which is exacted by the elevation of autonomy. Contrasting the different features of trust and autonomy, she notes, '[t]rust flourishes between those who are linked to one another; individual autonomy flourishes where everyone has "space" to do their own thing' (2002, p.25).

Rather than fostering trust between patients and professionals, it is argued that elevating autonomy pits the patient and professional against one another. In situations in which disagreements engender conflicts and disputes, these are increasingly referred to the courts or Fitness to Practice Committees to resolve. Such a narrow view of autonomy conceives of the obligations of health professionals in terms of what they cannot do. This reinforces the already widespread culture of demoralisation and fear of litigation which focuses the minds of health professionals on expedience, pragmatism and self-protection.

It must also be remembered that not all cultures adopt identical views of autonomy or take an individualistic view of the person (Blackhall, 1995; Gaylin and Jennings, 2003). Thus, while respect for autonomy may be in line with Western liberal thinking, it may be wholly alien to people from other cultural backgrounds.

While identifying important questions about the status accorded to autonomy, critics of the principle do not advocate a return to old-style paternalism. In Callahan's words, there cannot be a 'return to those good old days that understood doctors to be good old boys who could work out moral problems among themselves in the locker room' (1984, p.42). If autonomy is to be preserved and to have relevance, it is argued that a broader account is needed to provide substantive basis for decision making. One such account is described by George Agich as 'actual autonomy' which focuses on paying attention to concrete actions carried out in everyday shared social life (Agich, 2003, p.19). This perspective pays attention to the conditions which foster capacity, provides treatment or care plans from which patients choose, and tries to ensure that available options are meaningful to the patients involved. See Further Discussion for philosophical supports for, and critiques of, the notion of autonomy.

4.2 The Importance of Autonomy

Although the elevated role of autonomy can be criticised and the cultural context in which autonomy is valued must be recognised, the principle provides an important foundation for decisions about healthcare, including at the end of life. Autonomy is a more complex ideal than simply respecting the right to say no. The right to say no – to refuse interventions – is important but so too is the more positive right of autonomy in the sense of facilitating patients in exercising control over how they live and how they die. One practitioner recounts:

> I've yet to remember when a patient had full, you know, control over what they exactly wanted. We feel we're doing what's best for the patient and we do, we do what's best, but I don't know whether we question enough by asking the patient 'is this what you want'. So I think as yet patients haven't got great control over end-of- life decisions. (Quinlan and O'Neill, 2009, p.52)

The especially strong need for protection of autonomy in this broader sense in a hospital context is evident when we consider one of the practitioner responses recounted by Quinlan and O'Neill (2009, p.69):

> Once you put your foot in the door of the hospital as a patient you lose that power, that power you have as an individual. A hospital is an institution and it has to tick, it has to keep going, staff come and go, there's rotas, there's crises, there's personalities, there's conflict, there's tension. People who are dying usually want to go home and they want to die at home. The journey they have had with cancer – could have involved a number of hospitals – and then they end up let's say in this facility here. My experience of working here for nearly 2 years is that, and I'm sure it's no different to any other institution or hospital, a lot of stuff gets lost, the emotional stuff doesn't get dealt with. That could be because of a combination of family dynamics and ward dynamics and hospital dynamics. So my experience is that people lose an awful lot of autonomy and I've seen a lot of people die who have been totally disempowered […] and people have good deaths I'm sure as well – but it's kind of sad.

Autonomy in this sense might be seen as an aspiration or a goal. In many cases, it will not be possible for patients to be fully autonomous; the circumstances of their illness and their hospitalisation may limit this. But recognising that respect for autonomy and the empowerment of patients are important values is an essential component of an appropriate framework for end-of-life decision making.

5. The Legal Right of Autonomy

Autonomy is an important ethical principle. It is also a recognised and enforceable legal right. While the existence of a legal right does not, of itself, guarantee that an ethical principle will be respected, legal endorsement allows patients to make ethical principles enforceable in their individual situations (Donnelly, 2008, p.34). An understanding of the legal right is essential in order to appreciate health professionals' legal obligations. However, it is crucial that the legal right is not seen as the only relevant factor in providing appropriate protection for patients' autonomy. Respect for the right of autonomy also imposes positive obligations to enhance patient autonomy and to ensure that patients are able to control to the maximum extent possible their own living and dying.

5.1 The Scope of the Legal Right

The legal right of autonomy has sometimes tended to be viewed primarily as a right to say no; a right to refuse treatment rather than a positive right to appropriate treatment.

5.1.1 A Right to Refuse Treatment

The Irish Constitution protects the right to refuse treatment. This has been recognised by the Irish Supreme Court in a number of cases, beginning with the decision in In re a Ward of Court (1995). In this case, the Supreme Court recognised the right of a patient to refuse medical treatment. The right to refuse treatment was again recognised by the Irish courts in JM v Board of Management of St Vincent's Hospital (2003) and in Fitzpatrick v K (2008). Speaking in Fitzpatrick v K (2008), Judge Laffoy said that it 'could not be argued that a competent adult is not free to decline medical treatment'.

The right of autonomy is also protected under the European Convention on Human Rights. In Pretty v UK (2002), Mrs Pretty was an Englishwoman who suffered from motor neuron disease. She was concerned that a time would come when she would wish to end her life. She did not wish to die by withdrawal of ventilation – which she would be legally entitled to request – as she had a fear of suffocation and did not wish to die in this way. Instead, she wished her husband to assist her in bringing her life to an end. She was concerned because assisted suicide is against the law in England (as is also the case in Ireland). She was worried that, after her death, her husband might be prosecuted for assisting her. She did not wish this to happen and sought a reassurance from the public prosecutor that it would not happen. The prosecutor declined to give this reassurance because the law on assisted suicide in England did not allow for any exceptions. Mrs Pretty applied first to the English courts. She argued that the blanket prohibition on assisted suicide was a breach of her human rights arising under the European Convention on Human Rights. The English courts rejected her case and she brought her case to the European Court of Human Rights.

The European Court recognised that a person has a right of autonomy which is protected under Article 8 of the European Convention on Human Rights which protects the right to private and family life. The court also found that respect for the right of autonomy required that people have the right to refuse medical treatment. The court also accepted that the prohibition on assisted suicide was a breach of Mrs Pretty's right of autonomy (although, as discussed below, it found that interference with this right could be justified in the circumstances).

5.1.2. The Right in Practice

Perhaps the most striking feature of the Irish cases on the right to refuse treatment is that, in all cases, while the right to refuse treatment was recognised, the right did not actually apply in any of the cases (Donnelly, 2008, p.36). In In re a Ward of Court (1995), the woman had been in a near PVS for 23 years and evidently lacked decision-making capacity. Nor had she given any prior indication of how she would have wished a situation like this to be dealt with. The decision to withdraw ANH from the woman was made on the basis that withdrawal was in her best interests and not on the basis of her right to refuse treatment.

In JM v Board of Management of St Vincent's Hospital (2003), the woman had refused a blood transfusion on the basis of her religious beliefs (she was a Jehovah's Witness). The woman had made her views known and then she lost consciousness. The issue for the court was whether her advance instruction should apply. The woman's husband gave evidence to the court that the woman had converted to become a Jehovah's Witness on her marriage to him and that she did so because her cultural background meant that she was culturally disposed to adopt her husband's religion. On this basis, the court held that the woman's decision was not a 'real' or 'true' decision. Because the decision was not a real or true one, the court considered that it was not autonomous and therefore the woman's advance refusal of the blood was not upheld and a blood transfusion was administered.

Fitzpatrick v K (2008) also concerned refusal of a blood transfusion for religious reasons. Here, the woman, who had recently given birth, refused a blood transfusion. She suggested that her condition should be treated instead with tomatoes and Coca-Cola. Judge Laffoy found that the woman lacked the capacity to appreciate the seriousness of her situation and held that the administration of blood was justified in such circumstances. The role played by capacity and decision-making freedom in end-of-life situations will be discussed in more detail below. For present purposes, the important point is that the Irish courts have recognised the right of autonomy in the sense of the right of the competent adult to refuse medical treatment but, in practice, a case has not yet come before the courts in which the right has actually been held to apply.

5.2 Limits on the Legal Right

The legal right to refuse treatment is not absolute. The right of autonomy may sometimes be limited because of duties owed to other people – so, for example, it may be justified to interfere with a person's right to refuse treatment if the person has a contagious disease which may infect other people.

A more unusual example of duties owed to others may be seen in one Irish case, Re K (2006). Here, a woman was not permitted to refuse a blood transfusion on the basis of her religious beliefs (she was a Jehovah's Witness) because, if she died, her infant son would be left without a parent. Judge Abbott held that the child's welfare should take priority over the woman's right of autonomy. This case was later reconsidered by the Irish courts under the name Fitzpatrick v K (2008). Judge Laffoy found that the woman had, in fact, lacked the necessary capacity to make the decision to refuse the blood transfusion and for this reason her decision was not an autonomous one. This meant that there was no need to consider the question of whether or not the child's welfare should take priority over the woman's right of autonomy and Judge Laffoy did not consider the matter.

In Pretty v UK (2002), the European Court held that the protection afforded to the right of autonomy under the European Convention was not absolute. It was permissible to interfere with a person's right of autonomy if it was necessary for the protection of the rights and freedoms of others. The court held that the United Kingdom had made a reasonable case that its prohibition on assisted suicide was intended to protect the rights and freedoms of others (in particular vulnerable people who might feel pressured into ending their lives if assisted suicide were lawful). For this reason, the prohibition on assisted suicide was a permissible breach of Mrs Pretty's rights.

The effect of the decision in Pretty is that the right of autonomy does not extend to allowing a patient assert a right to die in the sense of a right to have active steps taken to end his or her life or to assist him or her in ending his or her life. Courts in Canada and the United States have reached similar conclusions on largely similar grounds (Rodriguez v British Columbia, 1993; Washington v Glucksberg, 1997; Vacco v Quill, 1997). It is highly probable that the Irish Supreme Court would reach a similar conclusion. This does not mean that a country could not bring in legislation to allow for assisted suicide. For example, the Netherlands, Belgium and Luxembourg (all of which are subject to the European Convention on Human Rights) have done this in recent years. However, this is seen as a matter for politicians, following public debate, and not for the courts.

6. Cases: Exploring Rights in Action

As is often the case with rights, it is one thing to state the existence of a right of autonomy, it is quite another to determine what it means in practice in end-of-life contexts. This can be made more difficult because legal conceptions of the right of autonomy are often developed in once-off, usually dramatic situations such as the Jehovah's Witness refusing blood products. This can create a very unrealistic view of what autonomy in practice means for most patients who are not proposing to make dramatic decisions or to refuse possibly life-saving treatments. Most patients are simply trying to find the best way possible to deal with their illness and the end-of-life decisions which they must make.

In the cases to follow, the practical application of the right of autonomy in end-of-life contexts will be explored. This includes an exploration of the way in which autonomy has operated in the law; the requirements for autonomy and how these may be used to further autonomy as a positive right as well as a right to refuse and a discussion of ways to preserve and protect autonomy even after a patient has lost capacity.

6.1 Case 1: Applying the Legal Right of Autonomy – Re B

This case, which is based on the facts of an English case which came before the courts in 2002, shows the strength of the legal right of autonomy in those cases where the right is held to apply. The case is concerned with the withdrawal of ventilation. There has not been a similar case in Ireland. In an unreported case in 2001, ventilation was not withdrawn from a pregnant woman because the withdrawal would have ended the life of the foetus also. Because information on the facts of the case is restricted (the newspaper report provides only limited information), it is not possible to draw any conclusions from this.

Re B (Adult: Refusal of Medical Treatment) (2002):

Ms B was a 43-year-old woman who was quadriplegic following a stroke which had occurred in the previous year. She also required artificial ventilation and had been hospitalised in an ICU since her illness began. She brought an application to court for ventilation to be withdrawn saying that she had decided that she did not want to live any longer in her condition. Ms B had earlier asked the court to have ventilation withdrawn. She had been severely depressed at the time and had been found not to have the capacity to make this decision. At the time of this case, however, there was no dispute regarding her capacity to make the decision.

The medical professionals caring for Ms B expressed some concerns about her decision. In particular, some carers pointed out that she had never had the opportunity to experience life outside of the restrictions of the ICU environment. There was a possibility that she could successfully complete a ventilation-weaning programme and that she would be able to live a much more independent life. Therefore, some of her carers argued that she had not had the opportunity to make an informed decision about her future and that her decision should not be respected until after she had had such an opportunity.

The English High Court held that the 'personal autonomy of the severely disabled patient' should be recognised and that Ms B should be permitted to have ventilation withdrawn. The judge asked Ms B to reconsider her decision but she said that she could not require Ms B to do so. Ms B remained committed to her decision and shortly afterwards she moved to another hospital because her carers could not bring themselves to participate in the removal of ventilation. She had ventilation removed and shortly afterwards, she died.

6.1.1 Discussion

Case 1 shows that, when the right of autonomy arises in the context of treatment refusal, it is a very powerful right. It takes priority even when the effect of the refusal is the death of the person. In these circumstances, the right to refuse treatment 'trumps' or outweighs the ethical principle of the sanctity of life. The nature of the legal right is perhaps best summarised by Lord Donaldson in the English case of Re T (1992) who stated:

An adult patient who … suffers from no mental incapacity has an absolute right to choose whether to consent to medical treatment, to refuse it or to choose one rather than another of the treatments being offered … This right of choice is not limited to decisions which others might regard as sensible. It exists notwithstanding that the reasons for making the choice are rational, irrational, unknown or even non-existent (1992, p.486)

The judge in Case 1 could implore Ms B not to refuse treatment and she did so in the strongest terms. However, because of Ms B's right of autonomy, she could not be forced to accept treatment which she did not wish to have.

Case 1 also shows that decisions which implement the right of autonomy can be difficult and painful. The judge and Ms B's carers were all very anxious that she should continue to live. Some of Ms B's carers strongly believed that her situation could improve in many ways and that she had not had the opportunity to avail of all the possibilities available to improve the life of a person in her situation. But ultimately, the court held that it was Ms B's decision whether or not to avail of these possibilities.

Case 1 also reminds us of the difference between engagement and discussion on the one hand and force on the other. There was nothing inappropriate in people caring about Ms B and wanting her to have the opportunity to experience life outside the unit. Indeed, it may be argued that Ms B's carers had an ethical obligation to engage with her and to seek to persuade her to continue to live (Mclean, 2009). Healthcare provision would be much poorer if health professionals did not have an interest in the person they cared for or if carers simply accepted decisions such as Ms B's without engaging closely with her and seeking to persuade her to change her mind. However, there is a very significant difference between engaging with, discussing, seeking to persuade and actually forcing a person to accept a treatment which the person rejects. In Case 1, Ms B's carers did the right thing in engaging with her decision but the ultimate decision was for Ms B to make and her carers were bound, both legally and ethically, to respect this decision.

6.1.2 Suggested Professional Responsibilities

- If a person seeks to refuse treatment, especially life-saving treatment, health professionals should consider whether the person has the capacity to make this decision (capacity is discussed further below). If in doubt about capacity, professionals should consult another professional with expertise in this respect (perhaps a psychiatrist or geriatrician). Ultimately, if doubt remains, legal advice should be sought.

- Professionals can and should engage with patients who refuse treatment. If professionals believe that it would be in the patient's best interests to have treatment, they can and should seek to persuade the patient to consent to the treatment. This attempt should be on the basis of dialogue and discussion which should be conducted in a way which is honest and which does not attempt to manipulate the facts.

- A distinction must be made between honest persuasion and force. While persuasion is legitimate, the use of force is not (unless the person lacks the capacity to make the decision).

6.2 Case 2: Informed Consent – Information in Practice

In order to be maximally autonomous, decisions must be fully informed. Tom Beauchamp (1997, p.194) describes informed consent as follows:

A person gives an informed consent … if and only if the person, with substantial understanding and in substantial absence of control by others, intentionally authorises a health-care professional to do something.

Ethicists Ruth Faden and Tom Beauchamp point out that informed consent requires the patient to be fully informed about the nature of the decision and also that any information of particular relevance to the patient should be available (1986, p.302). A patient who makes a decision on the basis of inadequate information cannot be said to have made an informed decision. This is especially true where the decision has life-changing consequences. For example, if a patient refuses life-saving treatment, he or she must be aware of the probable consequences of this decision and of the likelihood that this will occur.

However, simply providing information does not of itself comprise a complete basis for autonomous decision making. Nor is more information necessarily better (Manson and O'Neill, 2007). Neil Manson and Onora O'Neill argue that a narrow focus on the disclosure of information can serve to obscure the issue of 'effective communication and commitments between the parties' (2007, p.184). For this reason, we should not simply focus on disclosure of information in an end-of-life context, for example simply telling a person that he or she is terminally ill or providing information about treatment options, risks and outcomes. Instead, it is important to recognise broader issues of communication and engagement.

In some situations, also, failure to provide adequate information in respect of material risks in advance of consent to a medical procedure will leave a health professional potentially liable in the tort of negligence (Fitzpatrick v White, 2007). However, the legal duty to disclose information falls far short of what is required for genuine informed consent (Donnelly, 2002). The legal duty has focussed primarily on risks and has paid little attention to the other important information for a patient, such as side-effects or alternatives. There has also been a tendency to focus on the detail of the information conveyed without paying much attention to the method of communication. Respect for the positive right of autonomy requires that much greater effort at communication be made than is required under the law of negligence.

The importance of communicating information in the broader sense is evident is Case 2 which draws on a practitioner narrative provided in Quinlan and O'Neill (2009, pp.49–50):

I did have the experience of a gentleman, you know, I got a referral to say that he was, you know, quite anxious and, you know, he needed to speak to somebody. He wasn't really consenting to his treatment and, you know, I went to see him and his biggest thing was that he said he had got no information from the team as to what the treatment was, why he was getting it or what his outcome was going to be. Now he did say to me 'I understand it's not going to be good news but I'd rather know'.

I think if people know good or bad they'll find a way to deal with that or they'll find a way to cope with that, it mightn't be the best way but I suppose then you can come in and try and offer some support with that. But for that man, at that time, he just felt 'I don't know what they're talking about' and at the same time he had a sense, he knew it wasn't going to be good, 'but just tell me so I can get on with it', so those sorts of things.

I think just people being fully aware at all times of what's going on. I suppose that they feel that their wishes are respected, that we're not running off and ringing the family to say well 'they've said no but we really think ...', you know, and I would always feel that – I would always go and see a patient first and say to them 'listen, is it okay if I call such and such?', if they say 'no', that's fine, that's their decision and the team mightn't like that or, you know, a lot of people don't like that but that's – I feel that they should know that their wishes were respected. And then, you know, I suppose just the amount of dignity they have around that as well.

6.2.1 Discussion

This case as recounted by a practitioner shows a number of important issues in respect of the role of information in protecting patient autonomy. It reminds us that patients can respond in two different ways to lack of adequate information. Many patients will not object; they will go ahead with treatment and comply with their health professional's directions. But these are not autonomous decisions. Although the patient has given consent, the patient's positive right of autonomy is not being respected.

Patients may also respond like the gentleman in Case 2. He refused to consent. It turned out, when the practitioner investigated further, that the reason for the refusal was his lack of information. In a sense, he was using his refusal as a plea for information. However, not all patients will be as forthcoming as this gentleman. Some may withdraw or refuse treatment without ever explaining (or perhaps sometimes without even understanding) why they are doing do. If, in a case like this, the professional is not open and prepared to discuss with the patient and simply accepts the refusal at face value, the patient may continue to refuse treatment. If this happens, it would represent a failure to respect the patient's rights, including his or her right of autonomy. Thus, Case 2 reminds us that respect for the patient's right of autonomy requires more than simply not interfering with a patient who seeks to refuse treatment. In addition, respect for the right imposes a positive obligation to inform the patient and to discuss treatment options with him or her.

Communication (giving information and listening to patients) is central if patients are to be sufficiently informed about their diagnosis and prognosis. Lack of information and even mis-information can leave patients without power to make choices. One practitioner narrative notes 'it is not unusual that people are let out of here with misinformation because we use language like 'a shadow on the lung' and the patient doesn't know that he had lung cancer (Quinlan and O'Neill, 2009). It is not always easy to achieve good communication especially where a patient is dying. However, respect for patient autonomy requires positive efforts to be made. (The difficulties with honest engagement are explored in Module 2.)

A second notable aspect of Case 2 is the recognition, which this practitioner clearly shows, that autonomy is not a right respected in a once-off situation only, and that information is something which must be relayed on an ongoing basis. The practitioner says, 'I would always go to the patient first.' The positive right of autonomy in the sense of control over one's decision making requires more than once-off information. Facilitating autonomy in patients requires ongoing communication. Conversation to nurture autonomy is stressed as an indispensable ethical value in discussions on end-of-life care.

But good information and listening take time. There is a serious lack of time for communication with patients to find out their preferences, desires or wishes. Where this communication doesn't happen, staff can't help patients to be autonomous. Practitioners remind us that, 'if we're intent on nurturing and encouraging patient autonomy, then we need time to communicate with patients, with family and with each other on a ward' (Quinlan and O'Neill, 2009).

6.2.2 Suggested Professional Responsibilities

- In order to ensure that patients' decisions are as fully informed as is possible, health professionals must ensure that patients receive adequate information in respect of their condition.

- Health professionals should address broader issues of communication rather than focussing simply on the information communicated. This requires that they understand the emotional and social context in which the information is conveyed.

- Health professionals should recognise that information is not simply conveyed in a once-off way but that repeated efforts need to be made to engage with the patient.

- Adequate communication requires listening as well as speaking; each patient has unique informational concerns and these can only be addressed if the professional is aware of what these are.

6.3 Case 3: Capacity, a Pre-requisite for Autonomy? – Re C

Respect for autonomy principle is inherently linked to the requirement for capacity. The right of autonomy presumes that the person whose right is respected has the capacity to make the decision in question. Decision-making capacity is a requirement for the moral or ethical right of autonomy. It is also a requirement for the legal right. Legal capacity, in Buchanan and Brock's words, is 'a threshold concept, not a comparative one' (1989, p.27). The law sets the required standard for capacity and asks simply whether the patient reaches the designated threshold. This means that the law is not concerned with whether someone is a good decision maker as we might think of the concept in other contexts. The law does not ask whether the person is reflective and careful or impulsive and careless. The only matter of interest to the law is whether or not the person reaches the legal standard.

A person may lack the capacity to make decisions at the end of life for two reasons. First, she or he may be too young to make the decision or, secondly, she or he may lack the necessary decision-making abilities. This may be because the person is unconscious or because of intellectual disability, mental illness or dementia. In both cases, the law sets out a threshold point at which a person has capacity. In order to understand the legal right of autonomy, it is essential that these thresholds be appreciated. However, it is also important to remember that, just because a person lacks formal legal capacity does not mean that his or her views and preferences can simply be ignored. This point will be returned to in the Further Discussion.

First, however, it is necessary to consider Case 3. This case provides an example of the relevant threshold for legal capacity to make decisions for adults. This is based on an English case from 1993. In the Irish case of Fitzpatrick v K (2008), the Irish courts have held that the same standard applies in Ireland.

Re C (An Adult) 1993

Mr C had been detained in a mental hospital for many years. He developed gangrene in one leg and medical advice was that his leg needed to be amputated. Mr C resisted this and said that he would prefer to die with two legs than to live with one. Mr C also offered the view that God would save him and he referred to his own (delusional) belief that he was a world-famous surgeon.

The court held that Mr C had the necessary capacity to refuse the amputation even if the refusal would lead to his death. It was not relevant that Mr C had a mental illness. Everyone must be presumed to have capacity regardless of their underlying circumstances.

The test for capacity related to his capacity to make this particular decision and not to his overall situation. The court identified three questions as relevant in deciding if Mr C had legal capacity:

1. *Could he understand the information relevant to the decision (to refuse the amputation)?*
2. *Did he believe the information?*
3. *Could he use this information to make a decision?*

The court found that Mr C understood the information relevant to his decision – including that if he did not have the surgery, he could die. He was also found to believe this information 'in his own fashion' and to be able to use this information to reach a decision. Therefore Mr C was permitted to refuse the amputation.

6.3.1 Discussion

Although Case 3 happened in England, the test for capacity set out in Case 3 applies in Ireland as well. A bill on mental capacity is due to be published in late 2011 and this is likely to become law in 2012. The standard for capacity set out in the bill is likely to be more or less the same as that in Case 3. There are a number of features of the test for capacity as set out in Case 3 which merit further reflection in an end-of-life context.

First, all persons are to be presumed to have capacity. Just because a person is very old, or mentally ill, or intellectually disabled does not mean that they can be presumed to lack the capacity to make their own decisions. It is especially important to remember this when dealing with older patients or patients with intellectual disabilities. Quinlan and O'Neill (2009, p.48) note the following view offered by one practitioner:

I think the most obvious place where patient autonomy falls down is with ageism. If somebody is 30 or 40 or 50 we are much more likely to pay heed to what they're saying and involve them. If somebody is 70 or 80 or 90 we're much less likely to do so. As a sweeping statement I think patient autonomy tends to decrease with age and I don't think there's a good reason for that but I think that is the practice of what happens.

A second important aspect of the test for capacity as set out in Case 3 is that, in most cases, it will be health professionals who will decide if a patient has capacity or not. This places an onus on health professionals to acquaint themselves with the legal test. As Shaun O'Keefe notes, this also presents challenges for many professionals (2008, p.44) who may be unfamiliar with the test for capacity or who may be unsure of what exactly is required. Respect for the principle of autonomy requires that capacity be assessed in a way which is fair and appropriate and which is free from prejudices based on external factors such as old age, mental illness or intellectual disability (Donnelly, 2009b).

A final point about Case 3 is that capacity should be seen not just as a characteristic which must be assessed but as a characteristic which must be developed. This view of capacity is consistent with the positive right of autonomy which is put forward in this module. Research shows that patients' capacity can often be enhanced by quite simple steps, such as breaking down information into smaller 'bites' or making efforts to talk to patients in a way that they will understand (Gunn 1999, p.276). Clearly, this requires effort on the part of health professionals and, like many of the other efforts which delivering on the positive right of autonomy requires, this needs resource allocation. Time and commitment are crucial in deciding what can be achieved in terms of helping a person make autonomous decisions.

In relation to young people, the starting point for capacity is section 23 of the Non-Fatal Offences Against the Person Act 1997. This states that:

The consent of a minor who has attained the age of 16 years to any surgical, medical or dental treatment which, in the absence of consent, would constitute a trespass to his or her person, shall be as effective as it would be if he or she were of full age; and where a minor has by virtue of this section given an effective consent to any treatment it shall not be necessary to obtain any consent for it from his or her parent or guardian.

This means that once a person is 16 years old, she or he can consent to treatment and the consent of her or his parents is not required.

Section 23 does not mention the refusal of treatment. This leads to the question of whether a person aged 16 or more can refuse treatment in the same way as she or he can consent to it. This issue has not come before the Irish courts. It might be argued that consent and refusal are clearly two sides of the same matter and that the right to consent automatically includes the right to refuse treatment. However, the English courts, working with a broadly similar legal position, have held that the refusal of treatment is not the same as consent to treatment. This meant that a young person (below the age of 18) may have the automatic right to consent to treatment but does not have an equivalent right to refuse treatment. Instead, if a young person proposes to refuse treatment, the court must determine if this is in the best interests of the young person.

There is a strong possibility that the Irish courts would adopt a position similar to that taken by the English courts. In such a situation, the young person's views would have to be taken into account in deciding if treatment should be given.

6.3.2 Suggested Professional Responsibilities

- If a question arises in respect of whether a person has decision-making capacity, it is the responsibility of the professional/s involved to investigate capacity.

- If in doubt in this respect, the professional should seek a second opinion from another professional with expertise in the area of capacity assessment (perhaps a psychiatrist or a geriatrician depending on the circumstances).

- If doubts remain, legal advice should be sought.

- Professionals should familiarise themselves with the legal test for capacity as this is the relevant test to determine whether or not a person is legally entitled to make decisions.

- Professionals should presume that patients have decision-making capacity and should assess capacity in a way which is fair and free from prejudices based on old age, mental illness or intellectual disability.

- Professionals should seek to facilitate people of borderline capacity in making decisions for themselves insofar as this is possible. This may require breaking information down into more easily understandable 'chunks' and making efforts to talk to patients in a way which they can understand

6.4 Case 4: Voluntariness and Decision-Making Freedom – Families and Patients

Respect for the positive right of autonomy requires that necessary efforts are made to ensure that patients are free to make their own decisions. This does not mean that professionals should not engage with patients or seek to inform them. Nor does it mean that professionals should not offer their own views as to what is the most appropriate treatment option or seek to persuade patients in this regard. The positive right of autonomy requires professional engagement, not professional withdrawal. But, ultimately, the patient must be facilitated in feeling that he or she is free to make decisions and that decisions are not made simply to keep the relevant health professionals happy.

Interviews with hospital staff make clear that the role of family in decision making is among the most challenging of all ethical and legal topics. The challenges for a model of respect for autonomy of the patient while at the same time recognising the importance of families are evident in Case 4, which is taken from Quinlan and O'Neill (2009, p.59).

Families and Patients' Decision-Making Freedom

I can think of an example a few weeks ago where this man just used to do the answering for his wife and, you know, like he did respect her decisions but he kind of – she had a brain tumour and he kind of used to answer the question before you'd get a chance to hear her answer and when we were offering her – her balance was very unsteady and we were offering her a place in the hospice and he said 'no, no she can go home, we'll manage at home'.

And, you know, I suppose he was just not ready to let her go to the hospice and really keen to take her home and she went along with that but I felt that deep down, you know, if he was more open to the idea she'd have been more open to it as well because she was fearful that if she was at home the dogs would knock her over and that, you know, or that she'd be for periods on her own in the house – things like that.

6.4.1 Discussion

Keeping contact and communication with family is an essential component of a good framework for end-of-life decisions. Family input can be especially valuable with dementia patients. As one practitioner noted:

We depend a lot on the relatives, you know, for the information we receive as well. Communication with family is a big thing really in the elderly. They know the person better. And I think it's right that we listen to the family […] that's one good thing here, that the family are always welcome all day and they're involved a lot in the care. (**Quinlan and O'Neill, 2008**).

However, the position may not always be so straightforward. Another practitioner notes:

There's nieces an nephews who would know very little […] they turn up and make decisions that sometimes we know in our heart and soul the man would never have wanted.
(Quinlan and O'Neill, 2008)

Case 4 reminds us that sometimes family members can limit patient autonomy. This can sometimes have negative effects for the patient and can lead to a patient being deprived of treatment which could make his or her dying easier or more pain-free. One palliative care physician explains in Quinlan and O'Neill (2009) that family can exert pressure to the point of not allowing their relative access to palliative care because they pressurise physicians to agree not to tell patients their diagnosis (see Module 2). Patients in this situation may also be placed in a very lonely and frightening position with nobody to talk to about their concerns. Respect for the positive right of autonomy requires that efforts are made to engage with the patient him or herself as an individual and not simply to deal with the patient through family members.

6.4.2 Suggested Professional Responsibilities

- Professionals have an obligation to provide honest advice to patients, including about treatment options. However, advice should not be allowed to become coercive. Patients should not be in any doubt that decisions are his or her to make.
- Professionals should recognise the pressures which families can place on patients in end-of-life contexts. While recognising the importance of communication and engagement with family members, professionals should make efforts to ensure that the patient is not pressured into making decisions about end-of-life care which do not accord with what he or she wants or needs in order to keep family members happy.

Health professionals may need to reassure both the patient and the family that the primary duty is owed to the patient. While this needs to be done sensitively, it is essential that this primary duty is maintained and that all parties involved are aware of it.

6.5 Case 5: Preserving Patient Autonomy – Advance Directives in Practice

While the role of patient autonomy where a patient has capacity is fairly straightforward, the issue becomes more complex when a patient lacks the capacity to make healthcare decisions. A lack of capacity can arise in two circumstances. A patient who formerly had capacity to make decisions may have lost capacity, perhaps in an older patient due to conditions such as dementia or Alzheimer's disease. Other patients may never have had capacity to make decisions. These may include very young patients or patients who have significant intellectual disabilities.

For patients who once had capacity, it is possible in some circumstances to preserve patient autonomy, to a degree at least, even after a patient has lost capacity. There are two main ways in which this can be achieved. These are Advance Directives/Decisions and Enduring Powers of Attorney.

An Advance Directive or decision (sometimes known as a 'living will') is a decision made by a person while he or she has decision-making capacity regarding the medical treatment he or she would wish to receive (and more frequently not to receive) if he or she subsequently loses capacity. An Advance Directive may be stated in very general terms: i.e. 'I would not wish to receive treatment for cancer' or in much more specific terms: i.e. outlining specific treatments that a person would not wish to receive, for example a patient may request a DNR or do not resuscitate order to be placed on his or her notes stating that he or she would not wish to be artificially resuscitated in certain circumstances. Advance Directives are usually made in writing and this is advisable because it provides a clear indication of the person's wishes.

An Enduring Power of Attorney is a document, again drawn up when a person has legal capacity, which gives another person (sometimes known as the donnee of the power) the power to make certain kinds of designated decisions if the person who drew up the Enduring Power of Attorney subsequently loses capacity. The principle behind this model for decision making is that the substitute decision maker will act in a way which represents the views of the person who has lost capacity. In this way, the autonomy of the person is preserved even though he or she has lost decision-making capacity.

The advantage of the Power of Attorney model for decision making when compared with the Advance Directive model is that it allows for a more nuanced and complex approach to decision making. The person granting the power does not have to make firm advance decisions (although he or she may do so and communicate these to the person to whom the Power of Attorney is given) but can rely on his or her representative to act on his or her behalf. The substitute decision maker can take account of all the factors, including developments in medical science, past wishes and current attitudes and situations in order to reach a decision about healthcare, including when life-sustaining treatment should be withdrawn. Clearly, however, this model requires a good deal of trust to be placed with the person granted the Power of Attorney. Depending on the circumstances, he or she has enormous control over the health and possibly even the life of the person who now lacks capacity.

Legislation regarding Advance Directives has been commonplace in the United States since at least the mid-1990s. More recently, in England and Wales the Mental Capacity Act 2005 allows for advance refusals of treatment (but not for advance requests regarding treatment) and for the appointment of Enduring Powers of Attorney. There is no legislation in Ireland.

However, it is likely that in a non-contentious case, especially where a patient had a terminal illness, an Advance Directive would be considered to be binding. Certainly, there is a strong ethical imperative to respect the stated wishes of the person in the Advance Directive.

Three recent Irish reports have called for the introduction of Advance Directives in legislation (Irish Council for Bioethics, 2007; Law Reform Commission, 2008; Law Reform Commission, 2009).

This view seems to be shared by healthcare practitioners, one of whom says:

> *I actually think that we should start bringing in Living Wills, I really do because by the time it comes to the end of their lives, most of our patients don't have a say because they're either confused or they're not compos mentis. You will try and listen to the ones that are and if you can make it possible you will make it possible but I do think we should bring in some sort of Living Will.*
> (Quinlan and O'Neill, 2009, p.47)

The Law Reform Commission (2009) proposes the introduction of legislation dealing specifically with Advance Directives. The Commission's report sets out a draft Mental Capacity (Advanced Care Directives) Bill 2009. It proposes that this would apply to refusals of treatment only. However, the Commission recommends that a person should not be able to refuse basic care, which includes warmth, palliative care, nutrition and hydration. The draft bill also provides for the nomination of a healthcare proxy to carry out the wishes of the person.

Current Irish law does not permit Enduring Powers of Attorneys to be made in respect of healthcare decisions (although it does allow them in respect of property and welfare decisions). It is likely that a limited Enduring Power of Attorney to make healthcare decisions will be included in the forthcoming Mental Capacity Bill. However, it is unclear whether this will extend to decisions at the end of life.

As matters currently stand, very few people provide advance instructions as regards how they would wish to be treated towards the end of their lives (Weafer, McCarthy and Loughrey, 2009). One practitioner notes that 'a lot of people in Ireland don't discuss or think about end-of-life decisions. I haven't really had any experience where people have made a decision beforehand' (Quinlan and O'Neill, 2009, p.42). In fact, research in other countries shows that this is not a uniquely Irish phenomenon (Francis, 2001, p.561). In the United States, where legislation on Advance Directives has been in effect for many years, a relatively small number of people make Advance Directives.

There are many reasons why people, even people who are serious ill or elderly, may not choose to take this step. There may be an inherent privacy and reticence. Or there may be an understandable reluctance to face up to the unhappy prospect of death, serious illness or dementia. However, there are strong reasons why people who wish to make these kinds of decisions should be facilitated in doing so.

An Advance Directive allows patients to direct their care even beyond incapacity. As Case 5 shows, this allows patients a degree of control which would otherwise be impossible. Case 5 is based on the facts of an English decision.

Advance Directives in Practice

AK was a young man with progressive motor neuron disease. While he still had the ability to communicate, he made an Advance Directive setting out what should happen when he lost this ability. The directive stated that, when he signalled an intention – by blinking his eye in a particular way – this was a communication that ventilation should be withdrawn.
The English Court approved the directive and when AK indicated that ventilation should be withdrawn, this was carried out with appropriate palliative care.

6.5.1 Discussion

Case 5 is somewhat unusual in that AK did not lose the capacity to make treatment decisions, as is normally the case where Advance Directives are employed. Rather, he lost the ability to communicate these decisions. However, from a practical point of view, loss of the ability to communicate decisions is similar in effect to loss of the ability to make decisions.

Case 5 also reminds us that Advance Directives can serve to preserve life as well as decide when life should end. AK could have declined ventilation when it became necessary through a straightforward exercise of his right to refuse treatment. However, he was a young man who did not want to die at that time. He wanted to gain the maximum from his life for the time he had left. Because he could make an Advance Directive, he was able to avail of the possibilities for a longer life offered by ventilation while still ensuring that, at a time of his choosing, the treatment could be withdrawn. In this very sad situation, also, the knowledge that he had a means of control may have given the young man in Case 5 some consolation and fortitude and helped him to get the maximum benefit from the time he had left.

However, while Advance Directives are important tools in furthering patient autonomy, they are not without ethical, or indeed legal, complexity. The liberal legal philosopher Ronald Dworkin, himself a strong proponent of Advance Directives, uses an example based on a woman called Margo to explore the challenges to which Advance Directives give rise (1993, p.201).

In the example, Margo has Alzheimer's disease and has no long-term memory and minimal short-term memory. She is very contented and spends her days listening to music, reading (choosing pages at random) and painting pink circles. Her doctor described Margo as 'the happiest person I know'. Dworkin imagines that Margo has made an Advance Directive stating that if she develops Alzheimer's disease, she wishes to decline all medical interventions. He also imagines that Margo now develops a form of cancer which is easily treatable and for which treatment is relatively un-invasive and has a high likelihood of success. In other words, it is clearly in Margo's current best interests that she should receive treatment. He asks whether Margo should receive the treatment notwithstanding her Advance Directive.

Dworkin himself argues that Margo should not receive the treatment. He argues that her prior expressed wishes should take priority because respecting the autonomy of a capable person is the most important value. Other commentators such as Dresser (1986) disagree. She argues that Advance Directives are important but that they do not justify overriding the current best interests of a person who now lacks capacity. Dresser argues that the person lacking capacity should not be bound by the decisions of his or her former, capable self. Rather the current person's best interests should take priority over his or her previously expressed views. Court cases on advance refusals of treatment have tended to support Dresser's view rather than Dworkin's.

The 'Margo'-type situation is unlikely to occur frequently. Most of the time, in end-of-life contexts, there will not be a clear conflict between what a patient's Advance Directive proposes and his or her best interests. Rather, as in Case 5, the Advance Directive will dictate at a level of detail how the person should be treated. In this, Advance Directives can play an important role in allowing patients to retain control over their future care.

6.5.2 Suggested Professional Responsibilities

- Although the legal framework for advance decision making is still limited in Ireland, professionals should engage with patients where possible in order to ascertain the treatment they would wish to receive if they lose capacity.

- Most of the time, there will not be a clear conflict between the patient's wishes expressed while capable and his or her best interests. In such a situation, the professional should take account of the previously expressed wishes in making decisions about treatment.

7. Module 4 Further Discussion

Autonomy is an important legal and ethical principle. The view of autonomy taken in this module is of autonomy as a positive right to control together with the steps required to make this meaningful, as well as a negative right to refuse treatment. This ethical conception of autonomy is broader than the legal conception. But this broader view is more helpful in thinking about decisions at the end of life.

7.1 Implications of the Positive Right of Autonomy

Autonomous decisions must meet three requirements: the patient must have adequate information; he or she must have capacity; and he or she must act freely without undue pressures from health professionals, family members or others. In respect of each of these requirements, there is a positive obligation to assist the patient in making autonomous decisions. This means that autonomy requires a good deal from health professionals and a commitment to autonomy will require resources. It is much less likely that pressured staff with limited resources and facilities will be able to dedicate the time and energy necessary to deliver autonomy as a positive right.

7.2 Participation by People Lacking Capacity

An important final point to note relates to those patients who lack the capacity for autonomous decision making, whether because they are too young or because they have dementia or another capacity-impairing condition. It should not be presumed that, simply because a person lacks the capacity to make an autonomous decision, his or her views should simply be disregarded. Patients who lack decision-making capacity have a right to participate in decisions made about them.

As discussed in Module 3, the United Nations Convention on the Rights of the Child requires that children be permitted to participate in decisions in accordance with their age and maturity (Kilkelly and Donnelly, 2006). The United Nations Convention on the Right of Persons with Disabilities and Council of Europe Recommendation on Incapable Adults impose similar requirements in respect of adults lacking capacity. It is highly likely that the proposed Mental Capacity Bill will also include a requirement to this effect in respect of adults.

It is not always easy for professionals to find a way to facilitate participation in end-of-life decisions by patients lacking capacity. As one professional interviewed by Quinlan and O'Neill (2009, p.54) recounts:

A child who is on the cusp of having their own autonomy, you're looking at teenagers, and we see children here from premature babies up to 18, 19 and sometimes 20. We see children with intellectual disabilities as well and the whole role of autonomy for somebody with an intellectual disability and the challenges that poses, in terms of can they be autonomous? Are they allowed be autonomous? Whether that is from their parents' side of things or from the medical point of view or the child's own abilities. That's a huge challenge.

This professional identifies the challenges involved. However, there are ways in which patient participation can be facilitated notwithstanding the fact that a patient lacks capacity. The Code of Practice to the English Mental Capacity Act (2007) provides a useful resource in setting out ways to facilitate participation by adults lacking capacity. These include using simple language, speaking at the appropriate volume and speed, using appropriate words and sentence structure, breaking down information into smaller points, and using illustrations and/or photographs to help the person understand the decision to be made. Where a person has communication or cognitive problems, possibilities are offered by the use of picture boards, Makaton, signing, technological aids. For some people who are restricted to non-verbal methods of communication, their behaviour and, in particular, changes in their behaviour may provide indications of their feelings (Donnelly, 2009a).

In making end-of-life decisions for patients lacking capacity, it is also possible to take account of the patient's past wishes and preferences and to ask what the patient would have wanted if he or she had had capacity. Even if a person has not made a formal Advance Directive, there should be room for his or her prior preferences to be taken into account in determining what is in his or her best interests. In England, the Mental Capacity Act 2005 requires that, in making decisions about the best interests of a person lacking capacity, account should be taken of the person's past and present wishes and feelings (and in particular any written statement made by the person when he or she had capacity) and of the beliefs and values that would be likely to influence the person's decision if he or she had had capacity. It is likely that the proposed Irish legislation on capacity will contain a similar requirement.

It is not always easy to find ways to take account of the prior views of a person when these have not been formally stated in an Advance Directive. It is crucial to consult with families and friends as to what the person was like before this illness and to ask what he or she would have wanted in the situation that now arises. It is essential that a space be created where the person who is now without decision-making capacity can influence the process to the maximum extent possible (Donnelly, 2009a).

7.3 Traditional Views of Autonomy

Because of the significance attached to autonomy, respect for autonomous choice is a core element of many different philosophical and political theories. Two philosophers, the eighteenth-century German, Immanuel Kant (1724–1804), and the nineteenth-century Englishman, John Stuart Mill (1806–1873), have greatly influenced the way in which we understand what respect for autonomy involves.

7.3.1 Autonomy and Rationality

Kant appealed to the deontological belief that some things are intrinsically or inherently good, and that each person is intrinsically valuable or has unconditional worth because they have the capacity to be autonomous (See Module 1 for explanation of the deontological moral theory). For Kant, human dignity resides in the fact that each person has a free will which they can follow independently of their passions or desires. On his view, human beings can be distinguished from many other sentient creatures because, unlike animals, they are not wholly determined by their own immediate desires.

Believing that human beings are able to act freely and independently of personal desires, loves and hates, Kant argued that they are capable of prescribing general moral rules or principles for themselves to follow. They can legislate for their own conduct. The neo-Kantian Thomas Hill takes this to mean that:

> [T]he autonomy of a moral legislator means that, in debating basic moral principles and values, a person ideally should not be moved by blind adherence to tradition or authority, by outside threats or bribes, by unreflective impulse, or unquestioned habits of thought [...] must try not to give special weight to his or her particular preferences and personal attachments [...]. In other words, at the level of deliberation about basic principles, morality requires impartial regard for all persons. (Hill, 1991, p.45)

On the Kantian view, human beings have a capacity for free, rational and impartial decision making. This means that they are able to decide a course of action on the basis of careful reflection, and in the absence of coercion from authority or custom. In addition, they can decide the best course of action independently of their own personal preferences or inclinations.

It is on the basis of this kind of autonomous capacity that each human being has a special status that deserves protection and respect for Kant. In his terms, failing to respect a person's autonomy would involve treating that individual merely as a means to another's ends, and not in terms of their own ineliminable value:

So act as to treat humanity, whether in thine own person or in that of any other, in every case as an end withal, never as means only. **(Kant, [1785], 1993)**

7.3.2 Autonomy and Individuality

In his well-known thesis in *On Liberty* ([1859], 1991), John Stuart Mill also promoted respect for individual autonomy (or liberty), but on grounds different from those suggested by Kant. Mill viewed each person as worthy of respect, not because of their rationality or impartiality but because of their unique individuality. He appealed to the utilitarian view – that an action is morally good if it gives rise to more good than evil – to support his position (see Module 1 for an explanation of the utilitarian theory). For Mill, respecting individual autonomy gives rise to more good than evil; society ought to respect autonomy because, in the long term, society benefits from doing so:

> *The worth of a State, in the long run, is the worth of the individuals composing it . . . a state which dwarfs its men in order that they may be more docile instruments in its hands even for beneficial purposes – will find that with small men no great thing can really be accomplished.*
> (Mill [1859], 1981, p.187)

In other words, on the Millian view, individual freedom is compatible with, and contributes towards, the good of society as a whole. It follows that a person ought to be allowed to act according to their own life's plan and their own beliefs and values, whether or not their actions are considered wise or good or foolish by everyone else. (One needs to read Mill's text as referring to both genders when he uses the language of 'small men', etc.)

For Mill, autonomy is not an absolute right. On his view, a state or an individual is justified in interfering with a person's liberty when their action causes harm to others (this is known as the harm principle). He distinguishes between public and private morality, and between those actions which affect others in society – 'other-regarding' actions – and those which affect only ourselves – 'self-regarding' actions. This is a classic liberal position which holds that the freedom of the individual can be compromised only when it is in competition or conflict with the rights and freedoms of other individuals. Respect for autonomy requires, on this view, that we refrain from interfering with the self-regarding acts and decisions that people make.

> *[T]he only purpose for which power can be rightfully exercised over any member of a civilized community, against his will, is to prevent harm to others. His own good, either physical or moral, is not sufficient warrant. He cannot rightfully be compelled to do or forbear because it will be better*

for him to do so, because it will make him happier, because, in the opinions of others, to do so would be wise, or even right. These are good reasons for remonstrating with him, or persuading him, or entreating him, but not for compelling him, or visiting him with any evil in case he does otherwise. (Mill [1858], 1981, p. 68)

(See Module 7 for an example of the application of the harm principle in relation to patient confidentiality.)

7.4 Relational Autonomy

While the principle of autonomy is one of the cornerstones of contemporary bioethics, it is a highly complex and problematic one. Some thinkers repudiate the concept altogether, while others accept its value but dispute the meaning which has been attached to it. For example, some thinkers refuse to accept the concept of the autonomous self central to modern Western philosophy – namely, the depiction of the self in abstract, asocial terms as an independent and rationally self-sufficient individual – and demand a new conception of autonomy which recognises the inherently social nature of human beings (MacIntyre, 1981; Sherwin, 2008; Taylor, 1989). According to this interpretation, the self is essentially social:

We are not isolated atoms, or islands, or self-contained entities, but rather products of historical, social, and cultural processes and interactions. The existence of any person is dependent on the existence and social arrangements of many others. Our interests are discovered by and pursued within social environments that help to shape our identities, characters, and opportunities. […] relational autonomy […] requires us to examine the types of options on offer and ask questions about how these have arisen and also about options that are not available or accessible. (Sherwin, 2008, p.12)

One of the implications of viewing the self as profoundly social is to accept that one's actions are determined or influenced by one's social context. Secondly, one's social attachments may motivate one's actions, and, finally, one's very identity may be constituted by these social attachments (Barclay, 2000).

In the first of these senses, the relational autonomy position rejects the idea of autonomy as simply a matter of deciding what one wants or desires. Relational theorists insist that attention is paid to the social circumstances which inform or ground desires of any kind. Such social circumstances include social norms and oppressive patterns. The skills and competencies for the exercise of choice to begin with include self-trust, self-understanding, self-direction and self-worth – and these may be undermined or made possible in the company of others. On this view, the actions of individuals are framed and contrained by the opportunities available to them. In addition, the ability to imagine and pursue a course of action depends on options available.

Autonomous capacity, on the relational view, can be understood as the ability to negotiate the effects of socialisation by actualising certain capacities, including the capacity to choose preferences, goals and projects and make them one's own (Barclay, 2000, pp.54–5). The implication of this view for health professionals and organisations is to enable patients to develop their capacity to direct their care: autonomy is not simply something that is assessed but it is something that is developed (Barclay, 2000, p.57).

A second implication of viewing the self as social is to see the self as 'motivationally social'; that is, primarily motivated to act, not by rational self-interest or by a striving for self-sufficiency – as caricatures of the modern ideal of autonomy would suggest – but by a sense of solidarity and by deep attachments to other people (Barclay, 2000, p.60). This view is supported by international and Irish research with patients and families who are terminally ill and who often prioritise the interests of their loved ones over their own (Quinlan, 2009a; Weafer, McCarthy and Loughrey, 2009).

The third sense in which the self may be described as social – the 'constitutively social' self – involves understanding one's identity as a product of one's social relationships and attachments. On the view of the philosopher Michael Sandel, for example, the goals and ends which define us as who we are are not private, but shared; they are the goals and ends of the communities of which we are a part and they are formed by participation in these communities. We don't so much choose these ends as discover them when we reflect on who we are and what we aspire to (Barclay, 2000, p.65). For Sandel, the classic expression of the rational exercise of autonomy involves a person ranking their desires and choosing that plan of action which will satisfy as many of their principal desires as possible. Against this, Sandel argues that even the evaluation of our desires presupposes a set of socially-shared values which constitutes who we are; it is this set of 'constitutive values', rather than our desires per se, which forms the foundation for our choices and actions.

Finally, it has been suggested by feminists such as Barclay (2000) and Sherwin (2008) that the fact that our choices are socially determined and our identities are socially mediated opens up the possibility of change and liberates us to choose reflectively which values to endorse and which goals to prioritise. And this reflection upon which relationships and attachments we choose to promote does not undercut, but reinforces, the importance of the capacity for autonomy, understood as relational.

8. Module 4 Summary Learning Guides

8.1 The Nature of Autonomy

- The right of autonomy protects a person's interest in making significant decisions about his or her own life
- Autonomy is not just a negative right – a right to say no but also a positive right – a right to be facilitated in taking control of one's dying to the maximum extent possible
- Autonomy is especially important in a hospital setting
- Concern with autonomy is to some extent a cultural phenomenon which is especially associated with Western liberalism

8.2 The Legal Right of Autonomy

- This right is protected under the Irish Constitution and the European Convention on Human Rights
- The legal right is very often seen as a negative right – a right to refuse treatment
- As part of protection of the legal right of autonomy, capable adults have the right to refuse medical treatment even if the refusal leads to their death
- But there are some limits: duties to others may arise –the extent of these duties is not clear

8.3 Information is Key to Autonomy

- The positive right of autonomy requires that patients are informed
- 'Informing' in this sense requires more than simply passing on information: communication is essential
- 'Informing' is an ongoing process – it is not a once-off event
- Legal requirements in respect of information provision are insufficient in protecting a patient's positive right of autonomy

8.4 The Role of Decision-Making Capacity and Freedom

- Legal capacity is a prerequisite for the legal right of autonomy

- For adults, legal capacity requires that the person can understand information relevant to the decision, believe the information and use the information to make a decision

- Young people can consent to treatment from the age of 16

- There is still legal uncertainty regarding whether young people from the age of 16 can refuse treatment (if the refusal is not considered to be in the young person's best interests)

- To be autonomous, decisions must be freely made

8.5 Advance Decision Making

- An Advance Directive or 'Living Will' is a binding instruction made by a person with capacity about the treatment that the person would wish to receive or to refuse if he or she subsequently loses capacity

- There is no legislation in respect of Advance Directives in Ireland. However, the courts have approved Advance Directives in principle

- An Enduring Power of Attorney allows a person with capacity to designate a person to make decisions on his or her behalf if he or she subsequently loses capacity

- Although there is legislation on Enduring Powers of Attorney in Ireland, it does not currently include healthcare decisions

- Advance Directives and Enduring Powers of Attorney provide a means of preserving autonomy after losing capacity

8.6 Autonomy and the Person without Capacity

- The fact that a person lacks capacity does not mean that his or her views should be completely disregarded

- It is important that a person without capacity be facilitated in participating in decisions about end-of-life care where possible

- Efforts must be made to take account of the past preferences of a person without capacity and of what he or she would have wished to happen in a situation like this. Consultation with family and friends about what the person would have wanted is essential

9. Module 4 Activities

9.1 Recall the distinction between the positive right of autonomy and the negative right of autonomy:

a. Would you add anything further to these points on the distinction?

b. What actions on the part of health professionals are needed to give effect to a negative right of autonomy?

c. What actions on the part of health professionals are needed to give effect to a positive right of autonomy?

d. Which form of autonomy is easier to deliver?

e. Which form of autonomy is most important? Or are both equally important?

9.2 Reflect back on the particulars of Case 1:

a. In reading Case 1, jot down your first, unanalysed response to the facts set out.

b. Do you think that the woman in this case should have been required to experience life outside the confines of the ICU before her decision to have ventilation withdrawn was respected?

c. In your view, is there a conflict between health professionals' ethical duty to care on the one hand and legal duty to respect a patient's refusal of treatment on the other? If there is a conflict, how should this be resolved?

9.3 Reflect back on the particulars of Case 2:

a. In your experience do patients often actively seek information towards the end of life?

b. Why is information essential to the positive right of autonomy?

c. Set out the information which, in your view, is most important for patients to receive in order to help them make autonomous decisions

d. Do communication breakdowns occur often in practice? If so, what steps can usefully be taken to avoid this occurring?

9.4 Reflect back on the particulars of Case 3:

a. What are the requirements for the legal test for capacity? Do these requirements strike you as sensible? Try to imagine yourself applying these requirements to a real patient that you have met in the course of your work

b. Does it strike you as sensible that the law regards capacity as a threshold concept and not a comparative one? Can you see any reasons for the law's approach? Can you see any difficulties with applying this approach in practice?

c. In your view, do professionals in practice make assumptions about capacity in respect of certain categories of patient? If so, which categories?

d. Do you believe that a patient's capacity can be enhanced? If not, why not? If so, what in your view are the most appropriate ways to enhance patient capacity?

9.5 Reflect back on the particulars of Case 4:

a. In your view, is it ever possible for a patient to make a wholly independent decision? If not, why not? If so, why?

b. At which point, in your view, does a professional begin to exert an inappropriate degree of influence on patients in decision making at the end of life?

c. To what extent does a professional have an obligation to protect a patient against the pressures of family members? What difficulties do you think professionals experience in this kind of context?

9.6 Reflect back on the particulars of Case 5:

a. What role, in your view, should Advance Directives play in end-of-life care?

b. Reflect on the case of Margo. In your view, should Margo have had the treatment for cancer notwithstanding her express statement in an Advance Directive that she did not want this treatment? If so, why? If not, why not?

c. Do you think that many Irish people are likely to make Advance Directives? If so, why? If not, why not?

d. Which form of advance decision making do you think works best: Advance Directives or Enduring Powers of Attorney? What are the limitations in each model?

9.7. Read Chapter 3 of the Code of Practice to the Mental Capacity Act 2005 available at www.justice.gov.uk/guidance/mca-code-of-practice.htm

a. Is participation important even for patients who lack decision-making capacity? If so, why? If not, why not?

b. Can you think of ways to enhance the autonomy of adults who lack decision-making capacity?

c. Can you think of ways to enhance the autonomy of children who lack decision-making capacity?

10. Module 4 References and Further Reading

Agich, G.J. *Dependence and Autonomy in Old Age: An Ethical Framework for Long-Term Care* (Cambridge: Cambridge University Press, 2003)

Barclay, L. 'Autonomy and the Social Self', in C. MacKenzie and N. Stoljar (eds), *Relational Autonomy: Feminist Perspectives on Autonomy, Agency and the Social Self* (Oxford: Oxford University Press, 2000), pp.52–71

Beauchamp, T. 'Informed Consent', in R.M. Veatch (ed.), *Medical Ethics* (2nd ed.) (Sudbury, MA: Jones and Bartlett, 1997)

Beauchamp, T. and Childress, J. *Principles of Biomedical Ethics* (5th ed.) (Oxford and New York: Oxford University Press, 2001)

Beauchamp, T. and Childress, J. *Principles of Biomedical Ethics* (6th ed.) (Oxford and New York: Oxford University Press, 2008)

Blackhall, L.J., Murphy, S.T., Frank, G., Michel, V. and Azen, S. 'Ethnicity and Attitudes Toward Patient Autonomy', *Journal of the American Medical Association*, vol. 274, no. 10, 1995, pp.820–5

Buchanan, A. and Brock, D. *Deciding for Others: The Ethics of Surrogate Decision Making* (Cambridge: Cambridge University Press, 1989)

Callahan, D. 'Autonomy: A Moral Good, Not a Moral Obsession', *The Hastings Center Report*, vol. 14, no. 5, 1984, pp.40–2

Callahan, D. 'Individual Good and Common Good: A Communitarian Approach to Bioethics', *Perspectives in Biology and Medicine*, vol. 46, no. 4, 2003, pp.496–611

Council of Europe, The European Convention for the Protection of Human Rights and Fundamental Freedoms as Amended by Protocol No. 11 (ETS No. 155) (Rome: Council of Europe, 1950)

Council of Europe Committee of Ministers, Recommendation no. R (99) 4 of the Committee of Ministers to Member States on Principles Concerning the Legal Protection of Incapable Adults (Strasbourg: Council of Europe, 1999)

Department of Constitutional Affairs, Mental Capacity Act 2005 Code of Practice (London: TSO, 2007)

Donnelly, M. *Consent: Bridging the Gap between Doctor and Patient* (Cork: Cork University Press, 2002)

Donnelly, M. 'The Right of Autonomy in Irish Law', *Medico-Legal Journal of Ireland*, vol. 14, 2008, pp.34–40

Donnelly, M. 'Best Interests, Patient Participation and the Mental Capacity Act 2005', *Medical Law Review*, vol. 17, 2009(a), no. 1, pp.1–29

Donnelly, M. 'Capacity Assessment Under the Mental Capacity Act 2005: Delivering on the Functional Approach? *Legal Studies*, vol. 29, no. 3, 2009(b), pp.464–91

Donnelly, M. *Healthcare Decision Making and the Law: Autonomy, Capacity and the Limits of Liberalism* (Cambridge: Cambridge University Press, 2010)

Donnelly, M. and Kilkelly, U. 'Child-Friendly Healthcare: Delivering on the Right to be Heard', *Medical Law Review*, vol. 19, 2011, pp.27–54

Dresser, R. 'Life, Death and Incompetent Patients: Conceptual Infirmities and Hidden Values in the Law', *Arizona Law Review*, vol. 28, 1986, pp.373–405

Dworkin, R. *Life's Dominion: An Argument about Abortion, Euthanasia, and Individual Freedom* (New York: Alfred A Knopf, 1993)

Faden, R. and Beauchamp, T.A. *A History and Theory of Informed Consent* (Oxford and New York: Oxford University Press, 1986)

Fitzpatrick v K [2008] IEHC 104

Fitzpatrick v White [2007] IESC 51

Francis, L. 'Decision Making at the End of Life: Patients with Alzheimer's or Other Dementias', *Georgia Law Review*, vol. 35, no. 2, 2001, pp.539–92

Gaylin, W. and Jennings, B. *The Perversion of Autonomy: Coercion and Constraints in a Liberal Society* (Washington: Georgetown University Press, 2003)

Gillon, R. 'Ethics Needs Principles – Four Can Encompass the Rest – And Respect for Autonomy Should be "First Among Equals"', *Journal of Medical Ethics*, vol. 29, no. 5, 2003, pp.307–12

Gunn, M.J., Wong, J.G., Clare, I.C.H. and Holland, A.J. 'Decision-Making Capacity', *Medical Law Review*, vol. 7, no. 3, 1999, pp.269–306

HE v A Hospital NHS Trust [2003] EWHC 1017; [2003] 2 FLR 408

Health Service Executive, *National Strategy for Service User Involvement in the Irish Health Service 2008–2013* (Dublin: Department of Health and Children, 2008)

Hill, T.E. (ed.), *Autonomy and Self Respect* (Cambridge: Cambridge University Press, 1991)

Huxtable, R. 'Re B (Consent to Treatment: Capacity): A Right to Die or is it Right to Die?' *Child and Family Law Quarterly*, vol. 14, no. 3, 2002, pp.341–55

In re a Ward of Court [1996] 2 IR 79

In re Martin (1995) 538 NW 2d 399

Irish Council for Bioethics, *Is it Time for Advance Healthcare Directives?* (Dublin: Irish Council for Bioethics, 2007)

JM v Board of Management of St Vincent's Hospital [2003] 1 IR 321

Kant, I. *Groundwork for the Metaphysics of Morals* (trans. J.W. Ellington) (London: Hackett, 1993)

Kilkelly, U. and Donnelly, M. *The Child's Right to be Heard in the Healthcare Setting: Perspectives of Children, Parents and Health Professionals* (Dublin: Office of the Minister for Children, 2006)

Kukla, R. 'Conscientious Autonomy: Displacing Decisions in Health Care', *The Hastings Center Report*, vol. 35, no. 2, 2005, pp.34–44

Law Reform Commission, *Consultation Paper. Bioethics: Advance Care Directives [LRC CP 51–2008]* (Dublin: Law Reform Commission, 2008)

Law Reform Commission, *Bioethics: Advance Care Directives [LRC 94 – 2009]* (Dublin: Law Reform Commission, 2009)

MacIntyre, A. *Beyond Virtue* (London: Duckworth, 1981)

MacKenzie, C. and Stoljar, N. (eds), *Relational Autonomy: Feminist Perspectives on Autonomy, Agency and the Social Self* (Oxford: Oxford University Press, 2000)

Manson, N. and O'Neill, O. *Rethinking Informed Consent in Bioethics* (Cambridge: Cambridge University Press, 2007)

McLean, A. *Autonomy, Informed Consent and Medical Law* (Cambridge: Cambridge University Press, 2009)

Medical Council, *Guide to Professional Conduct and Ethics for Registered Medical Practitioners* (7th ed.) (2009), http://www.medicalcouncil.ie [accessed 20 November 2009)]

Mental Capacity Act 2005 (England and Wales)

Mill, J.S. *On Liberty* (Harmondsworth: Penguin, 1981 [1859])

Mill, J.S. in J. Gray (ed.), *On Liberty and Other Essays* (Oxford and New York: Oxford University Press, 1991)

Non-Fatal Offences Against the Person Act. No. 26/1997

O'Keefe, S. 'A Clinician's Perspective: Issues of Capacity in Care', *Medico-Legal Journal of Ireland*, vol. 14, 2008, pp.41–50

O'Neill, O. *Autonomy and Trust in Bioethics* (Cambridge: Cambridge University Press, 2002)

O'Neill, O. 'Some Limits of Informed Consent', *Journal of Medical Ethics*, 29, 2003, pp.4–7

Power of Attorney Act No. 12/1996

Pretty v UK [2002] ECHR 2346/02

Quinlan, C. and O'Neill, C. 'Practitioners' Narrative Submissions' (Unpublished) (Dublin: Irish Hospice Foundation, 2008)

Quinlan, C. and O'Neill, C. *Practitioners' Perspectives on Patient Autonomy at End of Life* (Dublin: Irish Hospice Foundation, 2009)

Re AK (Medical Treatment: Consent) [2001] 1 FLR 129

Re B (Adult: Refusal of Medical Treatment) (2002) 2 All ER 449

Re C (Adult: Refusal of Medical Treatment) [1994] 1 WLR 290

RE K Ex Tempore High Court Abbott J, 22 September 2006

Re T (Adult: Refusal of Medical Treatment) [1992] 3 WLR 782

Rodriguez v British Columbia [1993] 3 SCR 519

Sandel, M.J. *Liberalism and the Limits of Justice* (Cambridge: Cambridge University Press, 1982)

Schneider, C.E. *The Practice of Autonomy* (Oxford and New York: Oxford University Press, 1998)

Sherwin, S. 'A Relational Approach to Autonomy in Health Care', in S. Sherwin and The Feminist Health Care Ethics Research Network (eds), *The Politics of Women's Health: Exploring Agency and Autonomy* (Philadelphia: Temple University Press, 1998), pp.19–47

Sherwin, S. 'Whither Bioethics?' *International Journal of Feminist Approaches to Bioethics*, vol. 1, no. 1, 2008, pp.7–27

Taylor, C. *Sources of the Self* (Cambridge: Cambridge University Press, 1989)

United Nations General Assembly, United Nations Convention on the Rights of the Child, General Assembly Resolution 44/25 of 20 November 1989, http://www.un.org/documents/ga/res/44/a44r025.htm [accessed 2 August 2009]

United Nations General Assembly, Convention on the Rights of Persons with Disabilities, General Assembly Resolution A/RES/61/106 of 13 December 2006, http://www.un.org/disabilities/convention/conventionfull.shtml [accessed 2 August 2009]

Vacco v Quill, 521 US 793 (1997)

Veatch, R.M. 'Autonomy's Temporary Triumph', *The Hastings Center Report*, vol. 14, no. 5, 1984, pp.38–40

Washington v Glucksberg, 521 US 702 (1997)

Weafer, J. and Associates, *A Nationwide Survey of Public Attitudes and Experiences Regarding Death and Dying* (Dublin: Irish Hospice Foundation, 2004)

Weafer, J., McCarthy, J. and Loughrey M. *Exploring Death and Dying: The Views of the Irish General Public* (Dublin: Irish Hospice Foundation, 2009)

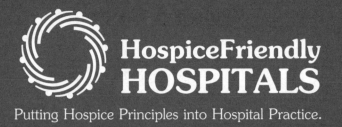

Module 5

The Ethics of Managing Pain

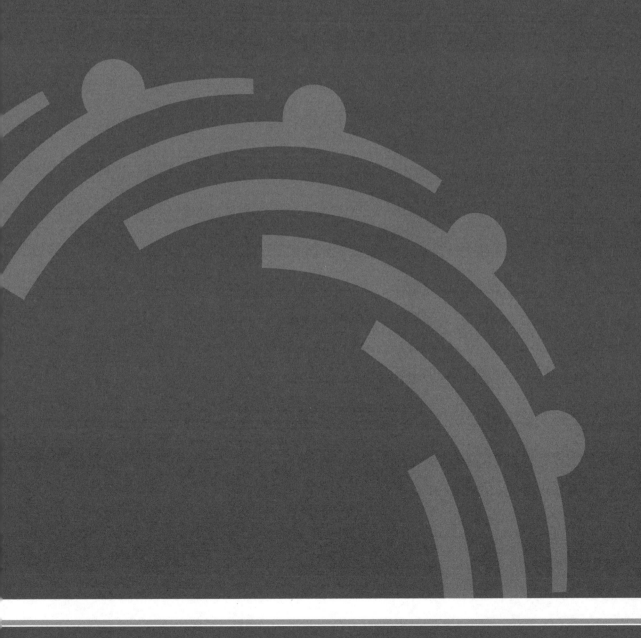

Module 5 Contents

1. Module 5 Key Points

1.1 Bad deaths:

often occur as a result of poor pain and symptom management, inadequate communication and the experience of abandonment and isolation. Very often bad deaths occur where there is inappropriate and, arguably, unethical active treatment and when obstacles prevent patients from accessing palliative care.

1.2 Comprehensive pain management:

includes not only specialised clinical programmes to control physical pain but also counselling and human support to minimise psychological pain and soul pain, family and community support groups to counter social pain and pastoral care resources to address spiritual pain. These aspects of pain are interrelated and sometimes hard to distinguish. If efforts to manage pain focus on one aspect to the neglect of the others, the patient may not experience genuine relief. This can lead to the patient developing anxiety and concern about the ability of staff to control their pain.

1.3 Family resistance to palliative care:

deserves a careful conversation with health professionals to see why they don't want their loved one to receive such care. At times families can strongly influence health professionals who might think that palliative care would benefit a patient. Doctors and nurses can come under considerable pressure from patients and families who have assumptions and preconceptions about palliative care, such as 'I'm going there to die' or 'I'll be drugged to my eyeballs' (Quinlan and O'Neill, 2009, pp.31–4). This resistance can abandon patients to unnecessary suffering.

1.4 Good deaths are more likely to occur:

when the beliefs, values, preferences and individuality of patients are respected and all pain management services are put in place. The experience of pain can diminish the energy and clarity of thought in attempts to exercise autonomy. Thus, the possibility of autonomy in practice is nurtured and enhanced by the management of a person's pain. Unrelieved pain experience is the most debilitating part of illness. In characterising a 'good death', the absence of pain is central.

1.5 Health professionals may fail to give patients adequate relief from pain:

for a number of reasons including: basic ignorance of the magnitude of the doses needed to relieve severe pain, an inappropriate fear of causing respiratory distress, a misplaced anxiety about the hazards of addiction or a fear of civil or criminal prosecution.

1.6 Patients often do not tell health professionals the extent of their pain:

The reasons for this vary according to gender, cultural background, religious beliefs, age etc. Patients also say they do not know how to describe their pain so as to get the right kind of help from health professionals. Their pain may be a combination of physical, psychological and soul pain. There are also concerns about being viewed as weak or a 'complainer', or the patient may observe that staff resources are low and think that time is simply not available to discuss pain relief.

1.7 The principle of beneficence:

or active concern for and promotion of patient well-being would rank pain relief and management among the most important objectives in caring for patients suffering from painful illnesses. Engaging the patient in discussion about their pain, about their concerns in relation to that pain and about what they hope for is reassuring for any person in the institutional setting of a hospital.

1.8 Slippery slope concerns apply to many areas of decision making:

The form of the concern is this. If we take a particular decision, even if it is a good decision, we need to ask: is it likely to lead to another decision which we would not desire or think is good? Slippery slope concerns in allowing competent patients to decline all life supports would be that we might slowly come to think it is justified to discontinue all life supports for patients lacking competence who seem to us to lack a good quality of life. One of the difficulties with slippery slope worries is that they can frustrate very good decisions out of fear that less desirable consequences will follow.

2. Module 5 Definitions

2.1 Euthanasia:

is a deliberate act or omission whose primary intention is to end another person's life. Literally, it means a gentle or easy death but it has come to mean a deliberate intervention by one person with the clear intention of ending the life of another. This is often described as 'mercy killing' of people in pain with terminal illness. Decisions to withdraw or discontinue life supports are not equivalent to euthanasia if they are validly authorised by a competent patient's consent or if a clinical decision is made that further life supports, based on all available evidence, would be futile – lacking in benefit for the patient and merely prolonging the dying process.

2.2 Life-Prolonging Treatment (LPT):

is any medical intervention, technology, procedure or medication that is administered to provide benefit for a patient and to forestall the moment of death. These treatments may include, but are not limited to, mechanical ventilation, artificial hydration and nutrition, cardiopulmonary resuscitation, haemodialysis, chemotherapy, or certain medications including antibiotics.

2.3 Palliative Care:

a comprehensive approach to treating serious illness that focuses on the physical, psychological, spiritual and existential needs of the patient. Its goal is to achieve the best quality of life available to the patient by relieving suffering and controlling pain and other symptoms associated with the particular illness of the patient.

2.4 Palliative Sedation:

is offered to patients if standard opioids are ineffective in managing their pain. It is used to induce an artificial coma especially in cases in which a dying person is experiencing severe, intractable suffering. The intention in using palliative sedation is to induce a state of decreased, or absent, awareness (unconsciousness) in order to remove the burden of suffering in an ethically acceptable way for patient, family and healthcare providers. The terms 'palliative sedation' or 'continuous deep sedation' have largely replaced the previously used term of 'terminal sedation'.

2.5 Physician-Assisted Suicide (PAS):

the act of assisting a person to die by providing the means for them to take their own life. A recurring example of PAS is the act of giving a prescription or supply of drugs to a patient who has requested this. The doctor providing the lethal dosage of drugs thus enables a patient to end his or her own life.

2.6 Principle of Double Effect (PDE):

an ethical rule which holds that effects of treatment which would be morally wrong if brought about intentionally are permissible if they are foreseen but unintended. The principle is often cited to explain why certain forms of care at the end of life which may risk and/or hasten death are morally permissible while others are not.

3. Module 5 Background

One of the classic themes of healthcare ethics concerns the moral acceptability of interventions to modify the dying process. Developments in the practice of palliative care give rise to new discussions about the ethical aspects of medical care at the end of life. This module focuses on these discussions.

3.1 Ethical Principles in Pain Management

3.1.1 Respect for Patient Autonomy (See Module 4, 4.2)

The moral principle of autonomy is pivotal in conversations with competent patients when considering options for pain management. The experience of pain can diminish the energy and clarity of thought to exercise autonomy. Thus, encouraging and fostering a patient's understanding and decision making in relation to these options through sensitive information sharing shows interest in the facilitation of patient autonomy. In fact, the possibility of autonomy in practice is nurtured and enhanced by the management of a person's pain (see Module 3).

3.1.2 The Principle of Beneficence

The active concern and promotion of patient well-being would put pain relief and management among the most important objectives in caring for patients suffering from painful illness. Engaging the patient about their pain, about their concerns with that pain and what they hope for is reassuring for any person in the institutional setting of a hospital.

Patients may have difficulties in speaking about their pain and seeking pain relief. This can apply to adults but applies especially to children. Describing pain is not easy and sometimes a patient may think they will be perceived as a complainer and incur the displeasure of staff (McCracken and Keogh, 2009).

One narrative recounted in an Irish hospital setting makes clear that some patients are assertive about their preferred pain relief methods:

Recently I became aware of a 90-year-old lady who is in long term care in a residential unit. The lady is as fun-loving and active as her physical abilities allow. The lady has terminal cancer. She has no relatives and receives weekly visits from the palliative care team. Approximately 6–8 weeks ago the lady decided that she had had enough of the pain medication as it wasn't helping her and she indicated she would prefer whiskey at night instead. The staff discussed this with her and she remained very clear that this was her wish. The palliative care team was in agreement.

Arrangements were made for a supply of whiskey to be on hand and the lady reported that the whiskey in her tea is a far more effective means of pain relief. She said she feels better in the morning as she is guaranteed a more peaceful night. (Quinlan and O'Neill, 2008, pp.26–7)

This amicable result came about not simply as a result of listening but by actively hearing what the patient was saying. The staff was flexible in responding positively to this request for 'whiskey therapy'. The 90-year-old lady was shown respect and her subsequent contentment showed her delight at this concern for her well-being. The staff's decision to provide whiskey heightened the patient's sense of self and allowed sleep and serenity. With this simple method of pain management for this lady, staff showed moral respect for her unique person.

The scenario that follows describes a less fortuitous outcome than in the case of the elderly lady above.

An 82-year-old lady with a diagnosis of COPD respiratory failure was being managed by the respiratory team. There were numerous requests from her for pain relief and symptom control. Inappropriate analgesia was prescribed and the patient was unable to swallow. While on night duty at 9.30 pm, I had to contact the Registrar on call and insist on analgesia, anti-emetics and hypocrite to dry secretions and promote comfort. The family were very distressed. The registrar came at 11.30 pm and spoke to the family and infusions were commenced. The patient was only comfortable at 12.30 am. When I looked at the Nursing and Medical Notes, this had been going on for four days. (Edited narrative, Quinlan and O'Neill, 2008, p.1)

It would seem that the pain suffered by the 82-year-old lady in this scenario is not all that rare internationally. Cassel (1999) claims that a great deal of pain is inadequately treated. He explains that 'too much suffering is unrelieved and undiagnosed, a situation more common now than a generation ago because current treatments keep people alive long enough to enter the chronic, terminal phase of their illness: the duration and severity of their suffering are thereby increased' (Cassel, 1999, p.531). He also traces the prevalence of untreated pain, in part, to deficits in physician training which focus on organs, diseases and aetiology rather than on persons as individuals with their unique fears and hopes.

The diagnosis of suffering is often missed, even in severe illness and even when it stares physicians in the face. A high index of suspicion must be maintained in the presence of serious disease, and patients must be directly questioned […] Often, questioning and attentive listening, which take little time, are in themselves ameliorative. […] The language that describes and defines the patient's suffering is different from the language of medicine – there is too often an actual disconnect between our case history and the patient's narrative [...] Physicians are trained primarily to find out what is wrong with the body – in terms of diseases or pathophysiology; they do not examine what is wrong with persons [...] when physicians attend to the body rather than to the person, they fail to diagnose suffering. (Cassel, 1999, p.531)

3.1.3 Nonmaleficence

The value of nonmaleficence, or 'Do no Evil', is closely linked to the objectives of pain management. Lack of adequate pain management causes harm to the patient. The harm, worry and, at times, consequent depression of painful suffering, and accompanying anxiety, needs no elaboration beyond the ethical and empirical research on end-of-life care (O'Shea, Keegan and McGee, 2002; Bon Secours Health System, 2007; German National Ethics Council, 2006). Unrelieved pain is the single factor accounting for patient experiences of a 'bad death'.

4. Resistance to Palliative Care

The discussion in this module shows that pain and suffering are not homogeneous realities and that the practice of thinking beyond the conventional limits of physical pain management serves patients well. Pain relief is one of the most important goals of palliative care where such care is universally understood as a comprehensive philosophy of care which includes pain and symptom management, support for patient and family and the opportunity to achieve meaningful closure to life (Deandrea, Montanari, Moja et al., 2008). A good death survey has shown that one of the elements in a good dying is skilled pain and symptom management and that lack of such skills ensures a 'bad death' (Steinhauser et al., 2000). If the elements of a good death call for good pain and symptom management, the provision of syringe drivers, the management of nausea and vomiting, and the establishment of good relationships between patients, families and health professionals, then the earlier palliative care can become involved with the patient the better.

4.1 Family Reluctance

The research conducted by Quinlan and O'Neill (2009) shows that adequate pain relief is sometimes not achieved because, for a variety of reasons, family members choose not to have their loved one receive palliative care. As one health professional interviewed commented:

> *I find on the ward that Palliative Care isn't brought in soon enough. I do feel that, especially with pain management because it's something I feel very strongly about. I still find that sometimes teams are resistant to involve palliative care for pain control. I don't know why, I just feel there's some resistance.* (Quinlan and O'Neill, 2009, p.35)

Another health professional observed:

> *[W]e would have patients who end up not seeing the palliative service because that's not acceptable to the family and there's been backwards autonomy in the first place, I mean that the autonomy has been given to the family – the family decides whether or not the patient is seen by Palliative Care. It should never arise […] and the family say 'well you've got to guarantee me you won't tell them that they have cancer otherwise I'm not bringing them in.*
> (Quinlan and O'Neill, 2009, p.68, see also p.27)

> *The role of families in healthcare decision making is a profoundly important issue. If family*

involvement in decision making is judged to be damaging to the well-being and proper care of a patient, then health professionals cannot, with good conscience, comply with family requests. The family may tend to claim proxy authority to decide for the patient, especially when the patient either lacks capacity or has declined to be involved in decision-making about pain management. However, there is a mandate here for staff to engage families and report the harm they are doing to their loved ones in denying them pain management or access to palliative care. Failure to seek palliative care often means that pain continues needlessly and the moral obligation of carers to provide for the well-being of patients is not met. Reluctance to use palliative services points to a very urgent need for education in palliative care for health professionals and the wider public.
(Randall and Downie, 2006)

4.2 Staff Collusion

But unfortunately, there can be unwitting collusion among some clinicians in a family's refusal to have palliative care for their loved one.

There is a patient who is at home who I know from the referring physician and [...] this patient is very unwell, needs the type of palliative support that we can offer and our community teams can offer but this patient went home and the doctor whose care they were under agreed not to tell them their diagnosis. They are now at home, the family isn't telling the diagnosis and the patient isn't being allowed access to palliative care because, we, palliative service, will not agree, if the patient asks us why this has happened, to not telling them the diagnosis. (Quinlan and O'Neill, 2009, p.63). See also Module 2, 6.1.1 and Module 4, 6.4.

5. Dimensions of Pain

Pain is an intriguing phenomenon and we have only begun to understand its complexity. Pain most often is multi-dimensional, consisting of a range of symptoms and types of suffering: physical, psychological, social, spiritual and 'soul'. In the cases that follow in this module, there is often a combination of different types of 'suffering', resulting in each patient's set of unique pains. The pain experienced in terminal illness is much more than physical. The combination of many dimensions of pain can overwhelm dying patients and weaken their sense of control, sense of purpose and meaning. It can also weaken their sense of connectedness to others. If effective patient care is to ensure pain relief, the patient needs to be seen in holistic terms as integrating emotional, physical, spiritual, cultural and social causes of pain. Michael Kearney uses the phrase 'total pain' to refer to the combination of the different pain components most often encountered (Kearney, 1996, p.24).

5.1 Physical Pain

Physical pain is the most obvious form of pain and major cause of suffering. It impairs physical functioning, mood, and social interaction. Physical pain serves as a clear warning that something is out of order in the normal functioning of the body. But, since pain affects the whole person, it can easily exceed its function as a warning signal. Severe pain can drive a person to request its removal at any price, even to the point of asking for death for oneself or for others.

5.2 Psychological Pain

Psychological pain often arises when facing the inevitability of death, losing control over the process of dying, letting go of hopes and dreams, or having to redefine the world one is about to leave in terms that never quite satisfy one's needs. Psychological pain is evident in the mood swings and strong feelings that often accompany terminal illness. (See Case 6.1)

5.3 Social Pain

Social pain is the pain of isolation. The difficulty of communicating what one is experiencing while dying creates a sense of aloneness at a time when companionship is most needed. The unwillingness or inability of others to keep company with the dying by visiting them, listening to their feelings and experiences or discussing the implications of what is happening to them only aggravate the isolation. The loss of a familiar social role is also painful. For example, letting go of the role of being a self-sufficient, caring parent and becoming the one who is dependent and cared for can be socially and psychologically painful (Ranger and Campbell-Yeo, 2008).

5.4 Spiritual Pain

Spiritual pain arises from a loss of meaning, purpose and hope. Despite society's apparent indifference to the 'world beyond this one', spiritual pain is inescapable and widespread. Everyone needs a framework for meaning – a reason to live. People who are dying often seek a larger landscape of meaning and therefore need to feel part of a community that shares that meaning. Some patients can find meaning and solace in a religious belief.

Spiritual pain endured by those patients with religious belief can arise from: 1) concern and anxiety about their relationship with their God; 2) worry that they might not remain steadfast in their faith while suffering pain and illness; 3) worry about whether a priest or chaplain will be with them when needed to offer spiritual companionship and religious solace.

Issues of faith are frequently mentioned by dying patients as integral to the overall healing at the end of life. This often becomes more important as the patient declines physically (Steinhauser et al., 2000). As evidenced by research with patients, spiritual pain can cause genuine suffering when patients are either denied spiritual companionship or have it provided without respect for their refusal (Quinlan and O'Neill, 2009, p.32).

5.5 Soul pain

Soul Pain is a particularly profound and excruciating form of pain. 'Soul' is here used in its more classical sense as meaning 'psyche' and is without religious connotations (Kearney, 1996, p.57). It is manifested in an all-pervading sense of emptiness, hopelessness and meaninglessness and characterised as anguished, tortured and restless (Kearney, 1996, p.62). Patients experiencing soul pain may request help to become unconscious, as seen in the following case.

(See Case 6.5)

6. Cases in the Ethics of Pain Management

6.1 Case 1: Psychological Pain of Anticipation – 'I Dread What May Come'

The following case illustrates the pain that can accompany psychological dread of what is to come.

> ### 'I Dread What May Come'
>
> *[...W]hen I was in a centre of adult Palliative Medicine, we came across Maurice, a young gentleman of 32, who was referred to us after he had attempted to commit suicide and he had thrown himself into the local river. The reason that he had tried to commit suicide was that he had a diagnosis of cancer which he'd lived with for about eight years at this stage but was developing increasing pain. He was worried that if his pain was so bad at this stage and not controlled, how bad was it going to be when he was closer to death? It was really his fear about symptoms, you know, not being controlled. So he was able to relay all this to us, and we then got his pain under control, relatively easily I suppose, it's what we do every day, and we were able to reassure him that his pain would never have to be out of control as it had been and thereby his suicidal ideation completely resolved.* **(Quinlan and O'Neill, 2009, p.34)**

6.1.1 Discussion

This case looks at the stressful reality of what we term anticipatory pain. Such pain is not uncommon even in ordinary life as we wait for the colonoscopy or go into the nursing home to see our failing elderly parent. What we call anticipatory pain comes under the heading of psychological pain. Psychological pain is indeed a form of authentic suffering. It is not illusory, nor is it simply 'in the mind'. Anticipating the real probability that one's manifest pain will increase in severity and regularity as one's disease progresses can exacerbate psychological suffering. Anticipatory suffering can be excruciating and requires relief using a variety of interventions.

Case 1 is a good news story in terms of the result for this patient and for the health professionals who listened to Maurice's desperate pleas for relief from his present pain and excruciating anticipatory pain. Maurice was not only saved from his attempted suicide but he was given an opportunity to speak openly about his dread of increasing pain.

He was given relief and hope, through being assured of ongoing pain management. This young man's act of attempted suicide secured for him the therapeutic pain management and compassionate conversations with staff that he needed. Health professionals responded when the patient demonstrated dramatically by means of a suicide attempt that he needed solace, communication, pain management and emotional support (Cassel, 1999).

The psychological pain for this man has at least three sources.

- He has lived with his cancer diagnosis for eight years and, given to reflecting on this reality, he experiences ongoing stressful pain. There is a belief among some patients with a diagnosis of cancer that it is only a matter of time before the cancer cells all go haywire (Steinhauser et al., 2000). The unique character of the person suffering certainly affects the nature, intensity and stressful nature of this prolonged pain of thinking 'how will this end, will I die in pain like this? What will it be like?' (Terry, Olson, and Wilss, et al., 2006, p.342).

- The second source of psychological pain was the fear and hopelessness that led to his attempted suicide in the local river. Again, the unique personal nature of his ever-present worries about his condition would have drained him of energy both physical and emotional. One difficulty with psychological pain is that the depression associated with it often leads the individual to believe (even subconsciously) that there is no solution. This is the essence of hopelessness and often can only be counteracted by human intervention. Persistent hopelessness is not a normal part of dying; it requires therapeutic attention (Cassel, 1999).

- A third source of psychological pain came for this patient with the measurable increase in his pain. With this increase, Maurice became very frightened and assumed that the cancer was all over his body.

This situation might have been prevented earlier if Maurice's family, GP or a trusted friend had heard about his pain, or had heard his concerns, however subtle, and encouraged him to seek help. An outpatient drop-in clinic for patients in need of pain relief, while quite uncommon in Ireland, would provide patients like Maurice with help in reviewing and monitoring his developing symptoms and give him reassurance. With help from hospital staff and ongoing sessions with his GP, Maurice might now continue living his days with his illness but in greater psychological security.

6.1.2 Suggested Professional Responsibilities

- Suicide is a cry for help and clear reaction to fear, frustration, sense of isolation and hopelessness. In a conversation with Maurice, the hospital team should find out if there was any previous history of suicide attempts or suicide ideation.

- A consultation with the clinician (preferably pain specialist) needs to give Maurice reassurance, as the case indicates, that any developing pain can and will be treated.

- An assessment can be offered to see what medicinal or other therapeutic help can be offered to Maurice for possible depression associated with his anxiety and anticipatory pain.

- A report of Maurice's attendance in hospital should be prepared and sent to Maurice's family doctor stating that the hospital clinician advised Maurice to see her within the next couple of weeks.

- Since Maurice's worries are linked to his fear of dying as pain increases, a careful assessment of Maurice's cancer condition should be arranged with the oncologist. This assessment can follow with a conversation about his cancer condition and specifically what therapeutic help can be offered to him.

- This consultation and recommendations for Maurice should be documented for the hospital records so continuity of care can be better ensured if or when Maurice returns to hospital.

6.2 Case 2: Interpreting Children's Pain – 'I Never Saw Anyone Suffer Like That in My Life'

Managing the pain of hospitalised children, even very young children, is one of the more profoundly challenging tasks in pain management. The ethical principles of the duty to benefit another (beneficence) and the duty to do no harm (nonmaleficence) oblige health professionals to provide pain management to all patients, including children, who are extremely vulnerable because of the constant developmental changes they undergo and the attendant insecurities of being ill and hospitalised in a strange setting (Kortesluoma, Nikkonen and Serlo, 2008, pp.143–4). Evidence also shows that we often underestimate the need to give room to a child's voice, failing to pay attention to verbal or bodily cues and therefore we fail to promote the child's incipient autonomy during hospitalisation (Royal College of Paediatrics and Child Health (RCPCH), 2008, p.9). Attentive observations of children by staff and regular conversations with parents can achieve significant insights into the uniqueness of children's experience of pain (Walco, Cassidy and Schechter, 1994).

'I Never Saw Anyone Suffer Like That in My Life'

During her last month of life, 4-year-old Madeleine lay on her bed in too much pain to watch her beloved Barney on TV. The little girl's pain was so great that she cried when her mom touched her, when she tried to speak to her, or when she turned on the lights. Just a few months had elapsed since Madeleine was first diagnosed with leukaemia.

'I've never seen anyone suffer like that in my life,' said her mother. Madeleine was given chemotherapy with the onset of the disease, and after a relapse, doctors proposed another round of chemotherapy treatments, which, if successful, would prepare her for a bone marrow transplant.

The doctors assured her family that the pain she experienced from the chemotherapy could be controlled.

But when the pain came, and it came within three days after the first treatment, her mother said nothing worked to alleviate it. It took Madeleine 5 minutes just to roll over in bed because each movement was so painful. When the family pleaded for relief for their daughter, doctors seemed slow to act. In addition, Madeleine had a serious bout of pneumonia that went undiagnosed for two weeks. Madeleine's mother reported that 'All they were interested in was the cancer and the [white blood cell] counts going up. They didn't look beyond that.'
On Valentine's Day 1999, five months after she was diagnosed, Madeleine died.
(adapted narrative from Linsker, 2000)

6.2.1 Discussion

The above case illustrates the need for focus, attentiveness and ongoing conversation in the relationship between the health professionals, Madeleine and her family. Were parents kept informed by doctors and/or nurses about the meaning of the diagnosis of leukaemia? Did the family understand its severity, the prognosis, how amenable it might be to chemotherapy and what methods of pain management are available? (See Module 2)

The emotional narrative of the mother needs to be heard. It is a narrative based on four years' experience of rearing Madeleine and interpreting her pain, her body language, her fatigue, her nausea, her effort to do the simplest thing (Lesho, 2003, pp.2429–30). Here, the mother is the proxy voice for Madeleine and listening to her story of knowing her daughter intimately and witnessing her pain is perhaps vital to diagnosing the child's pain. Through team effort and ongoing communication with Madeleine, a strategic plan might have been devised to try and relieve the child's distress, a strategy that would also require negotiating and engaging with the parents.

The alleviation of children's pain has been investigated through the eyes of health professionals and parents, but the children's own perspectives have largely been ignored. Children have their own descriptions and expectations for pain management interventions. The evidence shows that children themselves, perhaps somewhat older than Madeleine, should be regarded as experts on their own pain in order to maximise the options for pain management and provide high-quality care (RCPCH, 2008, p.9). Respecting the incipient autonomy of the small child in the case above calls for a concerted effort to communicate with the child by paying attention to all bodily cues available and any verbal signals provided by Madeleine. By focussing exclusively on her white cell count, the physicians may have focussed on the hopes for curative treatment and failed to diagnose and deal with the degree of Madeleine's suffering (Lesho, 2003, p.2430).

The ethical values of beneficence and nonmaleficence (Do No Harm) can be combined with the aim of respecting the incipient, developing, autonomy of this small girl as she suffers with leukaemia. Was another round of chemotherapy appropriate here? Was this treatment extraordinary for a dying four-year-old? Perhaps if active treatment for leukaemia stopped, the focus on pain management would yield more comfort and calm for the young patient (Linsker, 2000, p.2).

If the healthcare team had reasons to believe that further chemotherapy and possibly a bone marrow transplant would be beneficial, then this would need to be explained to the family. It seems from the information available in this case that the level of conversation and communication for understanding was deficient. Adequate pain relief in this case was not achieved and perhaps had even been thwarted by the focus on more aggressive treatment rather than on palliative care. One doctor's statement may sound a note of truth in relation to this case: 'As physicians, we are trained to cure, not trained to support the dying patient. We lack training in that and must acquire it on our own' (quoted in Linsker, 2000, p.1). The desire to cure is powerfully strong and is taught as a primary objective in medical training. In this case of Madeleine, cure was given precedence over care. As carer, her mother also needed care from health professionals for she failed to understand why white cell counts seemed more important to clinical staff than her daughter's experience of continuing pain.

- A thorough review of this case needs to be undertaken by the healthcare team who managed Madeleine and the concerns of her parents. The objective is to reflect on decisions taken and honest self-scrutiny about the human outcomes. What clinical evidence contributed to decisions taken?

- Team review of the management of Madeleine's case should consider it a priority to ask whether Madeleine's mother may have been correct: Was the medical management of this child's chemotherapy aggressive? If not, an explanation should have been offered to the parents for the recommendation of further chemotherapy and, possibly, a bone marrow transplant.

- Documentation needs to be provided for the records of any diagnostic tests conducted on Madeleine, team consultations, number and evidence basis for chemotherapy sessions and prognosis justifying considerations of a bone marrow transplant.

- Following Madeleine's death, attention can turn to comforting the grieving parents and efforts made to heal some of the rift in the family–health professionals relationship. Can the healthcare team honestly say to the parents that 'all that could be done was done'?

- The team might take time to reflect on the case and address the question: Was the manner of pain management in Madeleine's dying deeply regrettable and overtaken by the drive to 'cure' or 'keep alive' at all costs? If so, how, precisely, can a similar situation in the future be improved?

6.3 Case 3: The Principle of Double Effect – 'I Don't Want to Die. I Want to Be Without Pain!'

The patient in the following case is explicit about his excruciating suffering and asks for more pain relief.

'I Don't Want to Die. I Want to Be Without Pain!'

Paul is a 68-year-old man with metastatic small-cell lung cancer. He is suffering from excruciating bone pain and he is near death. Initially, he responded to a combination of chemotherapy and radiation and had a 3-year remission. His disease recurred four months ago and he decided to choose a palliative approach. Paul's pain from extensive bone metastases was initially well managed with high-dose, around-the-clock opioids supplemented by radiation and nerve blocks.

Paul prepared for death through talks with his partner, Tom, and clergy and felt he had no remaining 'unfinished business'. In the end stages, he weighed 80 pounds, was bed-bound, and his pain averaged 8 points on a 10-point scale. Paul had always loved life and even now did not want to die but he told his doctor and the nurses on duty that he was willing to accept the risk of an earlier death which might come from further increasing doses of opioids.

After a palliative care consultation, his doctor increased his total opioid doses by 25% each day until the pain was adequately controlled, or, if sedated, until he would appear comfortable. On the third day after this dose increase, Paul became very sleepy but arousable. He appeared relatively free of pain. The doctor shifted an equi-analgesic amount of opioids from oral to transcutaneous administration because Paul was unable to swallow reliably. Tom was with him as he became unresponsive, appearing comfortable, neither restless nor struggling. Paul remained in that state until he died 2 days later.

(Adapted narrative from Quill, Coombs Lee and Nunn, 2000a, p.490)

6.3.1 Discussion

In this case the doctor and Paul were both willing to accept the possibility of an earlier death as a result of the increased opioid dose. This was a foreseeable possible consequence of increasing the pain dosage. However, the health professionals caring for Paul reassured him that his suffering was severe enough to warrant taking the risk of a hastened death due to depressed respiration. The intention here to increase pain medication was consistent with the aims of palliative care: the compassionate and beneficent relief of Paul's suffering.

Principle of Double Effect (PDE)

One ethical rule, originally formulated in the Catholic tradition during the twelfth century and used in moral reasoning in defence of providing pain relief methods without incurring accusations of killing, is the principle of double effect (PDE).

The PDE permits an act which is foreseen to have both good and bad effects, provided:

a. the act itself is good or at least morally neutral (the act of providing pain relief);

b. the good effect must be the primary intention and not the effect of shortening a patient's life. The possible earlier demise of the patient is said to be 'foreseen' but not explicitly intended or desired;

c. the good effect is not caused by the bad effect (the relief of pain was not caused by Paul's dying but by adequate pain medication); (See Case 4)

d. a proportionate reason exists for causing the bad effect (shortened life justified by need for relief from pain).

According to the ethical rule known as the 'principle of double effect', the effects of treatment that would be morally wrong if caused intentionally are permissible if foreseen but unintended. This principle is often cited to explain why certain forms of care at the end of life that result in an earlier demise are morally permissible and others are not.

So, according to the principle: Administering high dose opioids to treat a terminally ill patient's pain may be acceptable *even if* the medication causes an earlier death than otherwise might have happened. This relationship (correlational, causal, contributory or otherwise) between opioids (correctly administered) and death is contested; it is of particular concern to specialists in palliative care and any health professionals involved in end-of-life care (Cherny et al., 2009, p.582).

By contrast however, the principle of double effect does not authorise practices such as physician-assisted suicide, voluntary euthanasia and some instances of foregoing life-prolonging treatment (Irish Association of Palliative Care, 2011b).

The discussion of this case should clarify that there are some relatively uncomplicated clinical situations in which the PDE can help clinicians overcome a hesitation to prescribe sufficient dosage of pain medication for a particular patient's suffering. The following text defends the use of the PDE when providing pain relief:

[T]he intensive use of painkillers is not without difficulties, because the phenomenon of habituation generally makes it necessary to increase their dosage in order to maintain their

efficacy [...] Is the suppression of pain and consciousness by the use of narcotics [...] permitted by religion and morality to the doctor and the patient (even at the approach of death and if one foresees that the use of narcotics will shorten life)? Yes. If no other means exist [...] In this case, of course, death is in no way intended or sought, even if the risk of it is reasonably taken; the intention is simply to relieve pain effectively, using for this purpose painkillers available to medicine. (Edited from O'Rourke and Boyle, 1993, p.223)

An expansion of Case 6.3 might allow us the licence to eavesdrop on an invented conversation among members of the team. Such eavesdropping may help in clarifying some distorted views of the PDE.

One intern, Colum, said he knew the principle of double effect and said 'we seem concerned here but, we're not wishing or aiming for Paul's death but we can't let him suffer in pain this way. I know this is ok.' However, another colleague, Clare said, 'yes, it's true that we're not giving this increased dosage to kill Paul but I have to admit that, under the circumstances, dying without pain for Paul would be a blessing, not a bad thing. If that were to happen, how do I know that the increased medication dosage I provide is not really my way of achieving Paul's death? Could I clear my conscience that I have not killed Paul?'

This exchange may not always be verbal or explicit. However, research indicates that these sentiments often cause health professionals to wonder about the clarity of their intentions and motivations in providing pain relief (Quill, 1993). Many clinicians have learned of the principle and, when administering pain medication, their 'lesson in PDE' sometimes resurfaces, causing them to wonder whether they are doing the 'right' thing and if they are being honest about their state of mind and intentions.

Returning to the scenario between Colum and Clare, if Clare thinks that Paul's passing may be a blessing, why should this be a source of concern or anxiety? This is a thoroughly normal thought in the presence of anyone who is suffering from serious illness. 'God would be good to take him' is a common utterance. It is not our compassion that brings about the person's death. Qualms of conscience expressed by Clare are not trivial and call for understanding from the medical team. If persistent qualms or scrupulous worries about excessive opioid provision are left to take hold of one's moral reasoning, the result is serious under-treatment of pain in suffering patients which is a concern of many health professionals when writing of pain management.

The more severe and intractable the patient's pain, the greater is the justification for risking an earlier death. Thus, the amount of opioid pain reliever that is given and the rapidity with which it is increased must be in proportion to the amount of pain and suffering. Some physicians have been reluctant to use sufficient doses of opioid pain relievers, even when their patients are dying, in part because of fears (both ethical and legal) about contributing to an earlier death. The rule of double effect has helped some physicians to overcome this hesitation. Yet other clinicians remain unwilling to prescribe sufficient doses in part because they do not distinguish morally or psychologically between actions performed with the intent to cause death and those performed with the foreseen possibility of causing death.' (Quill, Dresser and Brock 1997, pp.1769–70; See Further Discussion of PDE)

Utilising the concepts of adequacy and proportionality in making decisions about pain management prove helpful in the clinical setting and do not embroil one in the difficult task of making clear and distinct intentions that are, in fact, often unclear and ambiguous (Woods, 2007, p.40).

Adequacy and Proportionality

Palliative treatment relies on the twin concepts of adequacy and proportionality in order to try to verify the intention of a doctor or nurse and consider whether they are consciously and knowingly trying to cause the patient's death.

Utilising these concepts, an intervention like managing a patient's pain is justified when and if:

- the particular treatment used (type of medication and dosage) is adequate for the relief of pain in the case of this particular patient and,
- the particular treatment used is proportionate in its effect to the symptoms this particular patient is experiencing
- a patient's pain is responsive to opiates, in which case the appropriate aim is to stabilise the patient on a regime that keeps them comfortable with minimum side-effects
- a patient experiences pain while taking morphine, in which case the aim is to increase the dose progressively until the patient's pain is relieved (dose titration).

With this recognised method, even a large dosage of morphine can be proportionate to a particular patient's pain experience (Woods, 2007, pp.130–1). This manner of providing pain relief contrasts starkly with cases in which patients were administered a disproportionate dose of an opiate without ongoing reference to the patient's level of comfort or tolerance for the drug. The latter would not be morally justified under the condition of proportionality of treatment to the patient's pain. It is possible, with attention to adequacy and proportion, to ensure that a person can be kept pain-free and conscious on a dosage of morphine which would likely be fatal to a person naïve to the drug, indicating that even a large dosage of morphine can be proportionate and therefore morally justified (Woods, 2007, p.131).

In conclusion, the ethical justifications for providing the pain relief which ran the risk of hastening Paul's death are five-fold:

a. Competence is evident: Paul was clearly competent when expressing his wishes to increase the pain medication.

b. Imminently dying: Paul was unambiguously and 'imminently dying' and the relief of his pain is a widely acknowledged moral good to aim at even while recognising the prospect of hastening death.

c. Consent is given: Paul consented to this pain management decision and was clearly heard to say he wished to have an increased dose of medication administered.

d. No desire to die: The case describes Paul's love of life even as his health diminished. Paul was not seeking death and nor could he be accused of seeking 'euthanasia' by the back door through his request for pain management. The companionship of family and clergy gave Paul solace in his dying moments (Terry et. al., 2006).

e. Adequate dosage to relieve this pain: The healthcare team attending Paul were not complacent about the increase in Paul's dosage. They had discussed the dosage of opioids required to keep Paul comfortable. They believe an increased dosage was justified.

6.3.2 Suggested Professional Responsibilities

- The healthcare team should document the series of palliative decisions taken in Paul's case since the process and outcome proved sensitive to both patient and family needs. Included in the documentation should be Paul's understanding and consent to the pain management recommended.

- Palliative care specialists are a necessary resource in critical care settings and, if such a specialist is lacking, a recommendation for this resource should be made a priority. The assistance of a palliative care specialist insured a compassionate and expert response to Paul's pain. It was adequate and proportionate to the needs of Paul.

- A provision of comfort and privacy is essential when a patient, is in their dying days. Family and clergy need that space as much as the dying patient for whom noises in the environment can be especially stressful.

- It was fortunate that Paul remained conscious until near his death, thus facilitating solace and companionship with the priest and family.

- When Paul dies, attention and care can be given to his partner and other family members, asking if there are other ways they might be helped at this time.

6.4 Case 4: Proper Use of PDE or Euthanasia? – R v Cox

Reflecting on the key concepts of adequacy and proportionality can offer a health professional moral assurance or raise serious questions about legitimacy when giving large doses of opioids in the treatment of a patient's extreme suffering and intractable pain. The following case reflects a compassion to relieve pain but at the price of a lethal injection.

R v Cox

In 1992 Dr. Nigel Cox, a consultant rheumatologist, was convicted of attempting to murder Mrs. Lillian Boyes, one of his patients. Mrs. Boyes had been terminally ill with rheumatoid arthritis; she suffered from septicaemia and had abscesses and ulcers on her limbs. Her heart was calcified, her lungs were malfunctioning. She had gangrene and a number of fractures of the lumbar spine. There is no doubt that Mrs. Boyes was in excruciating pain. Dr. Cox had administered heroin in an effort to alleviate her suffering but to no avail. It was then that he injected her with potassium chloride and she died shortly thereafter.

Many people praised Dr. Cox for his humane act and expressed hope that they might be treated similarly by their doctors if in equally severe pain during the final stages of terminal illness. It is clear, however, that the criminal law in the UK views his behaviour quite differently since he was charged with murder and, the body having been cremated before a conclusive cause of death could be established, convicted of attempted murder.

(Edited case from Ferguson, 1997, p.368)

6.4.1 Discussion

The case of R. v Cox (1992) is a helpful illustration to show that it is sometimes possible to have objective evidence of the intention to hasten death. As the case explains, Dr Cox was convicted of attempted murder when his patient, Lillian Boyes, died following an injection of potassium chloride. A fundamental question that was asked at the time was: Were all other avenues of proportionate pain relief exhausted? It does not seem so.

Cox was convicted of attempted murder because his chosen means, potassium chloride, had no analgesic effect and had no therapeutic uses in the circumstances, thereby falling short of one of the sufficient conditions of a justified act. Dr. Cox may have tried but could not claim that potassium chloride had a double effect. **(Ferguson, 1997, p.368)**

One does not give an injection of potassium chloride to alleviate pain unless it is administered to alleviate pain by inducing death. Had Dr Cox killed Lillian Boyes with an opiate that was given in very high doses, then it is highly unlikely that his action would have resulted in a conviction (Woods, 2007, p.130). In this case, the evidence that Dr Cox used potassium chloride makes it clear that what he clearly intended was to relieve Lillian's pain by means of ensuring that her life ended (see third condition of PDE).

Case 4 is a clear case of euthanasia because if the intended goal is to relieve the patient's profound suffering, potassium chloride may work by causing death but it fails to fulfil the criteria of adequacy and proportionality which would give evidence of moral justification for the action. Potassium chloride is not an opioid for treating the suffering arising from rheumatoid arthritis.

There is a significant moral difference between ensuring that the natural process of dying is made as comfortable as possible and actively precipitating someone's death by employing known lethal means. The former is clearly compatible with a health professional's commitment to preserve life and relieve suffering – the latter is not.

The crux of the difference lies in the intention behind the act and use of appropriate and proportionate means consistent with that intention. It cannot be accepted as a policy guideline that doctors can consider death among their range of treatments to relieve suffering. This would make doctors equal to a profession of executioners (Thomson, 1999, pp.81–2). (For a discussion of ethical and legal positions on euthanasia see Module 6, sections 7.2 and 7.3.)

6.4.2 Suggested Professional Responsibilities

- The case of Lillian Boyes raises a fundamental question for discussion: Is adequate and specialist pain management available in acute care hospitals in Ireland?
  If not, how can a hospital address this important resource deficiency?

- Ensure that a palliative care specialist is available for consultation and advice in acute care settings where pain management is meeting with little success.

- Discuss with the palliative care specialist whether palliative sedation would be an appropriate pain remedy in the case of Mrs Boyes (see Case 5 following).

- In attempting to manage the pain of a patient, attention to the adequacy and proportionality principles are essential. Applying these principles requires that the healthcare team know the extent of pain suffered by the patient in order to respond adequately. Assessments need to be put in place to get to know the patient's depth of pain.

- Encourage patients not to be timid and to let health professionals know if their pain is not being relieved. Many patients fear if they speak up about their pain they may come to be known as a crank or constant complainer.

6.5 Case 5: Palliative Sedation – Soul Pain

As part of the skills and services of palliative care, health professionals need strategies for responding to the troubling problems of patients who develop intolerable suffering despite receiving excellent care. Comprehensive palliative care is highly effective but survey data show that 5% to 35% of patients, even in hospice programmes, describe their pain as severe in the last week of life, and 25% describe their shortness of breath as 'unbearable' (Coyle, Adelhardt, Foley et al., 1990). Understanding each patient's unique situation is the crux of palliative medicine and moral response.

Pain is usually understood as a sensation caused by physiological phenomena and so is deemed treatable with pharmacological agents such as opioid, hypnosis or other mechanisms. However, pain is not simply physiological. With analgesics one can relieve a great deal of pain but might not touch the 'soul suffering' an individual may experience. Michael Kearney understands soul pain as: '[t]he experience of an individual who has become disconnected and alienated from the deepest and most fundamental aspects of him or herself' (Kearney, 1996, p.60). The holistic experience of the dying that is 'total pain' combines physical, emotional, spiritual and social dimensions of pain. Soul pain finds emotional expression as fear and behavioural expression as the 'fight' of an agitated struggle to find a way out of the awful situation. Observing a patient in this 'total pain' puts impossible demands on carers of patients to do something, anything: 'Can't you see I'm in agony?' (Kearney, 1996, p.62).

Kearney explains that when a patient is in soul pain, this is accompanied by an all-pervading sense of emptiness, hopelessness and meaninglessness. In such situations, the clinical team may recommend 'palliative' or 'continuous sedation' – sedation to unconsciousness – until the patient dies, a decision which relieves the patient of his or her complex physical and psychological experience of the unique suffering termed 'soul pain'.

The following case illustrates respect for the uniqueness of Maura in administering palliative sedation for her soul pain (Rady and Verheijde, 2010).

Soul Pain

Maura was a music teacher in her early fifties known by all students and friends as 'bright, brusque and breezy'. A malignant tumour invaded the nerves in her leg and was treated with radiotherapy and painkillers. Yet, this did not relieve Maura's suffering, profound and deep soul pain. Maura was anguished, terrified, agitated and would not settle. Eventually her defences 'cracked in an eruption of uncontrollable fear, paranoia and pain. She writhed about in her bed as she groaned, hyperventilated and cried out, wide-eyed, for someone to help.' These symptoms were treated with a morphine infusion but no medical workup was done and no antibiotic treatment was given. As the dose of morphine was increased to try and relieve symptoms, the patient became delirious and agitated. When the dose was decreased, Maura became more lucid but was very uncomfortable. She asked the doctors and nurses to help her escape from her agony.

The team offered to sedate her to the point of unconsciousness and then withhold further treatment including intravenous fluids. The patient was reassured that the sedative dose would be increased until she appeared to be resting comfortably and that it would not be cut back until she died. The healthcare team, the patient and her family reached the consensus that this was the best of the available options. It would allow Maura to achieve the death that she saw was good for her without violating the law or forcing her to suffer unnecessarily. She was given a midazolam infusion which was titrated upward until she achieved a sedated state and was then maintained at that level. She died within 24 hours. **(Edited case variation from Quill, Coombs Lee and Nunn, 2000a, p.491 and Kearney, 1996, pp.22–4)**

6.5.1 Discussion

Palliative sedation, also known as continuous deep sedation, is sometimes provided in end-of-life care, e.g.

- in end-of-life weaning from ventilator support
- in the management of refractory symptoms at the end of life
- for psychological or existential suffering (also termed 'soul pain')

However, it is important to understand that it is not always restricted to end-of-life care. It may sometimes be used as a temporising measure in trauma, burn, postsurgical, and intensive care (Irish Association for Palliative Care, 2011b).

Although rendering a patient unconscious to escape suffering is an extraordinary measure, withholding such treatment in certain circumstances would be inhumane. Because most of the patients who receive heavy sedation are expected to recover, careful attention is paid to maintaining adequate ventilation, hydration, and nutrition. (**Quill and Byock, 2000, p.409**)

In these cases, while patients are sedated, all other life-prolonging measures are carefully maintained with a view to patients eventually recovering consciousness and recovering from their illness.

However, a small percentage of patients who are receiving care, such as Maura in Case 5, reach a point where their anguish, suffering and restlessness become severe and unremitting despite the unrestrained palliative efforts. Where the patient is close to death – a matter of hours, days or at most a few weeks – the following process is an option that is considered a last resort.

In the context of far-advanced disease and expected death, artificial nutrition, hydration, antibiotics, mechanical ventilation and other life prolonging interventions are not instituted and are usually withdrawn if they are already in place. These measures are withheld […] because they could prolong the dying process without contributing to the quality of the patient's remaining life (Quill and Byock, 2000, p.409).

Such was the decision in the case of Maura. The decision to administer palliative sedation to patients whose death is imminent is based on clinical reasons but it clearly has ethical implications.

The question of withdrawing artificial nutrition and hydration is often difficult to address with the patient and family because nutrition has such a high symbolic value. Withholding food can be perceived as neglect, abandonment, or hastening death. (**Lesage and Portenoy, 2001, p.124**)

Ethical concerns and challenges arise in cases where the clinical decision is that the patient will be sedated until his or her death. In many cases, the patient has already ceased artificial nutrition and hydration (ANH), antibiotics and other life-prolonging therapies before sedation is applied (Kahn, Lazarus and Owens, 2003). In other cases, life-prolonging measures may be withheld during palliative sedation (Raijmakers et al., 2011). Failure to keep the reasons for a decision on sedation distinct from the reasons for ceasing all life-prolonging measures can lead to concerns that the decisions taken together amount to camouflaged euthanasia or physician-assisted suicide (PAS). *(See discussion of euthanasia and PAS in Module 6, section 7)*

The following text emphasises the need to keep the decisions distinct:

> [T]erminal sedation can be distinguished from euthanasia and, furthermore, is an ethical alternative to euthanasia in countries where the general ethos is against euthanasia […] sedation ought to be considered a valid option at the end of life […] but I believe that the distinction between sedation and euthanasia is much harder to sustain when other decisions, for example to withhold hydration and nutrition, are not considered as distinct decisions in their own right.'
> (Woods, 2007, p.127)

In brief, Woods is stressing the reasoning that, when considering palliative sedation for a patient, there need to be clinical reasons why withholding other life-prolonging therapies (LPTs), such as ANH, are also indicated.

Reasons for this may be that LSTs such as ANH:
- have been refused by the patient when competent and not under sedation
- are futile – may not provide any benefit for the patient and do not contribute to the quality of the patient's remaining life
- intensify the patient's suffering
- may prove too stressful or burdensome for the patient's system to bear

(Woods, 2007, p.127; Quill and Byock, 2000, p.409).

In the two decisions (sedation and withdrawal of LPTs), it is not only essential that clear reasons for each be thought through but the process involved in making the decisions with accompanying clinical and ethical reasons needs to be documented. The need to document decisions of this nature can contribute to clearer, more reason-based decision making.

Palliative Sedation Remains Controversial
It is important to stress that palliative sedation still remains a highly controversial practice among acute care clinicians. Palliative care specialists are also concerned about the widening of indications that are cited for its use. The case of Maura discussed here poses one of the more problematic indications for palliative sedation: existential or soul suffering.

> Perhaps the most controversial indication for sedation is unresolved psychosocial or existential distress. As palliative care physicians we must reflect on whether the role of medicine is to relieve all human suffering. Suffering is an essential part of the human experience and may have meaning for patients and families […] refractoriness should be determined only after repeated

evaluations by a skilled clinician who has a professional relationship with the patient. This implies that a single psychiatry consultation to rule out depression or anxiety is insufficient. Involvement of a social worker, chaplain, and ethicist, including evaluation of the family and social circumstances, may also be needed before decisions are made. Existential distress is perhaps the most important place for intermittent or respite sedation: time for rest and reorganization may resolve some of the distress. (Hauser and Walsh, 2009, p.578)

Extensive ongoing debate about the medical and ethical indications for palliative sedation continues. Some authors express worries that the use of palliative sedation and discontinuation of ANH by a consenting, competent patient may, in effect, be physician-assisted suicide. Proponents of palliative sedation continue to clarify that 'the purpose of the medications is to render the patient unconscious to relieve suffering, not to intentionally end his or her life' (Quill and Byock, 2000, p.561). On this understanding some commentators claim that the Principle of Double Effect would apply in the careful use of palliative sedation. (See Case 2 for a discussion of PDE)

Three features of Case 5 give evidence of moral reasoning in the clinical judgement to use palliative sedation as a last resort to ease Maura's 'soul pain'. Are these sufficient? Do these reasons show that, with Maura's comprehension of and consent to palliative sedation, the case seems to be a clinical and ethically based decision to withdraw further life-prolonging treatments and provide adequate pain relief?

a. Maura's symptoms reveal genuine 'soul pain' – the case narrative illustrates 'soul pain' as it is described by palliative care physicians and patients alike (Kearney, 1996).

b. Competence to arrive at consensus: Maura appears competent and sufficiently lucid to participate in the consensus reached in conjunction with the healthcare team and her family that this method of relief from suffering is the best of the available options for her suffering even though it involves the withholding of nutrition and hydration (Irish Association for Palliative Care, 2011a).

c. Requesting help – exercising autonomy of choice: Some may worry that Maura's appeal to her doctors and nurses to help her escape from her agony may be a request for assisted suicide. However this worry might be alleviated with the realisation that a competent patient in the throes of terminal illness can, with moral legitimacy, exercise their autonomy and decline life-support therapies? One burning question for patients and professionals making such a decision in an Irish context is the status of nutrition and hydration – should it be considered as simply another medical treatment or should it be understood as universally obligatory basic care? (See Module 6, section 6.5 for more detailed discussion of ANH.)

The European Association for Palliative Care have carried out an extensive review of the use of palliative sedation in clinical settings (Cherny, Radbruch and the Board of the European Association for Palliative Care [EAPC], 2009). The following are only a few of the problem practices cited as cause for concern about misuse of palliative sedation.

Problem Practices in Use of Palliative Sedation

There are a number of ways in which patient care can be undermined by the injudicious, abusive or unskilled use of sedation. There is, unfortunately, strong data indicating the prevalence of abuse but little is known about the prevalence of substandard sedation practices. The following four practices are problems in the use of palliative sedation and undermine the credibility of therapeutic effectiveness when used ethically and expertly.

Abuse of palliative sedation: This occurs when health professionals sedate patients approaching the end of life with the primary goal of hastening the patient's death. This has been called 'slow euthanasia'. Indeed, some physicians administer doses of medication ostensibly to relieve symptoms but with a covert intention to hasten death. Others, on request from patients, would use palliative sedation as a method of performing assisted suicide.

Excess dosage of pain medication, for example, can compromise physiological functions such as spontaneous respiration and haemodynamic stability. These duplicitous practices represent an unacceptable and often illegal deviation from normative ethical clinical practice (Cherny et al., 2009, p.581).

Injudicious use of palliative sedation: This occurs when sedation is applied with the intent of relieving symptoms but in clinical circumstances that are not appropriate. This means that the patient indications are inadequate to justify such a radical intervention. What accounts for injudicious use of palliative sedation?

1. Instances of inadequate patient assessment where potentially reversible causes of distress are overlooked.

2. Before resorting to sedation, there is a failure to engage with health professionals who are experts in the relief of symptoms despite their availability.

3. The situation of an overwhelmed physician resorting to sedation because he or she is fatigued and frustrated by the care of a complex symptomatic patient.

4. Situations in which the demand for sedation is generated by the patient's family and not the patient him/herself. The family may be emotionally distressed watching the suffering of their relative (Cherny et al., 2009, p.582).

Substandard clinical practice of palliative sedation: Examples include inadequate communication with the patient and/or family to ensure understanding of the goals of the care plan, anticipated outcomes and potential risks.

In addition are substandard clinical practices of inadequate monitoring of symptom distress or adequacy of relief; inadequate assessment of psychological, spiritual or social factors that may be contributing to the patient's distress; use of inappropriate medications to achieve sedation (i.e. opioids). (See under Further Discussion for several other important EAPC guidelines.)

6.5.2 Suggested Professional Responsibilities

- Health professionals must be carefully trained in the methods and management of palliative sedation or have a palliative care expert give advice on use for a specific patient. It is advisable to get a second opinion regarding the decision to use palliative sedation with a particular patient.

- A diagnosis of a terminal condition must be given with a life expectancy of days to weeks.

- Competent patients must give informed consent based on conversation, information and reassurance.

- A documented advance directive must be sought if the patient needing sedation lacks capacity or competence.

- In the absence of an advance directive, the patient's family must be consulted to determine what is in the best interest of the patient. Discussion with the family should include an open discussion about the advantages and concerns associated with palliative sedation.

- Where appropriate, open discussion with family around the withholding of life - prolonging therapies should take into account the emotions and religious beliefs that may underpin perspectives on these procedures.

- In sedating the patient, the family should be present if possible; nasal oxygen should be provided as well as a single room in a quiet part of the hospital (Quill and Byock, 2000; Royal Dutch Medical Association, 2005).

- The reasons why a decision might be taken to discontinue life-prolonging therapies if these are to accompany palliative sedation should be documented separately.

- The family should be supported in their bereavement and reassured that nothing more could be done to provide a good dying for the patient.

- The healthcare team should facilitate discussion of any member's reluctance or queries in the use of palliative sedation.

- The European Association for Palliative Care recommended framework for the use of sedation in palliative care should be considered and reviewed.

7. Module 5 Further Discussion

7.1 The Ambiguity of Clinical Intentions in Pain Management

Palliative care consultant Dr Timothy Quill has written extensively on pain management, the principle of double effect and ambiguity of intentions. Quill claims that a common belief that our intentions are always clear, uncomplicated and transparent is a serious mistake. It is a mistake especially because many doctors and nurses realise that their intentions in pain management decisions are often complicated, and are not transparent or clearly obvious to them.

Nurses and doctors may believe that the lack of clear and uncomplicated intentions might mean that, in truth, they are aiming for the death of a patient, or committing euthanasia. On the other hand, believing strongly that euthanasia is not only illegal but unethical, they may seriously under-treat pain and suffering to avoid this, even when a patient is dying (Quill, 1993, p.1039). Indeed, uncertainty about intention should not discourage the potentially lethal use of drugs, provided that that use is strictly governed by what is necessary to palliate in a given case.

More than anything we may need to move away from an idealised ethical perspective which argues that intentions must be clear and distinct if we are going to be sure of our moral propriety. If we probe intentions in much of human life we find that they may be ambiguous, complex and often contradictory. It is useful to consider a quotation from Quill on this point, because it provides food for thought and helps tease out the complex reasons why many health professionals continue to under-treat pain and suffering. It explains the multilayered complexity of human life, the life that any person seeking to act morally must live. Quill writes of the ambiguity of intentions in treating suffering patients while urging realism in the process of moral reflection.

> [M]ulti-layered intentions are present in most, if not all, end-of-life decisions. To understand physicians' reluctance to stop life-sustaining treatment once it is started, or to prescribe adequate amounts of narcotics to patients who are dying and in severe pain, we would do well to look beneath the sanitized intentions espoused by many medical ethicists to the actual experience of doctors and patients.

- *If we do not clarify the ethical and legal status of such actions as prescribing barbiturates to terminally ill patients, with their inherent complexities and contradictions, then most physicians will remain too fearful to help patients with these delicate deliberations.*

- *If we do not acknowledge the inescapable multiplicity of intentions in most double-effect situations, physicians may retreat from aggressive palliative treatment out of fear of crossing the allegedly bright line between allowing patients to die and causing their death.*

- *Our current ethical thinking and legal prohibitions reinforce self-deception, secrecy, isolation, and abandonment at a time when the exact opposite is needed.*

- *Perhaps a key to humanizing medical ethics and the law, as well as clinical medicine, lies in being more forthright and explicit about our intentions and responsibilities in working with dying patients. (Quill, 1993, p.1040)*

7.2 Ethical Concerns over the Use of Palliative Sedation

Three concerns of an ethical and clinical nature merit scrutiny when deciding on palliative sedation.

7.2.1 Fear of Euthanasia

Recall that the intent of palliative care is to relieve suffering, even if treatments for pain relief hasten death. Intent matters in law and ethics, with the rule of double effect stating that foreseeable adverse consequences of treatment are acceptable only if they are unintended, i.e. not the explicit aim and goal of the treatment. For many palliative doctors it is a matter of great importance to draw a clear distinction between palliative care and euthanasia (Douglas et al., 2008, p.390). However, research that examines the intentions of doctors in palliative care settings is fraught with difficulties:

In particular, one needs to be sure that the distinction between intention and foresight has been recognized by respondents who report their own actions. Furthermore, intentions in the setting of end-of-life care may be multiple and ambiguous, and respondents may have limited insight into their own intentions, or may recall them inaccurately, particularly in light of societal pressures that approve some intentions and disapprove of others.

(Douglas, Kerridge and Ankeny, 2008, p.390).

7.2.2 Suppressing Patients' Consciousness

This concern arises in relation to the perceived importance of maintaining consciousness and awareness – even when one is suffering and dying. The question is whether it is justified to control, curtail or reduce considerably the experiences of awareness for a dying person, as happens in some cases of deep sedation. The emphasis here is on the importance of sustaining a level of mental awareness in order to allow for communication with loved ones, family or healthcare staff. On this view, the aim of maintaining a patient's awareness to the greatest degree possible should temper when and how sedation ought to be used.

Without awareness a person cannot avail of opportunities for reconciliation. Likewise, without awareness the patient may feel that they are being abandoned (Woods, 2007, p.126; Craig, 1994).

Woods reassures on this point:

> *Even if a patient were to be deeply sedated, they would still be cared for with respect and dignity; with someone watching over them, turning them, keeping them clean, going to the bedside, quietly and discreetly, to observe and so on.* (Woods, 2007, p.126)

In addition, for some religious believers, consciousness may be considered a necessary condition of spiritual reconciliation with oneself or one's god. In this regard, the following statement on pain relief from a religious perspective claims that health professionals need to take special care in considering suppression of pain and consciousness through sedation (Rady and Verheijde, 2010).

> *Is the suppression of pain and consciousness by the use of narcotics […] permitted by religion and morality for the doctor and patient (even at the approach of death and if one foresees that the use of narcotics will shorten life)? If no other means exist and, if in the given circumstances, this does not prevent the carrying out of other religious and moral duties. Painkillers that cause unconsciousness need special consideration.* (Cited in O'Rourke and Boyle, 1993, p.223)

The text concludes:
'It is not right to deprive the dying person of consciousness without a serious reason' (cited in O'Rourke and Boyle, 1993, p.223).

The fundamental emphasis on respecting the values of the patient when making clinical decisions arises here. Where patients either explicitly request the therapy of sedation or consent to it when it has been explained to them by a health professional that it is necessary in order to relieve suffering, anxiety and restlessness, then health professionals can proceed with confidence that it is one way that they can facilitate the autonomy and choice of the patient who is suffering.

Woods urges health professionals and families not to substitute their own values for those of a competent patient or one who has left an Advance Directive about their wishes. He claims that palliative sedation should remain a morally justified option for the patient who is competent to choose it.

> *Deliberately aiming to alter the experiences of the patient is a legitimate goal in the use of*

sedation […] the possible meaning that people may find in their experiences of coping with challenging situations is boundless. However, whatever the meaning this experience may have for a person, it is the meaning he or she alone finds in the experience that endows it with value […] Individuals may find meaning in suffering, and the principle may be a sound one, but to claim that there is virtue in the suffering of a person if they find no meaning or value in the experience is a corruption of the virtue. The patient's own testimony should be the main reference point when adjusting the pain relief (Woods, 2007, p.125).

7.2.3 Fear of the Slippery Slope

A further concern about palliative sedation is that one may too easily mount the slippery slope which involves a move from employing it as a method for alleviating the pain of those who are terminally ill to employing it in treating depressed patients or those who have simply lost meaning in life. Where some health professionals could justify its use with patients who are unambiguously dying, they could not morally defend its use for profoundly depressed patients who are not 'terminally ill' or near death but seek escape from their chronic and profound suffering.

This concern voices a legitimate worry about the use of palliative sedation to treat profoundly depressed patients who are not terminally ill but nevertheless seek escape from profound suffering. The concern about using palliative sedation when a person is not 'terminally ill' is very much debated since it is widely agreed that alleviation of suffering is one goal of medicine. If this is the case, it is not clear why such relief from suffering should be limited to the imminently dying. However, if sedation for chronic depression were considered, it is not morally justified also to discontinue all life supports unless there is clear evidence of a competent patient's refusal of such supports.

Out of respect for patient self-determination, such discontinuation of life supports would need serious consideration. The serious problem here is that a patient who is acutely or chronically depressed may lack the capacity to decide on life-prolonging treatment or palliative sedation. A decision to use alternative therapies for depression would be essential and a psychiatric consultation with the patient advised before depression is cited as a condition warranting palliative sedation.

7.3 European Association for Palliative Care Guidelines

To ensure consistency in practice and also to allow for the ongoing review of pain management decisions, the European Association of Palliative Care (EAPC) published a decision-making framework in 2009. The 10-item framework incorporates an extensive literature review of the practice of palliative sedation. Expert peer review of the initial draft was invited from a wide range of palliative care clinicians both within and outside of the EAPC. (Cherny et al, 2009)

Some of the points provided in this framework are discussed above under Case 5 where palliative sedation was used. Two other significant points which are rarely stressed in such guidelines documents include the needs of carers – family and medical professionals.

7.3.1 Care and Informational Needs of the Patient's Family

Families need extensive support to understand the decision-making process, and be clear about the goals and expected outcomes of palliative sedation. Identifying a family spokesperson (preferably one chosen by the patient) may help communication, especially for large, geographically scattered or conflicted families.

Without effective communication families may be left with feelings of profound confusion, guilt or remorse, which complicate their subsequent bereavement. For these reasons, evaluation and decision-making by a multi-disciplinary team skilled in palliatve care is essential prior to initiating [palliative sedation]. (Hauser and Walsh, 2009, p.577)

Further advice is offered from the EAPC to improve compassionate care and attention for families of patients undergoing palliative sedation.

A patient's family often experiences profound distress. If the patient is hospitalised, all efforts should be made to provide privacy for emotional and physical intimacy. To promote the family's sense of well-being and peace, consideration should be given to the aesthetics of the care environment including an opportunity to sleep in the room or nearby.
(Cherny et al., 2009, p.587)

The healthcare team should counsel the family in the ways that they can continue to be of help to the patient: by being with, talking to and touching the patient, providing mouth care, managing the atmosphere of the patient's care (providing patient's favourite music, scents, saying prayers or reading to the patient).

Families of sedated patients need to be kept informed about the patient's well being and what to expect. This includes appropriate notification that death is approaching and what can be expected in the dying process.

7.3.2 Care for the Health Professionals

Health professionals and healthcare staff may also express profound distress when a patient is sedated. This is particularly true if there is discord regarding the appropriateness of the intervention and in situations when the process is protracted. Staff distress can be mitigated if there is development of a culture of sensitivity to the emotional burdens involved in care. Sharing information and engaging in multidisciplinary discussions can offer the group or individuals opportunities to express their feelings. This context can be therapeutic for staff distress and address any confusion about the procedure of palliative sedation (Cherny et al., 2009, p.588).

> *Staff need to develop awareness of their own preferences about care of the dying, and the potential role of frustration, sense of failure and burnout in decision-making. Individual physicians personal and professional factors may influence the practice of [palliative sedation], including prevalence, determination of refractoriness, level of sedation used, and drugs employed.*
> (Huaser and Walsh, 2009, p.577)

7.4 Critics and Proponents of the Principle of Double Effect (PDE)

7.4.1 Critics of the PDE

Critics have criticised the principle of double effect because:

a. The analysis of intention used in the principle is problematic and inconsistent with other analyses of human intention. According to modern psychology, human intention is ambiguous, subjective, multilayered and often contradictory. The principle of double effect does not acknowledge this complexity (Quill, 1993, p.1040; Bennett, 2001; Davis, 2001; Foot, 2001; Marquis, 2001). In addition, the PDE claims that where there are two outcomes of an action, one good and one bad, the doctor must focus on the good end that she or he intends and realise that the other bad effect is not intended but only foreseen.

Critics claim that this distinction between intended and only foreseen effects of an action is unconvincing. We cannot splice up our mental 'intentions' in this way. What we foresee is likely to happen must be included in our overall intention for an action.

b. The principle is 'absolutist' in the rigour with which it specifies kinds of acts that are 'evil' or 'bad'. The evil of aiming for 'death' is seen to be a prohibition without exception. For some, death is not seen as evil in all circumstances.

c. The principle may be paternalistic. This is because the absolute prohibition against taking human life can be interpreted to mean that a doctor cannot accept a request from a competent, terminally ill patient who seeks to end suffering through the cessation of life-prolonging therapy. This interpretation would endorse a strong form of paternalism that is difficult to harmonise with respect for patient autonomy (Quill, Dresser and Brock 1997, pp.1768–71).

7.4.2. Proponents of the PDE

a. The PDE has desirable effects on clinical conduct.

The principle has reassured clinicians that prescribing high-dose opioids for pain in terminally ill patients is morally permissible and that is all to the good.
(Quill, Dresser and Brock, 1997, p.1770)

b. Theory is faulty but PDE is correct. Proponents acknowledge that PDE is based on an inadequate theory of human intention and actions. But they claim that we do not have to accept the theory of intention and action regarding foreseen but unintended consequences. Proponents believe they can concede deficiency in theory of action and yet argue that the fundamental thrust of PDE is correct: When the positive goal of alleviating human suffering is at stake, then the obligation of the doctor is to take adequate action that is proportionate to the needs of the suffering patient. This would always assume the action is within the law of the jurisdiction of medical practice.

c. Many physicians embrace it as a better option than active euthanasia or physician-assisted suicide, both of which are often motivated by poor pain relief. It is not a trivial matter that the PDE may be useful as a way of justifying adequate pain management and other palliative measures for dying patients.

d. The PDE is not perfect but it is a coherent doctrine of moral justification and, unfortunately, suffers from being misunderstood. These proponents make considerable effort to explain their position. One misunderstanding is the idea that PDE is absolutist in prohibiting some actions categorically. These proponents say that PDE does not specify what makes an immoral act immoral. Traditional teachings or ethical views have handed down certain actions as prohibited but any ethical theory that allows that there are kinds of acts which are good and bad could be consistent with the PDE and could make use of PDE (Boyle, 2001, pp.7–20; Woods, 2007, pp.129–35).

8. Module 5 Summary Learning Guides

8.1 Effective Pain Management is the Primary Objective in Patient Care

- Pain experience is cited in empirical studies as a central element in a 'bad dying', whereas successful pain relief is a primary element in a 'good dying'.
- Unrelieved pain can cause depression and hopelessness.
- The experience of pain in illness can distract from all other factors in one's life. Pain can diminish an individual's capacity for clarity of understanding and the possibility of companionship.
- Pain can hinder the ability to participate in conversations about one's treatment decisions.
- The encouragement and facilitation of patient autonomy is frustrated if pain management is not effective.

8.2 Principle of Double Effect (PDE)

- The PDE is one way for reasoning through the moral complexity of pain management.
- Accounts for actions which have two effects: one intended good effect (relief of pain) and one not specifically sought or willed (earlier death).
- An effect that might be morally wrong if caused intentionally (taking someone's life) is permissible if foreseen but unintended.
- Human intentions are complex and ambiguous. As a result, a person cannot always be completely clear or certain about the cluster of intentions they hold when deciding on pain management methods for a patient.
- The PDE does not authorise practices such as physician-assisted suicide or euthanasia.
- The PDE helps health professionals to overcome a hesitation to prescribe a sufficient dose of pain medication for a particular patient's suffering.
- Clinical evidence about the sincerity of one's intentions can be facilitated if one observes the criteria of adequacy and proportionality. To be morally justified, a particular medication and dosage must be adequate for and proportional to this particular patient's pain.
- The PDE can be a helpful tool in decision making but it is not a moral calculus to ensure ethically correct decisions if the decision maker is using the PDE in a cynical way.

8.3 Palliative Sedation

- Sedation to unconsciousness may be used as a temporising measure in trauma, burn, postsurgical and intensive care.

- Called 'continuous deep sedation' by some and 'palliative sedation' by others, this refers to the administration of high doses of sedatives normally given to patients who are imminently dying and are not expected to recover from sedation.

- Can be indicated when a patient is suffering severe and intractable suffering, often called 'soul pain'

- Soul pain = the experience of anxiety, restlessness and hopelessness in a person who has become disconnected and alienated from the deepest and most fundamental aspects of themselves.

- If palliative sedation for the dying patient is administered, the decision may be taken to discontinue all other life-prolonging measures as well. The reasons must be documented but the central rationale is that these life-support measures often do not improve the quality of the patient's remaining life and may be more stressful than beneficial.

- Competent patients (often involving family in the conversation) may consent to palliative sedation and discontinuation of all life supports.

- Where patients lack capacity and have not left an Advanced Directive stating their wishes, the clinical staff and family must discuss the adequacy and proportionality of palliative sedation for the relief of their loved one's pain and consider the factors that make this decision in the 'best interests' of the patient.

- Compassionate care and understanding for the bereaved family members remain important features in the humane use of palliative sedation.

9. Module 5 Activities

9.1. Review Case 1

and reflect on the experiences of Maurice with a diagnosis of cancer and suffering increasing pain.

a. What are particular features of 'psychological pain'?

b. What measures might have been taken by health professionals to prevent this patient's 'anticipatory pain'?

c. Maurice explained that he attempted suicide because he dreaded the continuing intensification of pain that had already begun. What clinical evidence would you look for to validate whether, in addition, the man may be depressed and need help for that affliction?

d. The reassurance to the patient that his pain would be managed brought relief. Given that Maurice is an out-patient, how can the staff now ensure effective pain management for him?

9.2 Re-read the particulars of Case 2:

a. Consider yourself the nurse or doctor in charge of Madeleine. Specifically, how would you deal with the mother's concerns about Madeleine's continued pain? Consider jotting down a conversation you might have with Madeleine's mother.

b. Although Madeleine is very young, how can the health professionals try to discern her level and quality of pain? Provide a few concrete suggestions as to how you would proceed.

c. Madeleine's mother is particularly annoyed with what she sees as an erroneous clinical focus on white cell count and further administration of chemotherapy while greatly minimising the need for effective pain management. Do you think the mother was correct and deserves to be heard? Write a few notes on how you would respond to the mother's annoyance and concerns for her daughter's suffering.

d. On a scale of 1–10, how would you rate the acute care hospital provisions (space, privacy, pain management, decoration, etc.) for the care of seriously ill children?

9.3 Reflect back on the particulars of Case 3:

In this case, Paul is suffering from end-stage metastatic lung cancer and the health professionals involved recommend palliative care.

a. From your experience of managing pain for patients, do you think that Paul would have had equally effective relief from his suffering if he had not chosen a palliative care approach?

b. Discuss your own experience of caring for terminally ill patients like Paul. Would you find that it is a common occurrence to have a conversation with a patient about the risk of an earlier death following adequate pain medication? Explain.

c. In situations like this case scenario, how would you go about determining the patient's competence or capacity to consent?

d. Paul was comforted by the presence of family and clergy. Explain how you might provide solace and companionship for a patient who is not so fortunate to have this emotional and spiritual support.

9.4 Case 4

is presented as an apparently clear example of euthanasia. Consider the details of the case and wonder:

a. Considering that Dr Cox has, with stated compassion, relieved Mrs Boyes of excruciating suffering, what is it about the action of Dr Cox that you think makes it morally objectionable in law? What is the law protecting here?

b. Would the Principle of Double Effect work as a moral defence in this case?

c. Do you think that euthanasia is ever morally (if not legally) justified? Why or why not?

d. If you were the doctor or nurse in care of Mrs Boyes, what alternative to an injection of potassium chloride would you have offered her to ensure pain relief?

9.5 Re-read Case 5

and reflect on the treatment offered Maura for her soul suffering.

a. Do you consider that the provision of palliative sedation was ethically warranted as a response to Maura's request 'to relieve her from her agony'?

b. Consider the query about whether relief of unresolved psychosocial or existential distress falls within the role of medicine. Discuss with your colleagues whether the removal of ANH for Maura was warranted. Try to write down your reasons why or why not.

c. Maura exercised her autonomous request to be released from suffering by agreeing to this process of palliative sedation. With such a serious degree of suffering, how would you ensure that Maura's capacity to make this decision is intact?

d. Discuss with your colleagues whether they think that this method for managing suffering is equivalent to physician-assisted suicide? Explain.

9.6 Recall the empirical research

discussed in this module where Quinlan and O'Neill document clinical and family scepticism about referring patients to palliative care.

a. What reasons would you give to explain the reluctance of health professionals to refer patients for palliative care?

b. Try and explain why some families are very reluctant to refer their loved ones for palliative care even though it would mean diminished suffering and improved quality of life.

c. Do you think this sceptical attitude toward palliative care is mistaken? If so, what are your reasons?

d. Using your creative thinking in the interest of better pain management, what would you do to try and moderate or correct this scepticism about palliative care?

10. Module 5 References and Further Reading

American College of Physicians Ethics and Human Rights Committee, 'American College of Physicians Ethics Manual', *Annals of Internal Medicine*, vol. 117, no. 11, 1992, pp.947–60

American Pain Society, New Survey of People with Chronic Pain Reveals Out-of-Control Symptoms, Impaired Daily Lives (1999), http://www.ampainsoc.org/whatsnew/release030499.htm [accessed 1 August 2009]

Back, A.L., Young, J.P., McCown, E., Engelberg, R.A., Vig, E.K., Reinke, L.F., Wenrich, M.D., McGrath, B.B. and Curtis, J.R. 'Abandonment at the End of Life from Patient, Caregiver, Nurse and Physician Perspectives', *Archives of Internal Medicine*, vol. 169, no. 5, 2009, pp.474–9

Battin, M.P. *Least Worst Death: Essays in Bioethics on the End of Life* (Oxford and New York: Oxford University Press, 1994)

Battin, M.P. Book review. 'A Midwife Through the Dying Process: Stories of Healing and Hard Choices at the End of Life', by T.E. Quill. *New England Journal of Medicine*, vol. 336, no. 25, 1997, pp.1842–3

Beabout, G. 'Morphine Use for Terminal Cancer Patients: An Application of the Principle of Double Effect', in P.A. Woodward (ed.), *The Doctrine of Double Effect: Philosophers Debate a Controversial Moral Principle* (Notre Dame, IN: University of Notre Dame Press, 2001)

Bennett, J. 'Foreseen Side Effects Versus Intended Consequences', in P.A. Woodward (ed.), *The Doctrine of Double Effect: Philosophers Debate a Controversial Moral Principle* (Notre Dame, IN: University of Notre Dame Press, 2001), pp.85–118

Biggar, N. *Aiming to Kill: The Ethics of Suicide and Euthanasia* (London: Darton, Longman, 2004). See especially Chapter 3

Bon Secours Health System, *Building a System-Wide Foundation for Palliative Care: Bon Secours' Journey* (2007), http://www.supportivecarecoalition.org [accessed 1 August 2009]

Boyle, J.M.J. 'Toward Understanding the Principle of Double Effect', in P.A. Woodward (ed.), *The Doctrine of Double Effect: Philosophers Debate a Controversial Moral Principle* (Notre Dame, IN: University of Notre Dame Press, 2001), pp.7–20

Brock, D. 'Medical Decisions at the End of Life', in H. Kuhse and P. Singer (eds), *A Companion to Bioethics* (Oxford: Blackwell Publishers, 2001)

Byock, I.R. 'When Suffering Persists', *Journal of Palliative Care*, vol. 10, no. 2, 1994, pp.8–13

Byock, I.R. 'The Nature of Suffering and the Nature of Opportunity at the End of Life', *Clinics in Geriatric Medicine*, vol. 12, no. 2, 1996, pp.237–52

Cassel, E.J. 'Diagnosing Suffering: A Perspective', *Annals of Internal Medicine*, vol. 137, no. 7, 1999, pp.531–4

Cherny, N.I. and Portenoy, R.K. 'The Management of Cancer Pain', *CA: A Cancer Journal for Clinicians*, vol. 44, no. 5, 1994(a), pp.263–303

Cherny, N.I. and Portenoy, R.K. 'Sedation in the Management of Refractory Symptoms: Guidelines for Evaluation and Treatment', *Journal of Palliative Care*, vol. 10, no. 2, 1994(b), pp.31–8

Cherny, N.I., Radbruch, L. and The Board of the European Association for Palliative Care, 'European Association for Palliative Care (EAPC) Recommended Framework for the Use of Sedation in Palliative Care', *Palliative Medicine*, vol. 23, no. 7, 2009, pp.581–93

Churchill, L.R. and King, N.M.P. 'Physician-Assisted Suicide, Euthanasia, or Withdrawal of Treatment', *British Medical Journal*, vol. 315, no. 7101, 1997, pp.137–8

Coyle, N., Adelhardt, J., Foley, K.M. and Portenoy, R.K. 'Character of Terminal Illness in the Advanced Cancer Patient: Pain and other Symptoms during the Last Four Weeks of Life', *Journal of Pain and Symptom Management*, vol. 5, no. 2, 1990, pp.83–93

Craig, G.M. 'On Withholding Nutrition and Hydration in the Terminally Ill: Has Palliative Medicine Gone Too Far?' *Journal of Medical Ethics*, vol. 20, no. 3, 1994, pp.139–43

Davis, N. 'The Doctrine of Double Effect: Problems of Interpretation', in P.A. Woodward (ed.), *The Doctrine of Double Effect: Philosophers Debate a Controversial Moral Principle* (Notre Dame, IN: University of Notre Dame Press, 2001), pp.119–42

Deandrea, S., Montanari, M., Moja, L. and Apolone, G. 'Prevalence of Undertreatment in Cancer Pain: A Review of Published Literature, *Annals of Oncology*, vol. 19, no. 12, 2008, pp.1985–91

Douglas, C., Kerridge, I. and Ankeny, R. 'Managing Intentions: The End-of-Life Administration of Analgesics and Sedatives and the Possibility of Slow Euthanasia', *Bioethics*, vol. 22, no. 7, 2008, pp.388–96

Ellershaw, J., Ward, C. and Neuberger, R.J. 'Care of the Dying Patient: The Last Hours or Days of Life. Commentary: A "Good Death" is Possible in the NHS', *British Medical Journal*, vol. 326, no. 7379, 2003, pp.30–4

Ferguson, P.R. 'Causing Death or Allowing to Die? Developments in the Law', *Journal of Medical Ethics*, vol. 23, no. 6, 1997, pp.368–72
Foot, P. 'The Problem of Abortion and the Doctrine of the Double Effect' in P.A. Woodward (ed.), *The Doctrine of Double Effect: Philosophers Debate a Controversial Moral Principle* (Notre Dame, IN: University of Notre Dame Press, 2001), pp.143–55

Frank, A.W. *The Wounded Storyteller: Body, Illness and Ethics* (Chicago: University of Chicago Press, 1995)

Ganzini, L., Goy, E.R. and Dobscha, S.K. 'Oregonians' Reasons for Requesting Physician Aid in Dying', *Archives of Internal Medicine*, vol. 169, no. 5, 2009, pp.489–92

Garro, L.C. 'Culture, Pain and Cancer', *Journal of Palliative Care*, vol. 6, no. 3, 1990, pp.34–44

German National Ethics Council, *Self-determination and Care at the End of Life* (Berlin: German National Ethics Council, 2006)

Gillick, M.R. 'Terminal Sedation: An Acceptable Exit Strategy?' *Annals of Internal Medicine*, vol. 141, no. 3, 2004, pp.236–7

Greenhalgh, T. and Hurwitz, B. *Narrative-Based Medicine: Dialogue and Discourse in Clinical Practice* (London: British Medical Journal Books, 1998)

Hasselaar, J.G.J., Verhagen, S., Wolff, A., Engels, Y., Crul, B.J.P. and Vissers, K.C.P. 'Changed Patterns in Dutch Palliative Sedation Practices after the Introduction of a National Guideline', *Archives of Internal Medicine*, vol. 169, no. 5, 2009, pp.430–7

Hauser, K. and Walsh, D. 'Palliative Sedation: Welcome Guidance on a Controversial Issue', *Palliative Medicine*, vol. 23, no. 7, 2009, pp.577–9

Irish Association of Palliative Care (IAPC), *Artificial Hydration in Terminally Ill Patients* (Dublin: IAPC, 2011(a)), http://www.iapc.ie [accessed 6 May 2011]

Irish Association of Palliative Care (IAPC), *Palliative Sedation* (Dublin: IAPC, 2011(b)), http:// www.iapc.ie [accessed 6 May 2011]

Irish Association of Palliative Care (IAPC), *Voluntary Euthanasia* (Dublin: IAPC, 2011(c)), http://www.iapc.ie [accessed 6 May 2011]

Jansen, L.A. and Sulmasy, D.P. 'Sedation, Alimentation, Hydration, and Equivocation: Careful Conversation about Care at the End of Life', *Annals of Internal Medicine*, vol. 136, no. 11, 2002, pp.845–9

Kahn, M.J., Lazarus, C.J. and Owens, D.P. 'Allowing Patients to Die: Practical, Ethical, and Religious Concerns', *Journal of Clinical Oncology*, vol. 21, no. 15, 2003, pp.3000–2

Katz, J. *The Silent World of Doctor and Patient* (Baltimore: Johns Hopkins University Press, 2002)

Kearney, M. *Mortally Wounded: Stories of Soul Pain, Death and Healing* (Dublin: Marino Books, 1996)

Keown, J. *Euthanasia Examined: Ethical, Clinical and Legal Perspectives* (Cambridge: Cambridge University Press, 1997)

Keown, J. *Euthanasia, Ethics and Public Policy: An Argument against Legalisation* (Cambridge: Cambridge University Press, 2002)

Kortesluoma, R.-L., Nikkonen, M. and Serlo, W. 'You Just Have to Make the Pain Go Away: 'Children's Experiences of Pain Management', *Pain Management Nursing*, vol. 9, no. 4, 2008, pp.143–9, especially p.145

Kubler-Ross, E. *Death: The Final Stage of Growth* (New Jersey: Prentice-Hall, 1975)

Lesage, P. and Portenoy, R.K. 'Ethical Challenges in the Care of Patients with Serious Illness', *Pain Medicine*, vol. 2, no. 2, 2001, pp.121–30

Lesho, E.P. 'When the Spirit Hurts: An Approach to the Suffering Patient', *Archives of Internal Medicine*, vol. 163, no. 20, 2003, p.2429

Linsker, S.W. 'The Longest Pain: The Suffering of Children with Cancer', *Rx Magazine* (2000), http://members.tripod.com/rx.magazine/eol__200000515.htm [accessed 19 August 2009]

Mangan, J.T. 'An Historical Analysis of the Principle of Double Effect', *Theological Studies*, 10, 1949, pp.40–61

Marquis, D.B. 'Four Versions of Double Effect', in P.A. Woodward (ed.), *The Doctrine of Double Effect: Philosophers Debate a Controversial Moral Principle* (Notre Dame, IN: University of Notre Dame Press, 2001), pp.156–88

McCracken, L.M. and Keogh, E. 'Acceptance, Mindfulness and Values-Based Action May Counteract Fear and Avoidance of Emotions in Chronic Pain: An Analysis of Anxiety Sensitivity', *The Journal of Pain*, vol. 10, no. 4, 2009, pp.408–15

McGuire, D.B., Yarbro, C.H. and Ferrell, B. *Cancer Pain Management* (Sudbury, MA: Jones & Bartlett, 1995)

Meisel, A. 'The Legal Consensus about Forgoing Life-Sustaining Treatment: Its Status and its Prospects', *Kennedy Institute of Ethics Journal*, vol. 2, no. 4, 1993, pp.309–45

Miller, F.G., Fins, J.J. and Snyder, L. 'Assisted Suicide Compared with Refusal Treatment: A Valid Distinction?' *Annals of Internal Medicine*, vol. 132, no. 6, 2000, pp.470–5

Nelson, H.L. *Stories and their Limits* (New York: Routledge, 1997)

New South Wales (NSW) Department of Health, 'Guidelines for End-of-Life Care and Decision Making' (2005) http://www.health.nsw.gov.au/policies/gl/2005/pdf/GL2005_057.pdf [accessed 1 August 2009]

O'Rourke , K.D. and Boyle, P. *Medical Ethics: Sources of Catholic Teachings* (2nd ed.) (Washington: Georgetown University, 1993)

O'Rourke, K.D. and Norris, P. 'Care of PVS Patients: Catholic Opinion in the United States', *Linacre Quarterly*, vol. 68, no. 3, 2001, pp.201–17

O'Shea, D., Keegan, O. and McGee, H. *End-of-Life Care in General Hospitals: Developing a Quality Approach for the Irish Setting. A Statement of the Irish Hospice Foundation* (Dublin: Health Services Research Centre, Royal College of Surgeons in Ireland, 2002)

Orr, R.D. 'Pain Management Rather than Assisted Suicide: The Ethical High Ground', *Pain Medicine*, vol. 2, no. 2, 2001, pp.131–7

Polomano, R.C., Dunwoody, C.J., Krenzischek, D.A. and Rathmell, J.P. 'Perspective on Pain Management in the 21st Century', *Pain Management Nursing*, vol. 9, no. 1, 2008 (Supplement 1), pp.3–10

Quill, T.E. 'The Ambiguity of Clinical Intentions', *New England Journal of Medicine*, vol. 329, no. 14, 1993, pp.1039–40

Quill, T.E. and Byock, I.R. 'Responding to Intractable Terminal Suffering: The Role of Terminal Sedation and Voluntary Refusal of Food and Fluids', *Annals of Internal Medicine*, vol. 132, no. 5, 2000, pp.408–14

Quill, T.E., Coombs Lee, B. and Nunn, S. 'Letters: Palliative Treatment of Last Resort and Assisted Suicide. In Response', *Annals of Internal Medicine*, vol. 133, no. 7, 2000(a), p.563

Quill, T.E., Coombs Lee, B. and Nunn, S. 'Palliative Treatments for Last Resort: Choosing the Least Harmful Alternative', *Annals of Internal Medicine*, vol. 132, no. 6, 2000(b), pp.488–93

Quill, T.E., Dresser, R. and Brock, D.W. 'The Rule of Double Effect: A Critique of its Role in End-of-Life Decision Making', *New England Journal of Medicine*, vol. 337, no. 24, 1997, pp.1768–71

Quinlan, C. and O'Neill, C. 'Practitioners' Narrative Submissions' (Unpublished) (Dublin: Irish Hospice Foundation, 2008)

Quinlan, C. and O'Neill, C. *Practitioners' Perspectives on Patient Autonomy at End of Life* (Dublin: Irish Hospice Foundation, 2009)

R v Cox (1992), 12 BMLR 38

Rady, Mohamed Y. and Verheijde, Joseph L. 'Continuous Deep Sedation until Death: Palliation or Physician-Assisted Death?' *American Journal of Hospice and Palliative Medicine*, vol. 27, no. 3, 2010, pp.205–14

Raijmakers, N.J.H., van Zuylen, L., Costantini, M., Caraceni, A., Clark, J., Lundquist, G., Voltz, R., Ellershaw, J.E. and van der Heide, A. 'Artificial Nutrition and Hydration in the Last Week of Life in Cancer Patients: A Systematic Literature Review of Practices and Effects', *Annals of Oncology*, 2011, http://www.annonc.oxfordjournals.org [accessed 10 May 2011]

Randall, F. 'Why Causing Death is Not Necessarily Morally Equivalent to Allowing to Die: A Response to Ferguson', *Journal of Medical Ethics*, vol. 23, no. 6, 1997, pp.373–6

Randall, F. and Downie, R.S. *Palliative Care Ethics: A Good Companion* (Oxford and New York: Oxford University Press, 1996)

Randall, F. and Downie, R.S. *The Philosophy of Palliative Care: Critique and Construction* (Oxford and New York: Oxford University Press, 2006)

Ranger, M. and Campbell-Yeo, M. 'Temperament and Pain Response: A Review of the Literature', *Pain Management Nursing*, vol. 9, no. 1, 2008, pp.2–9

Redmond, K. 'Organizational Barriers in Opioid Use' *Support Care in Cancer*, vol. 5, no. 6, 1997, pp.451–6

Rietjens, J.A.C., van Delden, J.J.M., van der Heide, A., Vrakking, A.M., Onwuteaka-Philipsen, B.D., van der Maas, P.J. and van der Wal, G. 'Terminal Sedation and Euthanasia', *Archives of Internal Medicine*, vol. 166, no. 7, 2006, pp.749–53

Rodin, G., Zimmermann, C., Rydall, A., Jones, J., Shepherd, F.A., Moore, M., Fruh, M., Donner, A. and Gagliese, L. 'The Desire for Hastened Death in Patients with Metastatic Cancer', *Journal of Pain and Symptom Management*, vol. 33, no. 6, 2007, pp.661–75

Royal College of Paediatrics and Child Health (RCPCH), *Advocating for Children* (London: Royal College of Paediatrics and Child Health, 2008)

Royal College of Physicians, *Concise Guidance to Good Practice: A Series of Evidence-Based Guidelines for Clinical Management. Number 12: Advance Care Planning: National Guidelines* (London: Royal College of Physicians, 2009)

Royal Dutch Medical Association (KNMG), *Guidelines for Palliative Sedation* (Utrecht: Royal Dutch Medical Association, 2005)

Ruland, C.M., Hamilton, G.A. and Schjødt-Osmo, B. 'The Complexity of Symptoms and Problems Experienced in Children with Cancer: A Review of the Literature, *Journal of Pain and Symptom Management*, vol. 37, no. 3, 2009, pp.403–18

Smith, D. 'Key Guidelines on End-of-Life Care and Palliative Care', unpublished study notes, Royal College of Surgeons in Ireland, Dublin, 2008

Steinhauser, K.E., Clipp, E.C., McNeilly, M., Christakis, N.A., McIntyre, L.M. and Tulsky, J.A. 'In Search of a Good Death: Observations of Patients, Families, and Providers', *Annals of Internal Medicine*, vol. 132, no. 10, 2000, pp.825–32

Taylor, R.M. and Lantos, J.D. 'The Politics of Medical Futility', *Issues in Law and Medicine*, vol. 11, no. 1, 1995, pp.3–12

Terry, W., Olson, L.G., Wilss, L. and Boulton-Lewis, G. 'Experience of Dying: Concerns of Dying Patients and of Carers', *Internal Medicine Journal*, vol. 36, no. 6, 2006, pp.338–46

Thomson, A. *Critical Reasoning in Ethics: A Practical Introduction* (London: Routledge, 1999)

Walco, G.A., Cassidy, R.C. and Schechter, N.L. 'Pain, Hurt, and Harm: The Ethics of Pain Control in Infants and Children', *New England Journal of Medicine*, vol. 331, no. 8, 1994, pp.541–4

Warnock, M. and Macdonald, E. *Easeful Death: Is There a Case for Assisted Dying?* (Oxford and New York: Oxford University Press, 2008)

Weissman, D., Ambuel, B. and Hallanbeck, J. 'Pain Management Case Studies: Adapted from Improving End-of-Life Care. A Resource Guide for Physician Education' (3rd edition) (2004), http://www.eperc.mcw.edu/Educational%20Materials/Case_studies/Case%20 Studies-Pain.doc [accessed 24 August 2009]

Woods, S. *Death's Dominion: Ethics at the End of Life* (Berkshire: McGraw-Hill, 2007)

Woodward, P.A. (ed.), *The Doctrine of Double Effect: Philosophers Debate a Controversial Moral Principle* (Notre Dame, IN: University of Notre Dame Press, 2001)

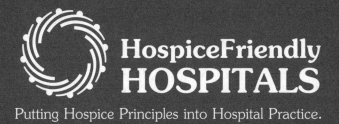

HospiceFriendly HOSPITALS

Putting Hospice Principles into Hospital Practice.

Module 6

The Ethics of Life-Prolonging Treatments (LPTs)

Module 6 Contents

Page

Module 6 The Ethics of Life-Prolonging Treatments (LPTs)

1. Module 6 Key Points

1.1 Advance care planning (ACP):

is at the centre of efforts to promote patient-centred care. ACP offers choice and respects the right of persons to consent to or refuse treatment and care offered. At present, legislation in Ireland covering advance care plans such as advance directives is not available, though in 2009 the Law Reform Commission published a report recommending that provisions be put in place to recognise validly drawn up advance directives. Nothing in ACP can authorise a health professional to do anything that is illegal.

1.2 Withholding and withdrawing LPTs:

such as ventilators, dialysis machines, chemotherapy and the sophisticated technology of the intensive care unit are ethically and legally accepted practices that should ideally be specified in advance care plans or directives.

1.3 Withholding a particular treatment:

for a particular patient is generally viewed as morally justified if the treatment is considered futile (without benefit) or unnecessarily burdensome. It is often recommended that decisions by a healthcare team to withhold life-supporting treatment require the consent of the patient and/or the patient's family. However, such a viewpoint about the obligation to achieve consent of patient and/or family is contested. This would especially be the case when the treatment under consideration is, on the basis of clinical evidence, deemed futile. However, where conversation with patient and/or family is pursued, an essential element in that conversation is that it must provide information on the nature of the treatment under consideration, the likely consequences of its use, and the benefits and/or burdens expected in the use of a particular LPT. This level of information is essential to help achieve patient and/or family understanding so that they are better positioned to give genuine and valid authorisation for refusal of LPTs.

1.4 Withdrawing treatment already begun:

is legally and ethically justified if it can be shown that the burdens of continued treatment for a particular patient outweigh the benefits. If a patient is competent and if they so wish, they should be central in the determination of what constitutes a 'burden'. Withdrawal is normally a decision taken with the patient and/or the patient's family through conversation about the patient's sufferings and prognosis. If a patient lacks capacity, then the health professional, usually in conjunction with any family or proxy, determines what is in the 'best interests' of the patient.

1.5 A common misconception on the topic:

of withholding and withdrawing LPTs is that it is morally more serious to stop an LPT than it is to withhold it. This perception is explained by the belief that 'stopping' a life support is an 'action' and 'withholding it' is only an 'omission'. Add to this perception the belief that 'actions' are much more serious than 'omissions' and we can see how misunderstandings occur. However, omitting a therapy can be morally just as serious as any action taken in treating a patient. Whether something is an act or an omission is never adequate to determine the morality of the action.

1.6 Judgements of 'futility':

of treatments in end-of-life care are part of everyday life, especially in ICU settings. Doctors have come to accept patients' rights to refuse treatment yet they have increasingly encountered patients, or more commonly the families of incompetent patients, demanding treatment that the health professionals judge to be futile.

2. Module 6 Definitions

2.1 Advance Care Planning (ACP):

is a process of discussion between an individual, their care providers and often those close to them about their values and preferences for ongoing healthcare. This process may lead to formulation of an advance directive, an advance decision to refuse treatment or the appointment of a personal proxy to help interpret a person's advance directive preferences.

2.2 Artificial Nutrition and Hydration (ANH):

is a term commonly used in medicine to refer to methods for preventing or treating malnutrition and dehydration where a patient has a problem taking fluids or food orally. ANH requires invasive procedures supplied through the patient's nose and throat (nasogastric tube), veins (IV line), stomach (gastrostomy), intestine (jejunostomy) or major vessel into the heart (hyper-alimentation). ANH is ethically controversial. Viewpoints differ about whether ANH is a form of universal human care and so always morally obligatory or whether it can be considered an optional treatment based on a benefit–burden judgement.

2.3 Cardiopulmonary Resuscitation (CPR):

is a group of treatments used when someone's heart and/or breathing stops. CPR was developed as a treatment intervention for cases of sudden unexpected cardiac or respiratory arrest. CPR is used in an attempt to restart the heart and breathing. It may consist of mouth-to-mouth breathing; chest compression, bag-and-mask positive-pressure ventilation, intubation and defibrillation. Electric shock and drugs are also frequently used to stimulate the heart.

2.4 Do Not Resuscitate (DNR):

a DNR order may generally be described as a note primarily written and signed by a doctor but which could involve the patient, healthcare team and family, stating that in certain circumstances should the patient suffer from cardiopulmonary failure, cardiopulmonary resuscitation (CPR) should not be attempted. Such an order is only relevant to not attempting CPR and not to the withholding of any other treatment.

2.5 Euthanasia:

is a deliberate act or omission whose primary intention is to end another person's life. Literally, it means a gentle or easy death but it has come to mean a deliberate intervention by one person with the clear intention of ending the life of another. This is often described as 'mercy killing' of people in pain with terminal illness. Decisions to withdraw or discontinue LPTs are not equivalent to euthanasia if they are validly authorised by a competent patient's consent or if a clinical decision is made that further life supports, based on all available evidence, would be futile – lacking in benefit for the patient and merely prolonging the dying process.

2.6 Life-Prolonging Treatment (LPT):

is any medical intervention, technology, procedure or medication that is administered to provide benefit for a patient and to forestall the moment of death. These treatments may include, but are not limited to, mechanical ventilation, artificial hydration and nutrition, cardiopulmonary resuscitation, haemodialysis, chemotherapy, or certain medications including antibiotics.

2.7 Physician-Assisted Suicide (PAS):

assisted suicide is the act of helping a person to die by providing the means for them to take their own life. An example of physician-assisted suicide is the act of giving a prescription or supply of a lethal dosage of drugs to a patient who has requested this. The doctor providing the lethal dosage thus enables a patient to end his or her own life.

2.8 Principle of Double Effect (PDE):

is an ethical rule which holds that effects of treatment which would be morally wrong if brought about intentionally are permissible if they are foreseen but unintended. The principle is often cited to explain why certain forms of care at the end of life which may risk and/or hasten death are morally permissible while others are not.

2.9 Principle of Proportionality:

states that whether or not a particular LPT for a patient is morally required should be evaluated in terms of its potential risks or burdens and probable benefits. If the risks or burdens to the patient outweigh the benefits, then the treatment is clinically inappropriate and not morally required. A fundamental ethical question in applying the principle concerns the issue of who takes part in any decision that determines the relative burdens and benefits of an LPT? If a patient has capacity and wishes to participate in decision making, then their input is important in any judgement about benefits and burdens of treatments proposed.

3. Module 6 Background

In times past, people died from minor illnesses because science had not yet developed medical cures. Today, an impressive range of medical therapies and life-support technologies offer not only amelioration of disease but, at times, a considerable extension of good quality of life. A key ethical challenge that these medical and technological advances present is to determine whether there is always an obligation to prolong human life simply because it is possible to do so.

In *The Patient as Person* (1970) Paul Ramsey claims that there are limits to our moral obligations to sustain life. Questions arise such as the following:

> *Must a terminal cancer patient be urged to undergo major surgery for the sake of a few months' palliation? What of fragmented creatures in deep and prolonged coma from severe brain damage, whose spontaneous cerebral activities have been reduced to those arising from the brainstem but who can be maintained 'alive' for years by a combination of artificial activators and by nourishment? Is there no end to the doctor's vocation to maintain life until the matter is taken out of his hands?* (Ramsey, 1970, p.115)

Admittedly, new treatments often benefit patients, restoring them to well-functioning lives. However, such treatments can also be used in situations where they may be neither a benefit to, nor wanted by, patients. Once pneumonia was an 'old man's best friend' and was one way that nature ended a life that had become debilitated. Now the technology of LPTs brings new ethical decisions to decide when such technology is warranted and respectful of patient autonomy. In considering decisions to prolong life, one is also considering postponing the dying process. If decisions about the use of LPTs are made without attempting to understand the values and preference of patients in this regard, then such use of LPTs may be imprudent, inhumane and certainly unethical in failing to respect the patient's own views of what should happen.

3.1 Autonomy and its Limits

In most European jurisdictions, it is well established that a patient with capacity has an unequivocal right to refuse medical treatment. This right of refusal is ethically defended by the principle of respect for patient self-determination or autonomy. Such a principle recognises that people have a right to act freely according to a self-chosen set of values and plan of life (see Module 4). This right to refuse treatment imposes limits on medical interventions and curtails judgements of clinicians to provide LPTs. Patients may request that a particular treatment not be given or, if it is already in place, that it should be withdrawn. The cases in this module illustrate this point.

Refusals by patients can be stressful for doctors and nurses, especially if their own judgement would indicate a contrary decision to that given by the patient. However, it is generally accepted that unless health professionals have concerns about a patient's capacity or consent, they should respect these refusals even contrary to their expertise, their best judgement and their emotional response.

Autonomy has its limits too. In law and to a great extent in ethics, the principle of autonomy confers mainly a negative right, a right to non-interference as explained in Modules 3 and 4. If patient autonomy were interpreted as conferring a positive right to treatment, this could entitle individuals to any requested treatment while ignoring medical advice and judgement and ignoring alternative claims for scarce healthcare resources (Gedge, Giacomini and Cook, 2007). A patient's request for LPT does not have to be granted if health professionals judge the request to be without benefit for this patient in this particular condition. In brief, the clinician does not have to grant what he/she judges 'futile treatment'. However, it is important that informative conversation with any competent patient be offered to ensure understanding of why a clinician refusal is given. Such communication is also an important opportunity to give hope to the patient and/or the family that a medical refusal of the patient's request for an LPT or other therapy does not mean that they will be abandoned by health professionals or left without optimal palliative care.

3.2 Advance Care Planning (ACP)

Advance Care Planning (ACP) has become the gold standard for patient-centred care. The ACP might include an advance statement of wishes and preferences (Advance Directive), and/or an advanced decision to refuse treatment (ADRT) in a predefined potential future situation. The ACP may also include the appointment of a personal-proxy representative who would interpret the stated wishes of a patient when/if they lose capacity. This personal representative is not currently part of an Enduring Power of Attorney in Irish legislation but could be an informal provision requested by a patient and/or their family. ACP has been strongly recommended by numerous societies and medical and nursing colleges. National UK guidelines published by the Royal College of Physicians (2009) state the role of ACP in achieving the ethical objective of patient-centred care.

At the core of current health and social care are efforts to promote patient-centred care, offer choice and the right to consent to or refuse treatment and care offered. This can be difficult to achieve when an individual has lost capacity – the ability to make one's own, informed decision. ACP may help in such scenarios. (Royal College of Physicians, 2009, p.2)

The objective of encouraging the use of ACP is not yet matched with reality in the uptake. In many countries, most deaths in intensive care are preceded by a decision to withdraw or withhold life support. However, clinicians, sometimes in conjunction with families, generally make the decisions about life support in intensive care as most patients are too ill to participate. Unfortunately, research indicates that few patients have ever discussed their life-support preferences with a family member or their family doctor. This means that decisions by proxy or surrogate decision makers about end-of-life care and use of life supports may not accurately reflect patients' wishes (Way, Back and Curtis, 2002).

3.3 Goals of Care

If healthcare decision making is to be truly patient-centred and respectful of a patient's wishes, then the goals of care must be clarified. The conversations toward patient consent discussed above are an essential part of establishing the goals of care. In fact, decisions about futility or starting or withholding life supports are impossible, in any case, without defining what the goals of caring for a patient are. It is necessary to consider such questions as: Should the focus be on pursuing curative therapies? On prolonging life? On palliating symptoms?

Determining the goals of care needs to consider the stage of a patient's disease or prognosis and uncertainties related to this. What are the realistic treatment options and, very importantly, does the patient understand what these options are? What are the personal hopes, values and understandings of the decision maker and the patient? The goals of care for any patient are not set in stone. They are dynamic and can change rather quickly. Ongoing reassessment of goals and ongoing documentation is necessary to ensure quality of care that is clinically judged feasible and in keeping with the particular patient's preferences.

4. Central Issues and Concepts in Decisions about LPTs

The moral concepts that are discussed in this section are guiding concepts in the process of making decisions at end of life. In the discussion of the concepts, readers may notice that there are certain recurring insights that reinforce elements of moral reasoning.

4.1 Starting and Stopping LPTs

Is the decision to stop an LPT morally more serious than the decision not to start an LPT? Health professionals sometimes feel morally uneasy about stopping a treatment that has been started. What explains this unease? In part, it is because stopping a treatment or therapy seems to 'feel' like 'killing' the patient. Stopping a treatment seems more akin to an active move that will certainly have consequences. In contrast, not starting a therapy or treatment seems more acceptable, apparently because it involves an omission rather than an action. Health professionals may believe that decisions to stop treatments are more momentous and consequential than decisions not to start them. Stopping a respirator, for example, seems to cause a person's death, whereas not starting the respirator does not seem to have this direct causal role. In fact, both actions and omissions can have a causal role in a patient's demise.

> If we adopt the view that treatment, once started, cannot be stopped, or that stopping requires much greater justification than not starting, then it is likely this view will have serious adverse consequences. Treatments might be continued for longer than is optimal for the patient, even to the point where it is causing positive harm with little or no compensating benefit. An even more troubling wrong occurs when a treatment that might save life or improve health is not started because the healthcare personnel are afraid that they will find it very difficult to stop the treatment if, as is fairly likely, it proves to be of little benefit and greatly burdens the patient. Fear of being unable to stop treatment can lead to failure to treat. Ironically, if there is any call to draw a moral distinction between withholding and withdrawing, it generally cuts the opposite way from the usual formulation: greater justification ought to be required to withhold than to withdraw treatment. (**President's Commission, 1983: 75–6**)

Morally speaking, then, in some circumstances it may be more serious to withhold than to withdraw treatments. It may be highly uncertain whether a particular treatment will have positive effects before it has been tried. Therefore, if we decide not to start a treatment for a particular patient who is not imminently dying, we may be losing the opportunity to glean evidence of patient response – perhaps even improvement from the treatment.

If a trial of therapy makes clear that it is not helpful to the patient, this is actual evidence (rather than mere surmise) to support stopping because the therapeutic benefit that earlier was a possibility has been found to be clearly unobtainable. (President's Commission, 1983: 76).

Feelings of reluctance about withdrawing treatments are understandable but 'not starting' and 'stopping' can both be justified depending on the circumstances of a particular case.

We conclude that the distinction between withholding and withdrawing is morally untenable and can be morally dangerous. Decisions about beginning or ending treatment should be based on considerations of the patient's rights and welfare, and, therefore, on the benefits and burdens of the treatment, as judged by a patient or authorised surrogate.
(Beauchamp and Childress, 2001, p.122)

4.2 Ordinary and Extraordinary Treatment

A Spanish Dominican theologian, Franciso De Vitoria (1486–1546), offered the first explicit treatment from the Catholic tradition about one's obligation to prolong life by providing food and medicinal drugs. However, it was Domingo Bañez (1528–1604) who introduced the terms 'ordinary' and 'extraordinary' into the discussion of morally obligatory and morally optional means of preserving life. In a short time after this terminology was introduced, the distinction became firmly established in both the Catholic moral tradition and secular contexts of medical practice. This distinction still operates today and is often used as a rule of thumb by health professionals.

4.2.1 Ordinary Means

Ordinary means are all medicines, treatments and operations which offer a reasonable hope of benefit and which can be obtained and used without excessive expense, pain, or other inconvenience. Such treatments would normally be considered morally obligatory. A medical treatment, usually considered ordinary, such as antibiotics or medically assisted nutrition and hydration, might be judged extraordinary for an individual because it will be ineffective or without benefit given the person's poor medical condition and dismal prognosis. The immanence of dying can render ordinary therapies extraordinary. The goal then moves to palliative care and accompanying the dying (Panicola, 2001, p.18).

4.2.2 Extraordinary Means

Extraordinary means are all medicines, treatments and operations which cannot be obtained and used without excessive expense, pain or other inconvenience or which, if used, would not offer a reasonable hope of benefit.

In conclusion, one is normally morally required to use only ordinary means – according to circumstances of persons, places, times and cultures: that is, means that do not involve any grave burden. Ordinary means must also give reasonable hope of benefit to a particular patient.

In the twentieth century it was the American Jesuit theologian Gerald Kelly (1902–1964) who studied the Catholic tradition on one's moral responsibility in end-of-life decisions. It is revealing that when clarifying the position, Kelly prefaced it by saying that ordinary and extraordinary means are always to be understood in terms of the patient's duty to submit to various kinds of therapeutic measures. (Kelly, 1950, p.550). The point here is that the interpretation of what treatments are ordinary or extraordinary, obligatory or optional is always patient-specific. There are no lists of treatments that are labelled 'ordinary' or 'extraordinary'. It is how proposed treatments are assessed vis-à-vis a particular patient that makes the judgement difficult. Kelly's emphasis is that the role of the patient in such decision making is primary. The reason for this emphasis is that, traditionally, the Catholic moral teaching on end-of-life decisions gives authority first to patients in decision making, then family members and finally health professionals.

4.2.3 Clinically Difficult Judgements

The concepts of ordinary and extraordinary treatment are indicators to be considered in making decisions but still rely firmly on the understanding and judgement of health professionals and patients where appropriate. While these concepts have a long tradition, they cannot be viewed as a facile method for determining precisely which means are obligatory and which optional. The determination of treatment obligations is clinically difficult in concrete cases. The reason for the difficulty is that included in the definitions of the concepts are several external factors, specifically relevant to a particular patient, that need to be considered, such as: circumstances of medical and personal information available, value considerations about benefits and burdens, information gleaned from available advance directives.

The distinction between ordinary and extraordinary means of treatment does not remove disagreements. The differences of interpretation are especially apparent on the issue of prolonging lives of patients with the use of artificial nutrition and hydration (ANH). These disagreements persist today, as we see in the discussions of ANH in case 6.5 below. On the topic of ANH in particular, a consensus is lacking among the general public, religious leaders and health professionals. It remains a matter open for discussion (Panicola, 2001, pp.20–1).

4.3 Principle of Proportionality

The principle of proportionality is a central principle when considering whether or not to utilise an LPT with a particular patient.

> *In clarifying goals, health professionals in conversation with patients or their proxies have the sensitive task of determining the benefits or burdens of procedures or treatments. This task requires a direct application of the proportionality principle. The proportionality principle states that a medical treatment is ethically mandatory to the extent that it is likely to confer greater benefits than burdens upon the patient.* (**Lesage and Portenoy, 2001, p.122**)

The text just quoted needs qualification: a medical treatment might be judged ethically required unless a competent patient has refused the treatment. The right of self-determination of a competent patient to refuse a medical treatment is a fundamental ethical value in Ireland, even if a clinician judges the treatment necessary to save the patient's life (see Module 3 and Module 4).

The principle of proportionality requires that the decision process about treatments should follow the general rule to maximise benefit and avoid undue burden. In conjunction with the ordinary/extraordinary distinction, this principle is widely cited as a moral rule of thumb as the basis for decision making about withholding or withdrawing LPTs.

4.3.1 Benefits and Burdens

While the principle of proportionality seems clear or perhaps self-evident, what is not obvious is that the patient with capacity should have a voice in determining (according to their values) what should be understood as a 'benefit' and what constitutes a 'burden' (General Medical Council, 2009).

If a benefit must accrue to one for a medical treatment to be considered morally obligatory, what constitutes a benefit? A holistic understanding of benefit means that one views the human person as a physical, psychological, social and spiritual being.

> *In the medical context, a treatment is considered beneficial if it restores one's health, relieves one's pain, improves one's physical mobility, returns one to consciousness, enables one to communicate with others and so on.* (**Panicola, 2001, pp.22–3**)

A claim that an LPT offers no hope of benefit simply means that the goods for which one seeks medical therapy are not forthcoming from the therapy. An 'excessive burden' means that any benefits forthcoming from use of a therapy are outweighed significantly by the burdens. Given the holistic view of persons, it follows that burdens may also be spiritual, psychic, and economic as well as physiological.

This holistic understanding of benefit and burdens has not been endorsed by everyone because it is too demanding in specifying the results of treatments. The effect of the holistic view would be that more physically or mentally impaired patients might have treatments withheld.

4.3.2 Competence and Incompetence

Where competent patients are involved, making a concerted effort to try and understand how they interpret 'burdens' and 'benefits' demonstrates respect and commitment to shared decision making with the patient whose life is at stake (see Case 3 and Case 5 below). Coming to know how a patient understands 'benefits' and 'burdens' is not the result of a single conversation with the patient. A patient's judgement of what is beneficial or burdensome may change over time, when the patient's medical condition either improves or increases in severity. Similarly, the goals of care are not set in stone but may change with the patient's experience of their condition.

Where the patient is not competent, the process of clarifying goals involves a process of communication and consultation between the healthcare team and the family to determine if any input about patient preferences may be relevant for a decision. Few decisions are more momentous than those to withdraw or withhold a medical procedure that sustains life. In some cases it is morally unjustified for surrogates and clinicians to begin or continue a therapy knowing that it will produce a greater balance of suffering and pain for a patient who lacks the capacity to choose for or against such therapy. Taking cognisance of any advance directive the patient may have aids understanding of a patient's values and preferences. In brief, what is required if the patient lacks capacity is a decision conforming to the 'best interests' of the patient (Joyce and The British Psychological Society, 2007; See Module 3 and Module 4).

4.4 Killing and Letting Die

Many distinctions and rules about LPTs derive from the distinction between killing and letting die.

The killing–letting die distinction often underpins distinctions between:

    1) suicide and foregoing treatment and,
    2) euthanasia and so-called 'natural' death.

'Killing' and 'letting die' are terms often used in bioethics literature as if they are clear and undisputed in their meanings. However, these terms are vague and widely contested, as the extensive amount of literature on the topic testifies. The concepts are discussed briefly here because they often arise in the context of decisions about LPTs as well as public policy debates.

Clarification may help to dispel some misunderstandings about 'killing' and 'letting die' in treatment decisions at the end of life.

4.4.1 Conditions of Judgement

'Letting die' is generally acceptable in medicine where one or more of the following three conditions apply:

a. Patients or their chosen surrogates have validly refused an LPT. A valid authorisation to refuse an LPT alters the obligation of the health professional to treat.

b. A best interest judgement is made by the healthcare team in cases where a patient lacks capacity and where a valid surrogate may or may not be present to contribute to the decision.

c. An LPT is judged to be 'futile' because it yields no benefit for a particular patient and only postpones an imminent dying. The task of giving reasons for the 'futility' judgement and discussing the judgement with the patient and/or family is the responsibility of the healthcare team. This condition is the most contentious of the three. What if a competent patient or authorised surrogate does not accept the health professional's or team's futility determination? If a patient is competent and does not accept the futility judgement, then it is usually advisable to continue the LPT and hope to glean further evidence that it is without benefit (see discussion of Futility below).

In these circumstances (a–c), letting a patient die (following a decision to withhold or withdraw LPTs) is normally considered legally and morally acceptable. If none of the three conditions above are satisfied, then letting a patient die following withdrawal of treatment may involve negligence and be a form of unjustified killing.

In conclusion: Valid authorisation by a patient, validly designated surrogate, or a reasoned argument from health professionals supporting a judgement of futility are conditions that morally justify a clinical decision to forego an LPT or to stop a treatment already begun.

> *Although the shortening of the patient's life is one foreseeable result of an omission, the real purpose of the omission was to relieve the patient of a particular procedure that is of limited usefulness to the patient or unreasonably burdensome for the patient and the patient's family or caregivers. This kind of decision should not be equated with a decision to kill or with suicide.*
> (O'Rourke and Norris, 2001, p.204)

Withholding LPTs without valid authorisation that result in a patient dying can be both as intentional and as immoral as actions that involve direct interventions to bring about death (and both can be forms of killing). Everything depends on other elements in the case and not whether the withholding or stopping of LPTs are omissions or actions.

The importance of 'valid authorisation' in assessing the morality of decisions at the end of life will be discussed below under Further Discussion. Suffice for now to conclude that the distinction between letting die and killing often suffers from vagueness and moral confusion.

- 'Letting die' is not always morally justified by saying it is an 'omission' of treatment.
- Neither is 'killing' always morally unjustified by saying it is an 'action' taken by the health professional to bring about death.

Nothing about either killing or allowing to die entails judgements about actual wrongness or rightness, or about the beneficence or non-maleficence of the action.

Rightness and wrongness depend on the merit of the justification underlying the action, not on the type of action it is.

Neither killing nor letting die, therefore, is wrongful per se. Accordingly, a judgement that an act of either killing or letting die is justified or unjustified requires that we know something else about the act besides these characteristics. We may need to know about the actor's motive (is it benevolent or malicious?), the patient's or surrogate's request, or the act's consequences.

These additional factors will allow us to place the act on a moral map and make a normative judgement about it. In short, whether letting die is justified and whether killing is unjustified are matters in need of analysis and argument, not matters that medical tradition and legal prohibition have adequately resolved. (Beauchamp and Childress, 2001, pp.141–2)

It is increasingly clear that laws and policies about end-of-life decision making are often vague and unclear because of the confusions discussed above about acts and omissions, killing and letting die. The discussion above is meant to clarify the ethical nature of these distinctions and is not making claims about the law (see Module 3 and Module 4).

4.5. Quality of Life Judgements

Thus far in these discussions, considerable weight is given to quality of life judgements in deciding whether treatments are ordinary or extraordinary, optional or obligatory, proportionate or disproportionate. The central premise in these discussions has been:

When quality of life is sufficiently low and an intervention is likely to produce more harm or burdens than benefits for the patient, it is morally justified to withhold or withdraw treatment. But such judgements require evidence based and defensible criteria of burdens and benefits in order not to reduce quality of life to arbitrary judgements of personal preference and the patient's social worth. (Beauchamp and Childress, 2001, p.136)

This latter point from Beauchamp and Childress is pivotal in understanding decisions based on estimated quality of life. It is also fundamental to objections to quality of life judgements. What worries all opponents of quality of life positions is that the view appears to define and prescribe the 'good life' in terms of the qualities necessary to live a minimal human and worthwhile existence. If this is an accurate reading of quality of life views, then the position becomes entrapped within the 'exclusionary' use of quality of life judgements. The lack of certain valued qualities in a patient's life becomes a way of positively excluding potential patients from the normal standards of medical and moral treatment (Walter, 2004, p.1391).

There is an apprehension and fear that decisions based on quality of life considerations could descend into an appraisal of a patient's place in a society, or discriminatory assessment of a patient's ethnicity or intelligence, etc. It is fundamentally important that the involvement of patients and/or authorised surrogates in decisions about LPTs can help to address concerns that clinical decisions in assessing benefits and burdens may discriminate against some patients.

Decisions based on quality of life considerations are judgements about what the likely outcomes (benefits or burdens) are for a patient if a particular treatment is given. It is impossible to determine what will benefit a patient without presupposing some quality of life standard and some conception of the life the patient will likely live after a medical intervention

Accurate medical diagnosis and prognosis are indispensable, but a judgement about whether to use life prolonging measures rests unavoidably on the anticipated quality of life, not merely on a standard of what is medically indicated. (Beauchamp and Childress, 2001, p.137)

Those who oppose quality of life judgements often propose a 'sanctity of life' position that emphasises the inherent dignity of every human being regardless of ability or status.

4.6 Sanctity of Life

The sanctity of life principle is associated with the major world religions. In the Christian tradition, the first book of the Bible portrays human life as having an intrinsic value independently of the individual's own view of it. Each life is viewed as unique, on loan, made in the image of God with an unrepeatable opportunity to praise God. Similarly, in the Islamic tradition, the Koran (Al-An'am, Verse 151) states that human life has intrinsic value, that it is made sacred by Allah. It is a divine trust, created to discover God's work and serve God's plan.

Historically, the sanctity of life position holds that the value of human life is not dependent upon its being valued by the individual themselves or by others or by the presence of certain functional capacities such as relationality or rationality. On this view, if the valuing of human life requires certain kinds of capacities, then their absence (for example, with patients who are considered to be in a persistent vegetative state) implies a different (lesser) kind of valuing. Conditions placed on the respect owed human beings results in an ethics of exclusion based on certain properties that some persons may lack through no fault of their own.

4.6.1 Challenges to the Sanctity of Life Position

A first challenge to the sanctity of human life commitment claims that it is intrinsically idolatrous. In talking of the 'sanctity' of human life this view overstates the nature of human essence in its insistence that human life is sacred and this is an attribute reserved only for God. Adherents of sanctity of life dispute this interpretation and claim that sanctity of human life only means that humans are set apart by God and are distinct in the created order. However, this response means that the special status attributed to humankind still requires a theological foundation and such religious reliance will not persuade those of different or no religious faith.

A second challenge to the sanctity of life view is the charge of medical vitalism:

> …the notion that all means must be utilized to keep a human being alive in the face of death. Because human life has incalculable worth a commitment is required to keep patients alive at all costs. Many critics of the sanctity of life perspective have assumed that vitalism is an inherent part of the tradition (Hollinger, 2004, p.1404).

However, those who propose the sanctity of life position reject vitalism as part of their position. They claim that there is a natural cycle to human life that must be accepted.

4.6.2 Inalienable Human Rights

A respect for the inherent dignity of human persons central to a sanctity of life view also supports communal life in society.

> *If laws were permitted to embody the idea that in some circumstances life loses its worth, or that some people lack sufficient worth to have their lives protected, individuals would no longer enjoy equal protection of the law so far as their lives are concerned.* (Hollinger, 2004, p.1404)

Others argue that religious arguments are not required to defend belief in the 'sanctity of human life'.

> *It is enough simply to say that all human lives are deserving of equal respect not because of what they have to offer or have offered or potentially will offer, but because they exist. The notion of inalienable human rights attributes force to the value of human life with the assertion that it needs no justification. This is the primary merit of the sanctity of life ethic – that a life requires no justification.* (Schwartz, Preece and Hendry, 2002, p.116)

The sanctity of human life position emphasises that medical termination of life does require justification. In this sense the principle acts as a powerful bulwark against the devaluing of human life. Article 3 of the United Nations Declaration of Human Rights asserts simply that: 'Everyone has the right to life, liberty and security of person' (Schwartz, Preece and Hendry, 2002, p.116).

4.6.3 Compatibility of Quality of Life and Sanctity of Life

If one removes a religious foundation as a requirement for acceptance of the sanctity of life view, then its essential meaning is compatible with quality of life judgements.

Human life needs no justification if we agree to the commitment that all human lives are accorded equal respect not because of what they can offer to society but because they simply exist. This respect for the dignity of human beings is harmonious with the belief that quality of life judgements are necessary when making decisions about LPTs. Those quality of life judgements deliberate on the possible efficacy or futility of LPTs in the life of the patient. Health professionals, in company with patients or authorised surrogates, can acknowledge when further life supports are greater burdens than benefits for a particular patient. This acknowledgment, in unison with expert palliative care, allows patients to achieve the dignity of a good dying.

5. Futility

Judgements of 'futility' of treatments in end-of-life care are part of everyday life, especially in ICU settings. Physicians have come to accept patients' rights to refuse treatment yet they have increasingly encountered patients, or more commonly the families of incompetent patients, demanding treatment that the clinicians judge to be futile.

Historically, the debate about what constitutes 'futile' treatments began with decisions relating to the stopping of cardiopulmonary resuscitation, but with increasing medical technology it has expanded to other forms of life-prolonging care. Paradigms of futile care often involve efforts to resuscitate a patient who is imminently dying as well as life-prolonging intervention for patients in a persistent vegetative state. Other paradigms include the use of aggressive therapy such as surgery, chemotherapy and haemodialysis for patients with advanced terminal illness and without a realistic expectation of improvement. Even the use of less invasive treatments such as intravenous hydration or antibiotics in near-moribund patients might be considered 'futile' treatment.

The impression may be that such judgements about futility are based on clinical criteria and can result in objective decisions that provide a certain and warranted basis for discontinuing further LPTs. The discussion that follows indicates that this is not the case.

5.1 Debates on the Meaning of 'Futility'
A central issue in the futility debate has been how to define futility.

> *Some try to narrowly restrict it [futility] to only those treatments known with certainty not to achieve their goal. The attempt is to eliminate value judgements from futility determinations and to make them only an empirical matter about which the physician should be expert. But others have pointed out that it is not possible to eliminate all value judgements. Others have more broadly characterised futility to include cases where the probability of benefit is considered too low, or the size of benefit too small, to warrant the burdens of treatment.* (Brock, 2004, p.1418)

'Futility' judgements are typically used to express a combined value judgement and scientific judgement. There is a considerable subjective element in judgements that further treatment is 'futile' – precisely because decisions that weigh up benefits and burdens are not based on rocket science. It is easy to see how clinicians and patients might disagree about whether or when further treatment is beneficial for improving one's function or one's quality of life. The value judgement seems in most cases appropriately left to the patient or surrogate, not the physician.

In some situations a physician can determine that a treatment is 'medically' futile or non-beneficial because it offers no reasonable hope of recovery or improvement or because the person is permanently unable to experience any benefit. In other cases the utility and benefit of a treatment can only be determined with reference to the person's subjective judgement about his or her overall well-being. As a general rule, a person should be involved in determining futility in his or her case. In exceptional circumstances such discussions may not be in the person's best interests. (Canadian Nurses Association, Canadian Healthcare Association, Canadian Medical Association and Catholic Health Association of Canada, 1999, p.4)

In discussing 'judgements of futility', it should not be people's lives that are judged futile. In making judgements of futility, a health professional (often in company with patient or family) is not (or should not be) making a value judgement about the significance or worth of this person's life. This point is most important to stress with family members where, for example, a do not resuscitate (DNR) has been signed. Respect for the patient's worth and concern to protect their dignity means that, if a patient has a DNR in their chart, they need reassurance that all pain management and compassionate care will continue.

5.2 Evolution of the Concept of Futility

What is beyond doubt is that the notion of futility is disputed and that it is very much a concept in evolution. For over twenty years now 'futility' has been debated in the hope that a clear and determinate set of criteria might be formulated that would help doctors make decisions about providing or withholding LPTs. The concept of medical futility surfaced in the 1980s largely in response to concerned families who insisted on LPTs for their loved ones while caregivers or health professionals deemed these treatments to be inappropriate. Clinicians felt providing futile treatment was cruel while studies of patients and families consistently stated that such care was valued and wanted (Burns and Truog, 2007).

The debate on 'futility' can be divided into three segments or three generations that mark the evolution of the concept.

1. A first generation was taken up with efforts to define futility in terms of definite clinical criteria. This process seemed guaranteed to give objectivity and certainty to futility judgements. However, these efforts failed because they recommended 'limitations to care based on value judgements for which there is no consensus among a significant segment of society' (Burns and Truog, 2007).

2. The second generation in the debates on futility offered a procedural approach that gave power to hospitals, utilising their ethics committees, to decide whether interventions

demanded by families were futile. However, this procedural approach failed as it seemed to try and distance the decision from health professionals by transferring it to ethics committees. Failure also resulted because it gave hospitals authority to make decisions that health professionals desired but any national consensus on what is 'beneficial treatment' remained under intense debate.

3. Burns and Truog (2007) predict the emergence of a third generation that should focus primarily on negotiation at the bedside and ongoing communication. This third view places importance on developing and deepening understanding between patients, families and professionals. In addition, it acknowledges that conflict can surface among health professionals if families demand what is judged futile treatment and wish 'all that can be done to be done'. While considerable stress can then be experienced by healthcare teams, Burns and Truog advise that, rather than initiate an adversarial encounter with the patient and/or their family, the health professionals should support each other to help deal with the stress of 'futility' judgements and ensuing conflicts (2007, p.1992).

5.3 Divergent Views about Futility Judgements

There are diverse approaches to making judgements that certain kinds of treatments are futile.

1. One position thinks that ambiguity is fostered by the use of the term to refer to both quantitative and qualitative components.

Those who question the use of futility judgements to limit the treatment options offered to patients often argue that what effects are deemed desirable or beneficial may depend on whether the patient's or the clinician's perspective is adopted. They express concern that assertions of futility may camouflage judgements about the comparative worth of patients' lives. It must be acknowledged that even seemingly objective claims about the likelihood that an intervention will produce some effect are tinged with uncertainty; for some patients, a vanishingly small probability of success will be viewed as preferable to foregoing the treatment.
(Centre for Bioethics, 1997b, p.5)

2. A second position about futility debates claims that it would be more helpful if we just abandoned the term 'futility' in preference for more concrete and precise descriptions of a clinical situation being considered. The amount of divergence in subjective, and even apparently objective, clinical estimates of futility should suggest that the resulting confusion can be remedied by more accurate accounts of specific situations where treatment seems contraindicated because earlier efforts at therapy indicate that no further patient benefit is expected.

The term 'futility' is used to cover many situations of predicted improbable outcomes, improbable success, and unacceptable benefit–burden ratios. This situation of competing concepts and great ambiguity suggests that we should generally avoid the term 'futility' in favor of more precise language. *(*Beauchamp and Childress, 2001, p.134)

3. A third area of diverging perspectives pertains to the obligations of health professionals to consult patients and/or their families in making decisions about the use of LPTs, most especially where there is clinical agreement that a particular therapy would be futile for the particular patient. Some clinicians and commentators on the topic of 'futility' judgements do not agree that a clinician must respond positively to a patient's insistence on a treatment that is judged to be without any discernible benefit. The argument is given that if a treatment is futile for a particular patient, this fact changes the doctor's obligations to seek agreement from patients or surrogates. Health professionals may not even have an obligation to discuss such a treatment as if it were a realistic option.

The physician is not morally required to provide the treatment (and in some cases may be required not to provide the treatment) and may not even be required to discuss the treatment [...] Increasingly hospitals are adopting policies aimed at denying therapies that physicians judge to be futile, especially after trying them for a reasonable period of time [...] respect for the autonomy of patient or authorized surrogates is not a trump that allows them alone to determine whether a treatment is required or is futile. (Beauchamp and Childress, 2001, p.134)

A recent study in one Dublin hospital seems to give credence to the above viewpoint that communication with patient and family is not always required when deciding on the use of LPTs that are considered futile. The research focussed on communication with families of patients in intensive care. The study of end-of-life care in one Dublin hospital by Collins, Phelan, Marsh et al. (2006) showed that the involvement of families with clinicians when making end-of-life decisions was low. Overall, almost a quarter of patients' families studied were not involved in the decision to limit life-prolonging therapy. Patients' input in the decision making was not discussed because all of the patients whose end-of-life condition was discussed lacked capacity.

The Collins et al. (2006) study explains that when a clinical judgement is made that further therapy or treatment would be futile because the patient is unresponsive to maximum medical therapy, health professionals tend not to consult a family about the possibility of providing such a treatment or discontinuing the treatment. The explanation given was that where a clinical judgement is made of acute physiological futility, consultation with family would be redundant. One might add that consultation with family may not even be obligatory. If a family were consulted and insisted on continued futile treatment, clinicians would face a serious conflict of conscience in believing that they would then have to provide futile treatment that may well harm the patient (Collins et al., 2006, p.318; See Cases 1, 2 and 4 below).

6. Cases: Decision Making Involving the Use of LPTs

6.1 Case 1: When is Treatment Futile? – Do Everything You Can

Do Everything You Can

Ms R., a 52-year-old woman with severe rheumatoid arthritis and chronic immobility, was brought to the emergency department. Her health was poor, although stable, until the morning of admission when she became disoriented and lethargic. She was admitted to intensive care and put on a ventilator while being treated for septic shock secondary to decubitus ulcers and for acute renal failure. On the day after admission she required increasing doses of vasopressor drugs and developed acute respiratory distress syndrome. Some members of the intensive care team became increasingly concerned about the 'futile' care they felt they were providing. The patient's family requested that the medical team 'do everything' to keep her alive.

After several days of observation of Ms R. and following conversations with the family, an ICU clinician agreed to meet with them to explain that Ms R.'s underlying immune suppression and general health was such that she was most unlikely to recover from the progressive septic shock but if improvement were not possible, the aim and value was to ensure patient comfort.

The clinician was sensitive to the family's anxiety, sense of impending loss and fear of Ms R.'s impending death. At the conference the family was asked to say how they understood the patient's condition. The team learned from the conversation that Ms R. was known for her energy and readiness to take on all challenges. The family expressed an unrealistic optimism about her condition and genuinely believed (or wanted to believe) that Ms R. could recover to an earlier mobile and healthy self. Careful listening by the clinician and expressions of interest about the person of Ms R. reassured the family that this conversation was not just a formality to be quickly concluded.

The team continued in their efforts to help the family to adjust their hopes to more realistic care goals for Ms R. The family were reassured that they would have time to think everything over. Life support would continue as long as the family believed it was what Ms R. would want. After a few days, the family decided Ms R. would probably not want ongoing life support. Here the team took time to explain the process of withdrawing life support while being careful not to alarm the family about Ms R.'s ensuing pain. All drugs were stopped for Ms R. except morphine and lorazepam, which were titrated to comfort during terminal ventilator discontinuation. Ms R. would be unlikely to survive for more than an hour after withdrawal. The team asked the family about spiritual needs and the family requested a chaplain. This was provided before extubation began. The family and chaplain were at Ms R.'s. bedside when she died thirty minutes later. (Adapted from Way et al., 2002, pp.1342–5)

6.1.1 Discussion

Many deaths in intensive care occur after withholding or withdrawing life support. In ICU situations, the decisions are often made by health professionals and families since the patient is frequently too ill to participate. But conflict can arise due to disagreements among healthcare staff in ICU or disagreements about treatment decisions by family members.

Conflict surrounding decision-making in intensive care units is common. Conflict can arise about issues such as communication styles, interpersonal interactions, pain control as well as about treatment decisions […] The evidence on the best way to resolve conflicts suggests that communication, negotiation and consensus building are the most important tools.
(Way et al., 2002, p.1343)

In Case 1, there is consensus on the part of the healthcare team that further provision of treatments aimed at cure would be futile.

The case here illustrates a general rule of thumb in ICU care: When diagnosis and prognosis is unclear, it is preferable to commence treatment and keep the patient under observation. Before an LPT is started, it is not certain whether it will bring the hoped-for benefits to the patient. Once it has been tried and it becomes clear that it does not produce the benefits sought, clinical evidence exists to justify stopping therapy that did not exist for not starting the ventilator. The principle supports the use of time-limited trials of LPT, with the understanding that if the treatment does not prove to be beneficial it will be stopped.

Few decisions are more momentous than those to withhold or withdraw a medical procedure that sustains life. But, in some cases, it is unjustified for surrogates and clinicians to begin or to continue therapy knowing that it will produce a greater balance of pain and suffering for a patient incapable of choosing for or against such therapy.
(Beauchamp and Childress, 2001, pp.135–6)

When the team observed the progression of Ms R.'s. illness, they may have clearly realised that continued ventilator support and increasing vasopressor drugs served only to prolong the dying process. Their responsibilities now were to provide appropriate palliative care for Ms R.

Justified 'Allowing to Die'?

A clinical decision to intentionally withdraw an LPT is often construed as a doctor's 'letting die' rather than killing. The argument is that if the decision is validly authorised then it is morally justified. A valid authorisation can often transform what might be a maleficent act of killing into a nonmaleficent (and perhaps beneficent) act of allowing to die. Normally valid authorisation is provided by a competent patient who refuses or perhaps requests continued life-support assistance. Ms R. lacks capacity to decide for herself or provide authorisation for a decision. The team's effort to involve the family in assessing benefits and burdens of continuing ventilator support demonstrates attempts to achieve surrogate authorisation for the decision to discontinue ventilation and commence palliative care.

Assessing the burdens and benefits of further LPTs for Ms R. involves reasonable medical judgements and quality-of-life judgements:

> *We conclude that competent patients and authorized surrogates can use controlled quality-of-life considerations with medical input to legitimately determine whether treatments are optional or obligatory.* (Beauchamp and Childress, 2001, p.139)

Abandonment

In conversations with the family of Ms R. an important point was stressed throughout; if some treatments were to be discontinued because they lacked discernible benefit for the patient, good care and pain management would continue to be provided. For example, therapeutic sedation to ameliorate symptoms of breathlessness and anxiety are essential in end-of-life weaning from ventilator support.

Families often fear abandonment by health professionals once a patient is no longer seen as curable or as responsive to LPTs. Expert guidelines on caring for patients at the end of life emphasise the importance of not allowing the patient to feel abandoned especially when the care plan includes withdrawal of disease-modifying treatment (Cherny, Radbruch and The Board of the European Association for Palliative Care [EAPC], 2009, p.581; Lesage and Portenoy, 2001, p.125). Non-abandonment has been cited as a primary tenet of medicine and a key value in professionalism. Despite the professed importance of non-abandonment to end-of-life care, surveys show that patients and family caregivers still experience abandonment around the time of death (Back, Young, McCown, et al., 2009, p.474).

The family of Ms R. felt their concerns were heard. The team did not appear rushed in their conversations and the family appreciated knowing the now revised care plans for Ms.R. Most of all, the family felt relieved that they had not been pressured into accepting withdrawal of life support.

6.1.2 Suggested Professional Responsibilities

- Communicate with the family to help them to realistically understand the clinical condition of Ms R., including likely prognosis.

- Give time and provide a proper atmosphere of privacy for the family to digest the reality of Ms R.'s illness. In this context, be aware of imminent grieving of family.

- Document in case notes the basis for a judgement that further 'curative efforts' were deemed 'futile'. This includes clinical and quality of life judgements about burdens and benefits for the patient.

- In an effort to minimise distress for the family and patient, the healthcare team can show they are partners with the family in trying to make the right decision for Ms R. When relatives feel the team are partners in the decision, they may feel less marginalised and/or burdened by guilt.

- Provide understanding and reassurance for the family that all comfort needs and pain management of Ms R will be carefully provided for in the dying process.

- Make every effort to accommodate the religious perspective of the patient and family.

6.2 Case 2: DNR and Family Disagreement – When God Might Intervene

Case 2 presents a rather ordinary situation of advanced and complex illness in an elderly gentleman. His wishes have not been expressed and his family voice their serious concerns about the clinician's suggestion that they agree to a do not resuscitate (DNR) order for their father.

When God Might Intervene

Mr W. is 82 years old and has many serious medical problems, including ischemic heart disease, hypertension and diabetes mellitus. He has had a series of debilitating strokes that have left him severely disabled and unable to communicate his wishes. His health care providers feel that he would not benefit from resuscitation attempts if he were to suffer a cardiac arrest and suggest to his family that a DNR be placed on his chart.

The devout Christian family is quite upset and reject this suggestion. They can't see that continuing to live is any burden on them or their father. They believe that God could still heal their father and they accuse the health care providers of trying to 'play God'. They ask to see the hospital Chaplain. (Smith, RCSI Residency Programme case no.12, 2008, p.52)

6.2.1 Discussion

Normally, unless a specific order to the contrary (e.g. DNR) has been recorded on the person's health record by the responsible doctor or a valid patient Advance Directive, CPR is used as a standard intervention in virtually all cases of sudden cardiac or respiratory arrest.

What is a DNR Order?

A DNR order may generally be described as a note primarily written and signed by a doctor but which could involve the patient, healthcare team and family, stating that in certain circumstances should the patient suffer from cardiopulmonary failure, cardiopulmonary resuscitation (CPR) should not be attempted. Such an order is only relevant to not attempting CPR and not to the withholding of any other treatment.

What is Involved in CPR?

Cardiopulmonary resuscitation (CPR) was first developed as a treatment intervention for cases of sudden unexpected cardiac or respiratory arrest. CPR includes chest compression, bag-and-mask positive pressure ventilation, mouth-to-mouth resuscitation, ventilation, intubation and defibrillation. During CPR the chest is pressed on forcefully. Electric stimulation to the chest and special medicines may be used. This is usually done for 15 to 30 minutes. A tube may also be put through the mouth or nose into the lung. This tube is then connected to a breathing machine (American Academy of Family Physicians (AAFP), 2000).

Judging Disproportionate Means

While very aware of the grief experienced by the family, the doctor explains to the family that prolonging life with CPR would not benefit their father and the distress of the process itself is sometimes more cruel than compassionate. In the case of Mr W., health professionals have judged CPR inappropriate and are relying on their benefit–burden judgement known as the principle of proportionality discussed above.

> *It needs to be determined whether the means of treatment offered are proportionate to the prospects for patient improvement. To forego disproportionate means is not equivalent to suicide or euthanasia: it rather expresses acceptance of the human condition in the face of death.'*
> (Ashley and O'Rourke, 1997, p.419)

The family disagree. They cannot see what is so burdensome about continued life for their father. They might believe that prolonging their father's life benefits him because:

a. Recovery of awareness by Mr W. is remotely possible, perhaps by a miracle;
b. Their father is better off alive than dead.

Here, as in Case 1, it is essential that the healthcare team engage in conversation with Mr W.'s family. This is not only out of respect for the family who are wondering about Mr W.'s condition but the conversation also needs to ensure that the family understands the CPR procedure as realistically as possible. This understanding is seldom the case with families.

In their research with practitioners in Irish hospitals, Quinlan and O'Neill (2009) found that patients and families often lacked knowledge and understanding about active treatments mentioned. They didn't know what was meant by 'PEG feeding', 'subcut fluids', 'defibbing' and 'shocking hearts back to life' (Quinlan and O'Neill, 2009, p.36). It is easy to see how patients or families end up confused and are intimidated about asking 'what does this mean?' when hearing abbreviated jargon from doctors or nurses.

Guiding principles about CPR and DNRs recur in statements offered by international medical and nursing associations (British Medical Association [BMA], Resuscitation Council UK, and Royal College of Nursing [RCN], 2007; General Medical Council, 2009; New South Wales Department of Health, 2005; Royal College of Paediatrics and Child Health, 2004).

These guidelines all agree that health professionals find it difficult to discuss CPR with their patients and part of that difficulty is a result of the point made above that it is a complex procedure and very dependent on the precise clinical condition of the patient (O'Keefe, 2001).

Some patients may ask that CPR be attempted should they arrest, even if the clinical evidence suggests that, in their case, there is only a very small chance of success. Health professionals may doubt whether the risks and burdens associated with CPR are justified with such a small chance of success but the individual – if properly informed, and whose life is at stake – may be willing to accept that chance.

Research continues to show that patients are not adequately informed:

a. Most patients are not aware or knowledgeable of possible risks and adverse effects of CPR in order to make an informed decision about whether or not they would want CPR.

b. Many people – patients, families and even some health professionals – have unrealistic expectations about the likely success and potential benefits of CPR and lack detailed understanding of what is involved.

c. This failure of understanding makes it very difficult to achieve genuine informed consent to a DNR or to CPR in the event of cardiac arrest (BMA, Resuscitation Council UK, and RCN, 2007).

In the health professional–family conversation, it is important to find out whether the family understands what is actually involved in CPR, what likely outcomes can be anticipated, and what possible suffering might be involved for Mr W. if it is attempted.
The potential benefits and risks of CPR need to be discussed with the family.

The Benefits of CPR
For a patient with an advanced life-threatening illness who is dying, the single benefit of CPR is that it may defer dying. CPR may prolong life if it's done within 5 to 10 minutes of when the person's heart stopped beating or breathing stopped.

The Risks of CPR
Attempted CPR carries a risk of significant side effects (such as sternal fracture, rib fracture and splenic rupture) and most patients require either coronary care or intensive care treatment in the post-resuscitation period. If there is delay between cardiopulmonary arrest and the resuscitation attempt, there is a risk that the patient will suffer brain damage. Some

resuscitation attempts may be traumatic, meaning that death occurs in a manner the patient and people close to the patient would not have wished (Sheikh, 2001, p.7).

These full, graphic details of potential risks of CPR may not have to be provided to Mr W.'s family but, on the other hand, without some explanation, the family may have a very unrealistic perception or image of what CPR involves. A possible misunderstanding such as this can obstruct a decision that could 'benefit' Mr W.

> *Information should not be forced on unwilling recipients and if patients indicate that they do not wish to discuss CPR this should be respected. All of these efforts in attempting to discover if the patient wishes to discuss CPR as well as the outcome of these attempts should be documented.* (BMA, Resuscitation Council UK, and RCN, 2007, p.2)

Based on interviews and narratives of Irish hospital staff, such conversations with patients and families to provide helpful information and aid understanding are uncommon occurrences. Documentation of such decisions with the circumstances and reasoning for the decision noted is also uncommon. Certainly, patient records do not show evidence of such conversations aimed at discovering patient wishes (Quinlan and O'Neill, 2009, p.37). The Irish Ethicus data with intensive care patients and families show that documentation of end-of-life decision making is sparse. This was especially the case with respect to CPR (Collins et al., 2006, p.317).

Ethical and Legal Status of DNR in Ireland

> *As is the case with many other areas of medicine, there is a serious lack of ethical and legal certainty regarding DNR orders. There exist no Irish medical guidelines and there is neither legislation nor judicial wisdom to assist medical practitioners in this emotionally sensitive and legally uncertain area of medicine.* (Sheikh, 2001, p.4)

In the absence of policy guidelines or legislation it is not surprising that health professionals may decide to 'walk slowly' if a patient arrests and CPR is thought to be a futile therapy for that individual. But in the absence of policies or legislation, families also have little recourse if they believe that they have been overlooked in a decision to provide or withhold CPR. The following report explains why a policy is required:

> *Because for every person there comes a time when death is inevitable, it is essential to identify patients for whom cardiopulmonary arrest represents a terminal event in their illness and in whom attempted CPR is inappropriate. It is also essential to identify those patients who do not want CPR to be attempted and who competently refuse it.* (Sheikh, 2001, p.6)

In the Best interests of the Patient

When patients and their families are consulted, decisions about attempting CPR raise sensitive and potentially distressing issues for patients and people emotionally close to them. Initially it is most important to determine the competence or incompetence of patients who are deciding on DNR or CPR. When an incompetent person's wishes are not known, treatment decisions must be based on the person's best interests, as discussed above. This best interests judgement is not solely a clinical or legal judgement that lacks reference to the particular patient. Quite the contrary: 'best interests' -based decisions need to take into account:

a. The patient's known or ascertainable wishes, including information about previously expressed views, feelings, beliefs and values and whether those views might still be the same.

b. Information received from those who are significant in the person's life and who could help in determining his or her best interests.

c. Aspects of the person's culture and religion that would influence a treatment decision.

As well as:

d. The likely clinical outcome, including the likelihood of successfully re-starting the patient's heart and breathing for a sustained period, and the level of recovery that can realistically be expected after successful CPR.

e. The risks involved with treatment and non-treatment.

f. The patient's human rights, including the right to life and the right to be free from degrading treatment.

g. The likelihood of the patient experiencing severe pain or suffering as a result of the treatment.

CPR can also be viewed as harmful and offensive to the dignity of a patient. The explanation above of the potential 'risks' involved in CPR is translated into reality in this anonymised Irish case cited in Quinlan and O'Neill (2009).

I'm a nurse on the resuscitation team and, to this day, a case still bothers me. An 84-year-old gentleman with end stage chronic obstructive airway disease (COPD) was admitted at night by a medical registrar who had not discussed this man's case with her consultant and had not discussed it with the anaesthetic consultant to review this patient. The patient was on maximum medical treatment and home oxygen. He would not have benefitted from his heart being shocked nor will he benefit from being put on a life support machine because, with end stage COPD, he would never come off the life support machine.

This gentleman was very skeletal and he had a pigeon chest as well. I arrived at the scene the same time as the anaesthetist and the medical registrar who called me [...]

I asked: 'Is this gentleman for resuscitation?' 'Yes.' So we were going through with it and all his ribs were cracking as we were doing the procedure. I said: 'God, this is very unethical!' Has this been discussed with the gentleman or relatives? The registrar said: 'No.'

(Quinlan and O'Neill, 2009, p.31)

This decision to apply CPR is made without the consensus from the healthcare team. It also shows no effort to consult the family. It appears to be an unjustified decision to apply CPR since it was, on all the medical evidence, futile treatment. Finally, even a brief consideration of benefits and burdens of the LPT for this gentleman would show that CPR is not only proving to be a 'futile' treatment; it is also harmful – the burdens are overwhelming. Justification for this medical decision is wholly lacking. This case provides a good example for documentation of all decisions in patient records. If documentation were provided, it would have required the clinical team to reflect on their actions and see if any warrant for their decision could reasonably be provided.

6.2.2 Suggested Professional Responsibilities

- Given the difference of perspective that exists between the healthcare team and the family in Case 2, it is important to allow time to observe the progress of Mr W's condition and continue conversations among health professionals and family.

- The nature, benefits and risks of CPR as they apply to Mr W's situation should be explained to the family.

- The family should be reassured that a DNR decision applies solely to CPR. All other treatment and care which are appropriate, including palliative care, are not precluded and will not be influenced by a DNR decision.

- All the health professionals in the team and the family members should be clear that while they have a duty to protect life, they must also balance this value with the obligation not to subject the patient to inhuman or degrading treatment.

- Any decision that CPR will not be attempted for an incapacitated patient should be documented on the patient's records and details given of components that went into the 'best interests' judgement.

6.3 Case 3: Requesting Ventilator Withdrawal – 'My Life has Lost Value for Me'

Decisions to apply a ventilator are difficult and, often in the busy days in ICU, patients may be ventilated as a stop gap until further review of the case can be provided. Research in Irish hospitals indicates that health professionals question the decision to provide ventilation in cases where the patient is 'trying to die':

> At the moment, a gentleman is ventilated up in ICU. He has been diagnosed with Motor Neurone Disease. He's ventilated and sedated. I suppose if things had been reviewed at the time when he was diagnosed, he probably would not have been put on the ventilator. Now that we're there, he's trying to die and just can't die. That ventilator is keeping him alive up there. He took a turn on Friday and is now on his second syringe driver and the wishes of his wife are that he wouldn't suffer any more. ICU is very curative and proactive. That's a huge dilemma, a huge ethical dilemma really for that patient. At Christmas when he was able to talk he clearly said 'I don't want anything else.' (Quinlan and O'Neill, 2009, pp.33–4)

Difficult challenges for health professionals are particularly acute when active or 'aggressive' treatment may be provided even when it seems inappropriate.

> A patient might be end stage COPD, and they're on continuous oxygen nebulizers and not able to do any kind of movement and then when they come in to ICU, they're ventilated and end up with a tracheotomy and maybe full care at that stage. And then down the road often they die from an infection. (Quinlan and O'Neill, 2009, p.34)

The case of Katherine that follows tells the narrative of a patient with capacity to request the withdrawal of the ventilator required for her to live. She makes a quality of life judgement about her life prospects and chooses to discontinue ventilation. Katherine's judgement is that this life support is posing a greater burden than any benefit for a functioning life that she wishes to live.

'My Life has Lost Value for Me'

Katherine Lewis is a single, 40-year-old woman suffering from Guillain-Barre's syndrome, a painful neurological illness that leaves its sufferers paralysed for unpredictable lengths of time. Many people recover from the syndrome more or less completely and live long, relatively healthy lives. However, Katherine's case became severe. She has been paralysed in her limbs for three years now. Ten months ago, it was recognised that she was having increased difficulty in swallowing and speaking.

The consultant had explained to Katherine that, due to swallowing difficulties, they may consider feeding intravenously or through a tube. Katherine was saddened to hear this but felt it was almost inevitable. She gradually found it was very difficult and painful to move or breathe on her own due to the extent of damage to her nerves and muscles. She now needs a ventilator to help her breathe.

You are a nurse on the ward who has come to know Katherine and develop methods of communicating with her during the night watch with her when all is quiet. You explain this prognosis to Katherine in a gentle but clear manner. Last week Katherine indicated that she wanted to communicate with you privately. She signals in her halting mode of communicating that she has considered her options and decided that she no longer wanted to continue living this way. She said her life held no value for her if it meant being in constant pain and without the freedom to move, eat or even breathe on her own. She said she discussed this with her family and they have accepted her wishes to have the ventilator removed.

(Edited from Schwartz et al., 2002, p.9)

6.3.1 Discussion

Ventilation is essential for life when a person cannot breathe on their own. Given the seriousness of this decision in Katherine's case, the withdrawal of ventilator support may well be ethically and clinically difficult for members of the healthcare team, family and even the patient.

For Katherine, life is no longer bearable. Ventilation is a burden and not a benefit to her. Katherine believes that, according to her values, continued use of the ventilator is futile. As discussed above, futility judgements are profoundly value laden, in part because the specification and choice of goals are so variable. The case of Katherine illustrates this subjective dimension of 'futility' judgements. What Katherine deems 'futile' is met with confusion and disagreement among health professionals. But Katherine does not see the goal of living with ventilator dependence as a positive personal value. The consideration that 'merely being alive' is a benefit would most likely not persuade Katherine to rethink her decision to remove the ventilator. Katherine seems to take the view that there is a profound difference between continued 'biological life' (merely being alive) and living a narrative of choices, relationships and opportunities that would be a 'biographical life'.

> *There is a deep difference between having a life and merely being alive. Being alive, in a biological sense, is [on its own] relatively unimportant. One's biographical life, by contrast, is immensely important; it is the sum of one's aspirations, decisions, activities, projects, and human relationships. [...] The doctrine of the sanctity of life can be understood as placing value on things that are alive [only in the biological sense]. But it can also be understood as placing value on 'lives' and on the interests that some creatures, including ourselves, have in virtue of the fact that they are subjects of lives. [...] The sanctity of life ought to be interpreted as protecting lives in the biographical sense, and not merely in the biological sense.* (Rachels, 1986, pp.24–7).

The value of simply being alive may be considered a 'benefit' to observers of Katherine's suffering. But it is Katherine who is making a judgement about the quality of her life, about her prospects for her future which concludes that living in this way is no longer a 'benefit'. The burden for Katherine is that, for her, this current existence is not a 'life'. It is biological endurance. Stress, frustration and relentless anxiety arise from the awareness that continuing to live in this way offers no prospect to make human choices, to relate to her family and friends outside the confines of her ventilatory context. In making the choice to request removal of the ventilator, the patient is effectively choosing her 'good dying'. A life of anticipated incapacity and unremitting pain is of negligible value for her. Having reflected for ten months on the continuing distress of ventilator reliance is not tantamount to a hasty or ill-thought-through decision.

It is understandable that, initially, if a doctor or nurse were faced with Katherine's request they might be reluctant to simply agree. Points that the healthcare team might discuss as a team are:

- If Katherine is not 'terminally ill' or 'imminently dying', should her refusal of the LPT be respected?
- If they agree to respect this patient's request to remove her ventilator, would they be complicit in assisted suicide?
- Because of the seriousness of this request, should they review the evidence that Katherine has capacity to consent to withdrawal of the ventilator?

There is no qualification such as 'imminently dying' on a competent patient's right to refuse life-prolonging therapies. Katherine's reasons for refusing the ventilator are important for the health professionals to discuss with her but ultimately they need to be assured of Katherine's valid refusal.

If Katherine's capacity to make this decision is in any way in doubt, one option would be to seek a consultation by an expert psychiatrist to assess Katherine's claimed competence. However, in this case the behavioural symptoms that Katherine shows would not normally cause alarm sufficient to request a psychiatric assessment. It is rather the doubts and possible disagreements of staff about her choice that begin to engender reluctance to accept it.

Is Ventilator Removal Assisting in Suicide?

In a situation such as the case of Katherine, there can be a lingering belief and emotional response from family and health professionals that this withdrawal decision (stopping the ventilator) is equivalent to actively taking the patient's life. The question may haunt health professionals: Is it always wrong to withhold or withdraw life supports such as a ventilator, artificial nutrition and hydration from a patient? Is this not euthanasia by omission?

> *Euthanasia must be distinguished from the decision to forgo so-called 'aggressive medical treatment', in other words medical procedures which no longer correspond to the real situation of the patient, either because they are by now disproportionate to any expected results or because they impose an excessive burden on the patient and the patient's family [...] [O]ne can in conscience refuse forms of treatment that would only secure a precarious and burdensome prolongation of life, so long as the normal care due to the sick person in similar cases is not interrupted [...] It needs to be determined whether the means of treatment available are objectively proportionate to the prospects for improvement. To forego extraordinary or disproportionate means is not the equivalent of suicide or euthanasia; it rather expresses acceptance of the human condition in the face of death.*
> (Ashley and O'Rourke, 1997, pp.419–20).

One objection to the removal of the ventilator might be that a ventilator is not medical treatment but basic humane care that is universally required. Denying basic and humane care, the argument claims, would be tantamount to physician-assisted suicide or euthanasia. However, this objection overlooks an important ethical and legal right of this patient. When a competent patient has refused the use of a life prolonging therapy, its use would be legally tantamount to assault and, morally, would be a denigration of the competent patient's liberty of choice and right to privacy and dignity. Katherine has the right, both legally and ethically, to refuse medical treatment even if such refusal leads to death. (See Module 4, section 5 for discussion on a competent person's right to refuse treatment.)

The support of the family for Katherine's decision is a positive feature of this case that the medical team can draw on to aid them in their understanding of Katherine's choice. Much of contemporary writing has spoken of autonomy in highly individualistic terms but this case illustrates how a woman like Katherine who is judged competent and autonomous has involved her family as supportive companions in her choice and her approaching death (Donchin, 2000). The form of autonomy illustrated in this case could be termed 'relational autonomy', which takes into account others who have been important in one's life and now, however haltingly, support one's choice to die (see Further Discussion, Module 4 for more on relational autonomy). The family have offered support and respect for Katherine's sense of the 'good life' that seems no longer available to her. While the family support is apparent, they will undoubtedly still need reassurance, comfort and support in the period when ventilator removal occurs.

Not everyone would agree with Katherine's decision and some would clearly voice the concern that compliance in this request is assisting suicide. In this case narrative, the patient wants to exercise control over her dying so some semblance of human dignity remains for her. The concept of human dignity encompasses a range of human sentiments with regard to people's place in this world, their relatives, the environment in which they live and their conception of the past, the present and the likely future. For sick people, the concept of human dignity includes a desire not to become a burden and the desire that their own suffering will not cause their loved ones to suffer (Cohen-Almagor, 2001).

Patients often express fear of developing dependency on others or on machines; they want their death to somewhat reflect the way they lived. Katherine chose to control the process of dying as much as possible. Perhaps she feared dying without control over her body and feared relentless suffering. Katherine's suffering was physical but also emotional and psychological in that she could anticipate the progression of her illness and knew what that would mean for her daily living. Health professionals who become poignantly aware of this can seek to reassure the patient that dying with dignity is a realistic possibility.

6.3.2 Suggested Professional Responsibilities

- In view of the seriousness of this decision and the healthcare team's commitment to respect human life, the health professionals should take measures to ensure competence, understanding and valid consent on the part of Katherine to withdrawal of the ventilator. It would also be reasonable for the clinician to encourage the patient to have a waiting period to see if her decision remains firm, reassuring her that this is not ignoring her distress and concerns but rather ensuring a careful and reflective decision.

- If Katherine continues in her determination to have the ventilator removed, then the healthcare team should agree to do this in moral recognition of her autonomy as a competent person to choose the meaning of her life in such illness. Health professionals need to show respect for Katherine's decision, even if they do not agree with it.

- The process of ventilator removal should be done with clinical care and expertise. Careful attention to pain management is vital if the patient is not to experience profound suffering from ventilator withdrawal. The process needs to be discussed with at least the family and, in this case, with the patient in order for them to achieve a clear understanding of what they are requesting but also to receive assurance that effective pain management will be provided.

- Given the stress that may be experienced by health professionals in situations such as this, it is important that collegial support be provided.

- Katherine and her family need to receive comfort, human presence and continued reassurance of care to company her in her dying days. It is important for Katherine that she does not feel abandoned by health professionals because of this choice she is making.

- For future reference in the healthcare unit, the full account of this decision needs to be documented. Included in such documentation is the evidence of the process seeking patient informed consent. Also for documentation are the specific measures taken to inform the family and patient of the actual process of removal of ventilator and promised follow-up care.

6.4 Case 4: Withholding LPT in a Neonatal Unit – A Low Birth Weight Baby

As with adults, decisions about the limitation of therapy and life supports for neonates are based on clinical prognoses but also ethical considerations about future suffering and profoundly diminished quality of life. The following case illustrates the clinical and ethical challenges involved in such complex decision making.

A Low Birth Weight Baby

Jan C. was admitted to the labour ward in advanced labour at 23 weeks gestation. This was her fourth pregnancy, the others having ended in miscarriages before 20 weeks. At 43 years of age she felt time was running out for her to achieve a successful outcome and Jan was desperate for this baby to survive. Baby C was born with a severe spina bifida, malformation of the brain stem, hydrocephalus, vocal cord paresis and severe deformities of the lower limbs. He was relatively unresponsive, had little spontaneous movement and had difficulty swallowing, sucking and breathing. If Baby C survived he would be unable to walk, be doubly incontinent, have no sexual function and probably require an artificial airway. He would certainly require multiple operations on his spine and lower limbs. The quality of his future life was estimated to be extremely poor.

The healthcare team agreed that no active treatment was warranted. Feeding was restricted to that on demand and the baby was given paracetemol and phenobarbitone. The consultant obstetrician told Jan C. and her husband that, given the prognosis of Baby C, the hospital's special care unit would not be able to offer more than basic care to the baby. In spite of the couple's pleas for everything possible to be done, when Baby C was born, weighing 400g, he was wrapped in a blanket and given to his parents to cuddle until he died about half an hour later.

(Tibballs, 2007, p.231. Edited variation on case of Baby M)

6.4.1 Discussion

Within the last few decades, developments in life-prolonging technology have meant that it is now possible to contemplate the survival of babies born at extremely early gestation and very low weight. However, clinical and family decisions to withhold or withdraw LPTs can be very stressful and challenging in these circumstances. Disagreements can occur between parents and health professionals, and within the healthcare team itself. In these circumstances, differences of ethical opinion and feelings of being emotionally overwhelmed are usually important factors that need to be addressed. This is especially clear in the case of Baby C.

While the healthcare team agree on withholding LPTs in the case of Baby C, the family do not have the background of neonatal experience that health professionals share. Moreover, the case of Baby C is particularly tragic for the parents since they have already suffered the grief of several previous miscarriages. A key challenge is that the health professionals do not usurp the parents' input into the decision but, at the same time, the parents cannot be left without the full details of the newborn's likely future.

The UK Royal College of Paediatrics and Child Health (RCPCH) (2004) suggests the circumstances that may involve the withholding or withdrawal of treatment in the case of children:

The Brain Dead Child – when brain stem death is confirmed the patient is, by definition dead. All life supports may be withdrawn with full emotional support for family and staff involved. (This condition does not apply to Case 4.)

The Permanent Vegetative State – in such circumstances treatment, inclusive of tube feeding, may be withdrawn while making the patient comfortable with nursing care. (This condition does not apply to Case 4.)

The 'No Chance' Situation – Prolonging treatment in these circumstances is futile and burdensome and not in the best interests of the patient; there is no legal obligation for a doctor to provide it. Indeed, if this is done knowingly it may constitute an assault or 'inhuman and degrading treatment' under Article 3 of the European Convention on Human Rights. An example would be a child with progressive metastatic malignant disease whose life would not benefit from chemotherapy or other forms of treatment aimed at cure. (The extent of serious impairment of Baby C would definitely be considered here as part of the clinical discussions with the parents.)

The 'No Purpose' Situation – In these circumstances the child may be able to survive with treatment, but there are reasons to believe that giving treatment may not be in the child's best interests. The child may not be capable now or in the future of mobility, speech or taking part in decision making and other self-directed activity. (This condition applies as it is a component of the 'best interests' judgement being discussed with Baby C's parents.)

'The Unbearable Situation' – This situation occurs when the clinician and family believe that further treatment is more than can be borne and they may wish to have treatment withdrawn or to refuse further treatment irrespective of the medical opinion that it may be of some benefit. (Parents in Baby C's case may not consider further treatment unbearable.) (RCPCH, 2004, pp.28–9).

In addition, European Specialists in Paediatrics offer the following ethical principles to guide decision making:

1. In the event of futile treatment, the primary obligation of the paediatrician is to counsel the parents and let the patient die with minimal suffering. The decision lies primarily with the physician.

2. The opinion of parents should be included in all medical decisions. Doctors treating the sick infant first should come to the conclusion on the basis of comprehensive facts. This should then be discussed with parents in thoughtful dialogue.

3. In the case of unclear situations or controversial opinions between members of the healthcare team and parents, a second expert opinion can be helpful.

4. Every form of intentional killing should be rejected in paediatrics. However, giving medication to relieve suffering in hopeless situations which may, as a side effect, accelerate death can be justified.

5. Decisions must never be rushed and must be based on evidence as solid as possible (Sauer, 2001, pp.365–7)

Recent research indicates that supports and values that parents find most important during neonatal decision making regarding use of LPTs are religion, spirituality, hope and compassion. These supports and values are not routinely acknowledged or incorporated by physicians. Parents in this research needed doctors to convey hope and compassion when discussing resuscitation options even when the infant's outcome was likely to be poor (Boss et al., 2008, p.585).

Physicians who were perceived as providing hope were not necessarily more likely to predict survival; in fact, some of the physicians whom parents described as hopeful predicted nearly certain death. These physicians gave parents hope because they expressed emotion and showed the parents that they were touched by the tragedy of the situation. [...] Expressing their own emotions during intense patient interactions can be uncomfortable for physicians. Nevertheless, there is evidence that parents value physicians' emotional reactions when the physicians communicate bad news. **(Boss et al., 2009, p.586)**

6.4.2 Suggested Professional Responsibilities

- The healthcare team may need to reiterate to the family how they determine the likely burdens and benefits that make up a judgement to withhold LPTs and promise provision of optimal palliative care.

- With the decision to withhold and withdraw treatments, all members of the healthcare team should have an opportunity to voice their opinions and feelings. The final decision should be made in consultation with parents though the team must take the main responsibility for the decision. This can help alleviate the burden of guilt that some parents feel.

- If the family disputes the decisions being taken, a procedure needs to be made available for another opinion (another independent clinician, the hospital ethics committee, etc.)

- Baby C's parents need time to be with their baby. They also may need reassurance that withholding LPT does not make them complicit in euthanasia.

- Withholding LPT signals a change of focus to palliative care and the parents need to feel that they are not abandoned in their grief and their efforts to understand why this happens.

- The family should be asked if they would like a member of the clergy or other spiritual support to be available.

- With a view to keeping ongoing records for occasional review by the healthcare team, the decision taken needs to be documented and the actions evaluated. The evaluation should include not simply the decision but the manner in which the decision was made and the follow up with parent(s).

- Following the death of the baby, the consultant in charge and the nurse most involved should offer to see the parents, to discuss the death and the result of the post mortem examination if it were available.

- Given the parents' history of multiple miscarriages, the healthcare team should offer suggestions about professional assistance for infertility difficulties.

6.5 Case 5: Artificial Nutrition and Hydration (ANH) – Is PEG Feeding Optional?

Is PEG Feeding Optional?

Nora is 62 years old and has had multiple sclerosis for 25 years. Initially the disease followed a relapsing and remitting course and Nora would have long periods of good health in between months of various disabling side-effects, such as temporary paralysis and visual problems. For the past ten years, however, her condition has become more disabling and Nora has had to move into a nursing home. The staff are friendly and she is well cared for. However, as a result of the insidious effect of her illness, most of her bodily functions have ceased to work. She is doubly incontinent. On the days when she is well enough to be aware of her surroundings, she finds her condition extremely distressing. She is embarrassed by her lack of bodily control and the fact that she has to have 24-hour nursing care. Her swallowing is unsafe and the decision was made a year ago to feed her via percutaneus endoscopic gastrostomy (PEG). She gets no pleasure from eating or drinking.

She does not have relatives or visitors. Some days she is described as barely conscious. Staff had a conference yesterday to discuss the continued use of the PEG tube wondering if withdrawal of ANH would be right. Wouldn't comfort care be more compassionate and appropriate? There was no consensus among the staff about withdrawal: some felt that providing ANH was a gesture of solidarity and wanted to ensure that Nora would not be abandoned. Others wondered if there is a moral or legal obligation to maintain life at all cost regardless of the quality of the life?

(Edited case from Johnston and Bradbury, 2008, p.161)

6.5.1 Discussion

An important consideration throughout the discussions on LPTs thus far is that any judgement about withholding or withdrawing treatments including ANH must be patient-specific. Abstract principles alone will not be sufficient. Even accepting this advice, health professionals and ethicists differ on the moral evaluation of ANH.

There is broad consensus that, if a patient is able to take food in the conventional way, then food should be offered and the patient encouraged to eat. However, when a patient is no longer able to take food in a conventional way, the difficult issue of deciding on ANH arises.

In Case 5, Nora has had the PEG tube in place for a year so the question is about whether this form of ANH should be removed. Case 5 is especially challenging because Nora's competence is diminished though she experiences intermittent awareness and lucidity. Some days she is described as barely conscious and when she is aware of her environment, her lack of bodily control is a cause of distress and embarrassment. The questions that arise include:

1. Why do clinical doubts arise, after a year, about the wisdom of continuing the PEG tube?
2. Is the withdrawal of ANH justified in this case?
3. Is it in the 'best interests' of Nora to continue or withdraw ANH?
4. Is withdrawal of ANH equivalent to euthanasia?

1. Why question the continuing of the PEG tube after a year?
   The health professionals notice Nora's distress with her disability and general condition. On days when she has intermittent awareness she seems particularly embarrassed by the 'insidious effect of her illness'. Chronic disability makes her daily life a struggle and she is often 'barely conscious'. With the PEG tube she derives no pleasure from eating or drinking. The reasons the health professionals wonder about continuing ANH are not obvious and there is not consensus among the staff about withdrawal. They need to continue their conversation about their reasons for considering withdrawal of ANH at this point in Nora's life. Comfort care might be more compassionate and perhaps even more comforting, but in what sense is it more appropriate? Withdrawal of ANH will result in the death of Nora within a relatively short time, perhaps 10 days to two weeks.

2. Is withdrawal of ANH justified?
   One issue that looms large in the debate about the ethics of feeding and often influences individuals in objecting to withholding or withdrawing of feeding is the powerful symbolism of feeding the hungry and giving drink to the thirsty. Feeding the hungry has been cited as the most fundamental of all human relationships and a perfect symbol of the fact that human life is inescapably social and communal. Food and water are undoubtedly powerful symbols of comfort and human care in our society. Through their provision we communicate such care and concern for others. Some people feel concern that withholding or withdrawing artificial nutrition and hydration will undermine our commitment to the values of comfort and care in medical institutions and society at large. On this view one would find it difficult to justify withholding feeding even if in the form of ANH (Centre for Bioethics, 1997a).

However, a focus on the symbolic value of providing food and water might mask several important differences. ANH is provided to treat malnutrition and dehydration. But these medical conditions are not invariably accompanied by hunger and thirst. In addition, hunger and thirst can sometimes be treated without having recourse to ANH, e.g. the sensation of thirst associated with a dry mouth can be alleviated by moistening the patient's lips and mouth with glycerine swabs or ice chips (Meidl, 2006, p.335). Importantly, ANH requires invasive procedures that strain the symbolism of offering food and drink to those in need.

For patients unable to take food or liquid orally, feeding and hydration are often supplied through the nose and throat (nasogastric tube), veins (IV line), stomach (gastrostomy), intestine (jejunostomy), or major vessel into the heart (hyperalimentation). All of these options highlight the profound difference between feeding the hungry with a meal and receiving nutritional support. It is also shown in some patients that withholding or withdrawing ANH may actually contribute to their sense of comfort. In brief, withholding or withdrawing ANH should not too readily be equated with 'starving the patient to death'. It may even be considered by some to be a form of compassionate treatment (Meidl, 2006).

3. Is it in Nora's 'best interest' to continue or withdraw ANH?
   This method requires the decision makers to consider what the 'best course of action' is for a particular (incompetent) person in a particular situation. See Case 2 above and Module 4 for a discussion of 'best interests'.

Special Legal Challenges in Ireland
In the Ward of Court case in Ireland (1995), a central ethical and legal issue that arose was the question of whether it was justified to discontinue the ANH that was being provided to the Ward via a PEG tube. The moral reasoning involved in that case highlights the contentious terms of the ethical and legal debate about ANH.

After a High Court judgement that allowed withdrawal of the PEG tube from the Ward, an appeal followed with a Supreme Court judgement upholding the High Court decision. The removal of ANH was defended by Justice Lynch in the High Court as a 'best interests' judgement. In their decisions to withdraw ANH from the Ward both the High Court and the Supreme Court took the view that ANH was equivalent to medical treatment and, as such, could be justifiably withdrawn because it was considered to be ineffective and burdensome.

However, following the Supreme Court Judgement, the Irish Medical Council and Nursing Board issued statements that ANH is an ordinary and humane requirement of care and they claimed that it was a duty of their members to continue the provision of nutrition and hydration. In 2009, the Irish Medical Council updated its position statement on feeding.

The Medical Council new guidelines offer more qualified and nuanced advice than that provided in 1995.

Nutrition and hydration are basic needs of human beings. All patients are entitled to be provided with nutrition and hydration in a way that meets their needs. If a patient is unable to take sufficient nutrition and hydration orally, you should assess what alternative forms are possible and appropriate in the circumstances. You should bear in mind the burden or risks to the patient, the patient's wishes if known, and the overall benefit to be achieved. Where possible, you should make the patient and/or their primary carer aware of these conclusions.

(Medical Council, 2009, p.20)

The 1995 statement of the Nursing Board has not been updated as yet and remains as follows:

The ethical principle requires that so long as there remains a means of nutrition and hydration of this patient it is the duty of the nurse to act in accordance with the Code and to provide nutrition and hydration. In this specific case, a nurse may not participate in the withdrawal and termination of the means of nutrition and hydration by tube. In the event of the withdrawal and termination of the means of nutrition and hydration by tube the nurse's role will be to provide all nursing care. (An Bord Altranais, 18 August, 1995, cited in Dooley and McCarthy, 2005, p.284). (See Module 4, section 5.1.2 for reference to the Ward of Court Case and ANH.)

4. Is withdrawal of ANH equivalent to euthanasia?
   If the decision to remove ANH is made with the clear intention of hastening Nora's death, then there is reason to pause and consider that this may be an act of euthanasia, a deliberate act or omission whose primary intention is to end another person's life.

   However, decisions to withdraw or discontinue life supports are not equivalent to euthanasia if they are validly authorised by a competent patient's consent or if a clinical decision is made that further life supports including ANH would, on the basis of all available evidence, be futile – lacking benefit for the patient and merely prolonging the dying process.

The following text offers one method of reasoning for decisions on ANH:

We should not assume that all or most decisions to withhold or withdraw medically assisted nutrition and hydration are attempts to cause death. To be sure, any patient will die if nutrition and hydration are withheld. But sometimes, other causes are at work. For example, the patient may be imminently dying, whether feeding takes place or not, from an already existing terminal condition. At other times, although shortening of the patient's life is one foreseeable result of an omission, the real purpose of the omission was to relieve the patient of a particular procedure that is of limited usefulness to the patient or unreasonably burdensome for the patient and the patient's family or caregivers. This kind of decision should not be equated with a decision to kill or with suicide. (O'Rourke and Norris, 2001, pp.205–6)

The position of O'Rourke and Norris combines application of the principle of double effect, the principle of proportionality as well as the ordinary–extraordinary distinction. The text does not provide an answer about the decision in the case of Nora but it highlights the questions that health professionals must reflect on and provide some answers for before a decision is taken and before they are confident that they can morally defend a decision to remove ANH.

The above arguments, reasoning and questions about the morality of ANH are representative of an expanding literature on this topic. The following sources offer an opportunity to reflect on viewpoints that are widely discussed among theologians, ethicists, doctors and nurses alike (Center for Bioethics, 1997a, 1997b; GMC, 2009; Dooley and McCarthy, 2005; Lesage and Portenoy, 2001; Meidl, 2006; Meisel, 1992; O'Rourke and Norris, 2001; Panicola, 2001).

6.5.2 Suggested Professional Responsibilities

- The intermittent awareness that Nora experiences is mostly dominated by the distress felt in relation to her condition. During the brief periods when Nora might show partial awareness, a conversation could be initiated with her about possible withdrawal of the PEG tube. However, such a conversation might be very distressful and may not provide reliable evidence of Nora's capacity to take part in this decision.

- In the absence of family or designated proxies, an assessment of Nora's 'best interests' should be made. For a patient with an advanced life-threatening illness who is dying, there may not be many benefits. Admittedly, continued existence might be seen by some as an important 'benefit'.

- The burdens of providing ANH in Nora's case should be assessed. There is always a risk to a patient being fed through a feeding tube. Feeding tubes may feel uncomfortable. They can become plugged up, causing pain, nausea and vomiting. Feeding tubes may also cause infections.

- Any disagreements that may arise within the healthcare team should be aired and constructively resolved based on careful evaluation of benefits and burdens of continuing ANH in Nora's case.

- The decision in terms of the process and the final determination made about continuing or withdrawing ANH should be documented.

7. Module 6 Further Discussion

7.1 Euthanasia and Physician-Assisted Suicide

'Euthanasia' derives from the ancient Greek, 'eu', meaning good and 'thanatos' meaning death, thus a 'good death'. Today, the term 'euthanasia' refers to the administration of death, the active intentional ending of life.

In the medical context, 'active euthanasia' is the act of purposely ending the life of someone. This might be done by a health professional injecting a patient with a lethal dose of drugs that directly causes his or her death.

The withholding or withdrawal of LPT is sometimes described as 'passive euthanasia'. However, it is argued that describing the withholding/withdrawing of treatment as passive euthanasia is not accurate. In such cases, it is argued that the person involved is not killed in the usual sense, nor is the death of the person intended by the withholding of additional treatment. Terms such as 'allowing natural death' are increasingly used as an alternative to 'passive euthanasia'.

Consent for euthanasia would be said to be voluntary if it were carried out at the patient's request.

If someone does not explicitly request euthanasia this does not mean that they do not want it; it would be reasonable, however, to assume that they do not. Euthanasia in such a case would be involuntary, and, even more obviously, it would be if someone had clearly expressed a wish to live as long as possible, whatever the circumstances.

Newborn babies do not yet have, and comatose or severely brain-damaged adults have lost, the capacity to request or refuse euthanasia. In such cases neither consent nor the lack of it can be said to be a factor, so euthanasia, if considered, is neither voluntary nor involuntary but non-voluntary.

Assisted suicide is defined as the act of helping a person to die by providing the means for them to take their own life. An example of physician-assisted suicide is the act of giving a prescription or supply of a lethal dosage of drugs to a patient who has requested this. The doctor providing the lethal dosage of drugs thus enables a patient to end his or her own life. The patient or individual may never use the drugs to end their life but it is suggested that having the means at their disposal offers a patient the security of knowing they have the means to end their life and suffering if they choose.

The following discussions consider the legal and ethical implications of euthanasia and physician-assisted suicide (PAS). International discussion of these topics has not abated but there are still relatively few countries that have legalised the practices. Reasons of public interest and threats to physician integrity are raised as justifications for unwillingness to legally endorse the practices. In the legal discussions (7.2; See Module 5, section 6.4. for discussion of the R v Cox case) that follow, the position in law on euthanasia and PAS is explained for a selection of countries.

In the ethics discussion (7.3 and 7.4) positions are distinguished that (1) offer reasons and arguments that serve to morally justify the practices of euthanasia or PAS and (2) offer reasons and arguments to show that moral justification is lacking for the practices.

7. 2 Legal Positions: Euthanasia and Physician-Assisted Suicide

7.2.1 The Law – Ireland

In Ireland, any person who takes active steps to end the life of another person is in breach of the criminal law. In this respect, a distinction may be made between assisting a person in ending his or her own life – perhaps by providing medical assistance – and actually taking the final step of ending the patient's life. The first situation involves assisting the suicide of the person. Under Irish law, suicide ceased to be a criminal offence under the Criminal Law (Suicide) Act 1993. However, the act states that anyone who 'aids, abets, counsels or procures' the suicide of another person commits a criminal offence which is punishable with a possible maximum sentence of 14 years.

The situation which is sometimes termed 'euthanasia' involves the deliberate action of ending the life of the person. Under Irish law, this is legally categorised as murder. The law does not allow a person to consent to his or her own death and, for this reason, the fact that the patient has consented to, or even requested, the action is irrelevant. A person who is convicted of murder is punishable on conviction by a mandatory life sentence. This means that the court cannot choose to give a lesser sentence because of a person's underlying motivations.

There have been no prosecutions of Irish health professionals in relation to either assisted suicide or euthanasia. It is thought that the position taken in the English case of R v Cox (1992) is likely to be followed in Ireland, effectively legally prohibiting euthanasia. (See Module 5 for discussion of the R v Cox case.)

A number of efforts have been made in other countries, including the US, Canada, the UK and under the European Convention on Human Rights, to assert a legal right to die through the courts (see Module 4, section 5.2 for discussion of the UK Ms Pretty case involving an attempt to receive assurance that an act of assisted suicide would not be prosecuted).

7.2.2 Switzerland

Although the law in most countries legally prohibits suicide and active euthanasia, there have been some moves in recent years to introduce measures to permit one or both practices. Both practices are permitted in Switzerland where they are not contrary to the criminal law and are largely unregulated. Because of the liberal regime in Switzerland, this is the most common country for people to travel to in order to avail of euthanasia. However, recent reports claim that the Swiss government is considering restricting or even banning organised assisted suicide in an attempt to reduce so-called 'death tourism'. Concerns stated that their current laws on assisted suicide could be open to abuse. A study in 2008 suggested more and more people seeking help to die in Switzerland did not have a terminal illness (Pidd, 2009).

7.2.3 The Netherlands

Both euthanasia and physician-assisted suicide have been permitted by legislation in the Netherlands since 2001, in Belgium since 2002 and in Luxembourg since 2008. In these countries, the practices are more regulated than in Switzerland. In the Netherlands, for example, the Dutch Criminal Code states that a physician who terminates a patient's life or who assists a patient's suicide will be exempt from criminal liability provided that he or she complies with two conditions. These are: first, he or she must practise in accordance with the due care criteria and, secondly, he or she must report the cause of death to the municipal coroner.

The due care criteria apply to both euthanasia and physician-assisted suicide. These criteria require that the attending physician must:

- be satisfied that the patient has made a voluntary and well considered request
- be satisfied that the patient's suffering is unbearable, and that there is no prospect of improvement
- have informed the patient about his or her situation and prospects
- have come to the conclusion, together with the patient, that there is no reasonable alternative in the light of the patient's situation
- have consulted at least one other physician, who must have seen the patient and given a written opinion on the due care criteria referred to above, and
- have terminated the patient's life or provided assistance with suicide with due medical care and attention.

7.2.4 United States

Physician-assisted suicide is also permitted in the American states of Oregon since 1996 and Washington since 2008, although in much more restricted circumstances than in the European models. In Oregon, the Death with Dignity Act 1996 requires that the patient must have a terminal illness with a life expectancy of less than six months. The act also requires the patient to have made two separate requests for assisted suicide and imposes a 15-day delay between the first and second requests.

7.2.5 United Kingdom 2009: The case of Debbie Purdy

Debbie Purdy, from Bradford was 46 and was diagnosed with MS in 1995. As her condition progressed and she knew of the likely prognosis, she considered going to Switzerland to end her life. However, she feared that her husband might be charged on his return to the UK. She wanted assurances from the DPP that her husband, Omar Puente, would not be prosecuted.

Ms Purdy believed that, unless the law was clarified, she might be forced to end her life earlier than she planned because her husband would be unable to help her, without risking prosecution, if she became totally dependent. If the risk of prosecution was sufficiently low, she could wait until the very last minute before travelling with her husband's assistance. If the risk of prosecution was high, Ms Purdy would have to go earlier while she was still fit enough to travel without assistance.

Purdy took her case to the House of Lords after the High Court and the Court of Appeal held that it was for parliament, not the courts, to change the law which makes assisted suicide illegal in the UK. The offence of assisting suicide is a criminal offence under Section 2(1) of the Suicide Act 1961 and carries a maximum penalty of 14 years' imprisonment. The Act defines assisting a suicide as 'aiding, abetting, counselling or procuring' the suicide of another. Committing or attempting to commit suicide is not a criminal offence. No individual to date has been prosecuted for assisting a suicide in relation to suicides committed abroad, including the Dignitas clinic in Switzerland.

The Law Lords agreed that changes were a matter for parliament but upheld Ms Purdy's argument that the DPP, Keir Starmer QC, should put in writing an 'offence-specific policy' identifying the facts and circumstances he would take into account in deciding whether it was in the public interest to prosecute under the Suicide Act.

The director of public prosecutions, Keir Starmer QC, has called for public participation in a 12-week consultation on the factors he had identified which will be taken into account when considering whether prosecutions will be brought for the offence of assisting a suicide. Starmer stated:

> *Assisting suicide has been a criminal offence for nearly fifty years and my interim policy does nothing to change that. There are also no guarantees against prosecution and it is my job to ensure that the most vulnerable people are protected while at the same time giving enough information to those people, like Ms Purdy, who want to be able to make informed decisions about what actions they may choose to take.* (**Crown Prosecution Service, 2009**)

Details of the interim policy on prosecuting assisted suicide can be found on this Crown Prosecution Service website: www.cps.gov.uk/news/press_releases/144_09/.

7.3 Ethical Positions: Euthanasia and Physician-Assisted Suicide

Consciously deciding to end a person's life is a profound and grave matter and actions which do, while motivated by compassion, are widely, intensely and heatedly considered and debated around the world. They engender strong feelings about

- the right to demand one's choice of dying

and

- that life is so precious there is a duty to preserve it at all costs
  (Watson Lucas, Hoy et al., 2009, p.14).

Considerable professional and public attention has focussed on voluntary euthanasia. This has partly been spurred by the publicity of the practice of euthanasia in the Netherlands and it is considered in this section.

7.3.1 Arguments in Support of Euthanasia

In general there are two kinds of arguments that support euthanasia. The first kind is a duty-based argument:

- Public support for euthanasia reflects recognition that the same values of patient self-determination and well-being that have been accepted as guiding treatment decision making in general, and decisions about LPT in particular, can, in some cases support voluntary euthanasia as well. For example, it is argued that permitting (voluntary) euthanasia respects patient autonomy and provides a more peaceful and humane death for some patients than they would otherwise have.

The second kind of argument appeals to anticipated (likely good) consequences of permitting euthanasia in addressing the fear and the reality of suffering.

- In significant part, the public interest in and support for euthanasia reflects fear of loss of control and dignity while dying.
- This fear includes concerns that, especially in acute care settings, aggressive use of life-prolonging technologies would allow one to linger in a semi-comatose state, unable to relate to others or communicate the extent of one's suffering.
- There is strong belief that, even with the best of palliative care, pain cannot be fully relieved in terminal illness.

The belief is that the availability of euthanasia will contribute to lessening these kinds of fears and concerns.

7.3.2 Arguments Opposing Euthanasia

In general there are also two kinds of arguments that oppose euthanasia. The duty-based argument usually takes the following form:

- Any individual instance of euthanasia is morally wrong because it violates the duty not to kill innocent human beings. For some, even the consent of the one killed does not make the killing permissible.

The second kind of argument appeals to anticipated (likely bad) consequences of permitting euthanasia. On this view:

- Although it might be morally justified in some individual cases, it would nonetheless be bad public policy to permit voluntary euthanasia. Among potential bad consequences opponents cite are: its seeming incompatibility with the proper aim of medicine to protect life in all its frailty; the erosion of the trust of patients in their caregivers; the erosion of the social commitment to provide appropriate care to the dying if euthanasia is seen as an acceptable alternative; the fear that providing voluntary euthanasia would, in time, lead to involuntary euthanasia or non-voluntary euthanasia of incompetent patients.

Evaluating and assessing the relative seriousnessness or likelihood of these consequences of permitting voluntary euthanasia is both controversial and difficult.

7.4 Physician-Assisted Suicide (PAS)

The difference between active euthanasia and aiding in a terminally ill patient's suicide is essentially that in active euthanasia the doctor determines the eventual course of action, whereas in PAS she merely assists the patient to realise his decision to end his life.

It should be said at the outset that some commentators claim we should change the terminology of PAS and refer rather to physician-assisted death (PAD) in order to clearly distinguish it from the usual meaning of suicide. Others like Debbie Purdy ask why assisted suicide should be only physician assisted?

It is sometimes said that, similar to the distinction between 'active' and 'passive' euthanasia described above, withholding or withdrawing LPTs from a patient who has capacity to request this is equivalent to PAS. However, it could be argued that this is placing an emotive label on an action that is legally and morally valid. When a society prohibits PAS and a case of discontinuing LPT is labelled PAS, both the doctor and competent patient seem implicated in a legal and moral offence. However, the point to be noted is that, based on a fundamental respect for a person's autonomy, competent patients have the moral and legal entitlement to discontinue LPT (see Module 3 and Module 4). If such decisions are labelled as PAS, this could be viewed as disrespecting the competent patient's right to refuse unwanted treatments.

7.4.1 Arguments Supporting PAS

Arguments in support of PAS include those that are put forward in support of euthanasia. They centre on respect for patient autonomy and are perceived to address some patients' fears about the possibility of a painful, distressful and/or undignified death.

- Specifically, supporters of PAS argue that the provision of PAS is consistent with the aim of medicine which is to: respect the patient's autonomy; ease the patient's suffering; and do what is in the best interests of the patient (Dieterle, 2007).

- It is also claimed that PAS differs greatly from the wrongful killing of innocent persons. Proposals to allow PAS do so on the assumption that the patient requests the medication – usually a number of times – the patient is terminally ill with less than 6 months to live and the patient is convinced over time that death would be far preferable than the life he or she is living. In brief, death is not a harm to those who seek and are granted PAS' (Dieterle, 2007, p.138).

The philosopher Tom Beauchamp claims that PAS may be a morally justified action. On his view, valid requests and authorisation for assistance in dying can legitimate PAS. This means that a doctor would not be obligated to honour all requests but that valid requests make it morally permissible for them, or some other person, to lend aid in dying. A doctor might refuse to honour a particular request if there is good moral reason for doing so: autonomy of the person seeking PAS may be impaired; excessive influence is being exerted on the individual requesting; the desire to avail of PAS is not stable over time; public trust in doctors would suffer, etc:

If letting die based on valid refusals of treatment does not wrong or harm persons or violate their rights, how can assisted suicide or voluntary euthanasia harm or wrong a person who died? In each case, persons seek what for them in their bleak circumstances is the best means to the end of quitting life.

(Beauchamp and Childress, 2001, p.148)

7.4.2 Arguments Opposing PAS

Arguments against PAS are, similar to euthanasia, duty based and consequential.

A first duty-based argument opposing PAS derives from the perceived aims of medicine in the same way as the argument supporting PAS does. On this view, the intent of the doctor is said to offer grounds for rejecting PAS:

- Doctors should not kill; this is prohibited by the Hippocratic Oath. The doctor is bound by their profession to save life, not take it. The idea behind this argument is that the intent of a doctor should be always to heal or cure.

A second argument considers the inherent wrongness of killing.

- Killing an innocent person is inherently wrong. The doctor indirectly kills the patient in cases of PAS by providing the lethal medication. So the doctor does something inherently wrong.

One of the most common forms of argument against PAS (similar to euthanasia) cites the possible negative consequences of the practice as a reason not to legalise it. These arguments rely on empirical claims about the future and, as a result, their persuasiveness depends on how likely it is that the predictions will be realised.

Seven consequences are most typically cited as the basis for opposing legalisation of PAS and similarly would be cited to claim that PAS could not be morally justified.

1. PAS could start us on a slippery slope to non-voluntary euthanasia.
2. Abuses of the law would be likely: patients might be pressurised by family to seek PAS and vulnerable groups would be more susceptible to persuasion to accept PAS.
3. Allowing or encouraging PAS would corrupt medicine and health professionals.
4. Acceptance of PAS would weaken the prohibition on killing.
5. Patients would give up too easily and abandon hope.
6. Improvements in palliative care would cease or diminish.
7. Citizens would begin to fear hospitals and health professionals.

In some research which assessed this list of possible consequences against the backdrop of the legalisation of PAS in Oregon (US) and the Netherlands, it was found that the overwhelming majority of predicted consequences of PAS laws have not come to pass (Dieterle, 2007). This does not mean that concerns about the consequences of legalising PAS have no basis in reality because these findings may be contested by findings from other research. What is important to note is the contribution that empirical research can make to informing ethical and legal debates on euthanasia and PAS.

7.5 Insights from Oncologists on Euthanasia and PAS

One robust piece of research, carried out in the US in 2000, surveyed 3,299 oncologists on the subject of euthanasia and PAS. Four insights were gleaned from the study:

1. Concern among oncologists about performing euthanasia or PAS may limit their willingness to prescribe opioids, thereby leading to inadequate pain management. This reticence may reflect fear that increasing opioid dose increases the risks for respiratory depression and death and might be construed as a form of euthanasia. (See Module 5)

2. There seems to be a relationship between the likelihood of performing euthanasia and PAS and the inability of physicians to obtain adequate end-of-life care for their patients. Worry was voiced that inadequate access to palliative care might make euthanasia and physician-assisted suicide attractive alternatives.

3. Physicians who reported receiving better training in end-of-life care seemed less likely to perform euthanasia or physician-assisted suicide.

4. Results suggest that among US oncologists support for PAS and euthanasia has decreased substantially. Between 1994 and 1998, oncologists' support for PAS declined by half, from 45.5% in 1994 to 22.5% in this study (Emanuel, Fairclough, Clarridge et al., 2000). This decline may reflect expanding knowledge about how to facilitate a 'good death', making PAS and euthanasia no longer appear as necessary or desirable (Emanuel, Fairclough, Clarridge et al., 2000).

Cognisant of the arguments to support PAS that suffering and inadequate palliative care are often contributing factors, the Irish Association for Palliative Care strongly recommends the continued appropriate development of specialist palliative care services throughout Ireland. It is the clear duty of the doctor to ensure that a patient dies with dignity and with as little suffering as possible (Irish Association for Palliative Care, 2011b). In addition the Irish Association holds the position that the legalisation of euthanasia has potential adverse effects on the patient–health professional relationship, society's expectations of health care and resources available to address serious illness (Irish Association of Palliative Care, 2011c).

8. Module 6 Summary Learning Guides

8.1 Central Issues and Concepts in Decisions about LPTs

- Decisions to start or stop treatment should be based on the benefits and burdens of the treatment, as judged by a patient or authorised surrogate.

- The distinction between ordinary and extraordinary treatment is often used as a rule of thumb by health professionals to distinguish between medicines, treatments, and operations which offer a reasonable hope of benefit without excessive pain or other inconvenience and those which do not.

- The principle of proportionality requires that the decision-making process about treatments should follow the general rule to maximise benefit and avoid undue burden.

- The meaning of the distinction between killing and letting die is widely contested and often underpins distinctions between: 1) suicide and foregoing treatment and, 2) euthanasia and so-called 'natural' death.

- It is impossible to determine what will benefit a patient without presupposing some quality of life standard and some conception of the life the patient will likely live after a medical intervention.

- Historically, the sanctity of life position holds that the value of human life is not dependent upon its being valued by the individual themselves or by others or by the presence of certain functional capacities such as relationality or rationality.

8.2 Futility

- The notion of futility is a disputed concept that is still evolving.

- The debate about what constitutes 'futile' treatments began with decisions relating to the stopping of cardiopulmonary resuscitation but it has expanded to other forms of LPT.

- Futility judgements are typically used to express a combined value judgement and scientific judgement.

- There is a considerable subjective element in judgements that further treatment is 'futile' – precisely because decisions that weigh up benefits and burdens are not based on rocket science.

- The debate on 'futility' can be divided into three approaches:

  the first defines futility in terms of definite clinical criteria.

  the second is a procedural approach that gives power to hospitals, utilising their ethics committees, to decide whether interventions demanded by families were futile.

  the third approach focuses primarily on negotiation at the bedside and ongoing communication with patients, families and the healthcare team.

9. Module 6 Activities

9.1. Reflect back on the particulars of Case 1:

a. Ms R. was put on a ventilator when she was admitted to intensive care. The family asked that everything should be done to keep their loved one alive. Do you agree with the ICU team that further LPTs for Ms R. would be 'futile'?

b. The team took time (a few days) to provide life support and ongoing conversation with the family. In what way was this process therapeutic for the family?

c. Based on your experience caring for patients, what is it in the procedures of the hospital setting that might contribute to a patient's sense of abandonment?

9.2 Reflect back on the particulars of Case 2:

a. Mr W.'s life is in the balance: Would CPR provide benefit?

b. The family of Mr W. are experiencing the grief of potentially losing their loved one. They believe that providing CPR may give them a reprieve from this grief. What information or conversation would you provide that might give the family of Mr. W. reason to believe that CPR might be more harmful than helpful for their loved one?

c. Can you understand how the family of Mr W. think that biological life can be construed as a benefit even if there is no realistic opportunity for Mr W. to continue having a biographical life?

d. From your clinical experience, what is the likely outcome for Mr W. if CPR proceeds?

e. What means would you suggest for resolving the disagreements between the family, doctors and nurses? When faced with continued resistance to clinical advice, is it ever legally or morally justified to simply go ahead and write up a DNR without family consent?

9.3 Re-read Case 3

where Katherine requests removal of the ventilator and discuss the following with your colleagues:

a. Even if Katherine is competent, given the seriousness of this request, are there any further complications among health professionals that you anticipate?

b. You are the clinician in charge where Katherine is a patient. Explain what kind of information or understanding you would want to provide for Katherine. Since she had already approached a staff nurse about her desire to discontinue ventilator use, what conversation would you have with her?

c. Who should participate in the decision: Family? The entire clinical team? Hospital ethics committee? On-site hospice clinician?

d. How would you explain your choice of participants?

9.4 Reflect back on the particulars of Case 4:

a. In this time of grief and desolation, can you suggest further clinical advice for Jan and her partner who have already experienced three miscarriages before 20 weeks?

b. What appropriate after-care for the family's grief can be provided in the confines of the hospital setting? Is this available in your work context?

c. Based on your experience and study, who do you think should be responsible for final decisions about CPR and DNR?

d. Are guidelines for CPR and DNR available in your work context? If so, what do they include? If not, is there a reason?

9.5 Reflect back on the particulars of Case 5:

a. How would you evaluate the benefits and burdens of continuing ANH for Nora?

b. In your experience, how would a clinical team deal with a case such as Nora's? Who would be involved in the decision making on the case?

c. Do you think there is realistic basis for clinical disagreement about what is in the 'best interests' of Nora?

10. Module 6 References and Further Reading

Ackerman, R.J. 'Withholding and Withdrawing Life-Sustaining Treatment', *American Family Physician*, vol. 62, no. 7, 2000, pp.1555–64

American Academy of Family Physicians (AAFP), *Cardiopulmonary Resuscitation (CPR)* (Chicago: Institute for Ethics at the American Medical Association, 2000)

Ashley, B. and O'Rourke, K. *Health Care Ethics: A Theological Analysis* (4th ed.) (Washington DC: Georgetown University Press, 1997)

Back, A.L., Young, J.P., McCown, E., Engelberg, R.A., Vig, E.K., Reinke, L.F., Wenrich, M.D., McGrath, B.B. and Curtis, J.R. 'Abandonment at the End of Life from Patient, Caregiver, Nurse, and Physician Perspectives', *Archives of Internal Medicine*, vol. 169, no. 5, 2009, pp.474–9

Beauchamp, T. and Childress, J. *Principles of Biomedical Ethics* (5th ed.) (Oxford and New York: Oxford University Press, 2001)

Beauchamp, T. and Childress, J. *Principles of Biomedical Ethics* (6th ed.) (Oxford and New York: Oxford University Press, 2008)

Boss, R.D., Hutton, N., Sulpar, L.J., West, A.M. and Donohue, P.K. 'Values Parents Apply to Decision Making Regarding Delivery Room Resuscitation for High-Risk Newborns', *Pediatrics*, vol. 122, no. 3, 2008, pp.583–9

British Medical Association (BMA), *Withholding and Withdrawing Life-Prolonging Medical Treatment: Guidance for Decision-Making* (London: BMJ Books, 1999)

British Medical Association (BMA), Resuscitation Council UK and Royal College of Nursing (RCN), *Decisions Relating to Cardiopulmonary Resuscitation: A Joint Statement from the BMA, the Resuscitation Council (UK) and the Royal College of Nursing* (London: Resuscitation Council (UK), British Medical Association and the Royal College of Nursing, 2007)

Brock, D.W. 'Life-Sustaining Treatment and Euthanasia', in S.G. Post (ed.), *Encyclopaedia of Bioethics* (3rd ed., vol. 3) (New York: Macmillan, 2004), pp.1410–20

Burns, J.P. and Truog, R.D. 'Futility: A Concept in Evolution', *Chest*, vol. 132, no. 6, 2007, pp.1987–93

Canadian Medical Association (CMA), 'Joint Statement on Resuscitative Interventions' (1995), http://www.cma.ca/index.cfm/ci_id/33236/la_id/1.htm [accessed 24 August 2009]

Canadian Nurses' Association, *Joint Statement on Resuscitative Interventions: Policy Statement* (Ottawa: Canadian Nurses' Association, 1994)

Canadian Nurses; Association, Canadian Healthcare Association, Canadian Medical Association and Catholic Health Association of Canada, 'Joint Statement on Preventing and Resolving Ethical Conflicts Involving Health Care Providers and Persons Receiving Care' (1999), http://www.cma.ca/index.cfm/ci_id/3217/la_id/1.htm#princ [accessed 7 December 2009]

Caplan, A.L. and Synder, L. 'The Role of Guidelines in the Practice of Physician-Assisted Suicide', *Annals of Internal Medicine*, vol. 132, no. 6, 2000, pp.476–81

Center for Bioethics, *Reading Packet on Withholding or Withdrawing Artificial Nutrition and Hydration* (Minneapolis: University of Minnesota, 1997a)

Center for Bioethics, *Reading Packet on Termination of Treatment of Adults* (Minneapolis: University of Minnesota, 1997b)

Cherny, N.I., Radbruch, L. and The Board of the European Association for Palliative Care, 'European Association for Palliative Care (EAPC) Recommended Framework for the Use of Sedation in Palliative Care', *Palliative Medicine*, vol. 23, no. 7, 2009, pp.581–93

Churchill, L.R. and King, N.M.P. 'Physician-Assisted Suicide, Euthanasia, or Withdrawal of Treatment', *British Medical Journal*, vol. 315, no. 7101, 1997, pp.137–8

Cohen-Almagor, R. *The Right to Die with Dignity: An Argument in Ethics, Medicine and Law* (New Jersey: Rutgers University Press, 2001)

Collins, N., Phelan, D., Marsh, B. and Sprung, C.L. 'End-of-Life Care in the Intensive Care Unit: The Irish Ethicus Data', *Critical Care and Resuscitation*, vol. 8, no. 4, 2006, pp.315–20

Council on Ethical and Judicial Affairs, American Medical Association, 'Medical Futility in End-of-Life Care: Report of the Council on Ethical and Judicial Affairs', *JAMA: Journal of the American Medical Association*, vol. 281, no. 10, 1999, pp.937–41

Criminal Law (Suicide) Act No. 11/1993

Crown Prosecution Service, 'DPP Publishes Interim Policy on Prosecuting Assisted Suicide', http://www.cps.gov.uk/news/press_releases/144_09 [accessed 8 December 2009]

Curlin, F.A., Nwodim, C., Vance, J.L., Chin, M.H. and Lantos, J.D. 'To Die, To Sleep: US Physicians' Religious and Other Objections to Physician-Assisted Suicide, Terminal Sedation, and Withdrawal of Life Support', *American Journal of Hospice and Palliative Medicine*, vol. 25, no. 2, 2008, pp.112–20

Curtis, J.R. and White, D.B. 'Practical Guidance for Evidence-Based ICU Family Conferences', *Chest*, vol. 134, no. 4, 2008, pp.835–43

Deep, K.S., Griffith, C.H. and Wilson, J.F. 'Changes in Internal Medicine Residents' Attitudes about Resuscitation after Cardiac Arrest over a Decade', *Journal of Critical Care*, vol. 24, no. 1, 2009, pp.141–4

Dieterle, J. 'Physician-Assisted Suicide: A New Look at the Arguments', *Bioethics*, vol. 21, no. 3, 2007, pp.127–39

Donchin, A. 'Autonomy, Interdependence, and Assisted Suicide: Respecting Boundaries/Crossing Lines, *Bioethics*, vol. 14, no. 3, 2000, pp.187–204

Dooley, D. and McCarthy, J. *Nursing Ethics: Irish Cases and Concerns* (Dublin: Gill & Macmillan, 2005)

Emanuel, E.J., Fairclough, D., Clarridge, B.C., Blum, D., Bruera, E., Penley, W.C., Schipper, L.E. and Mayer, R.J. 'Attitudes and Practices of Cancer Doctors in the United States Regarding Euthanasia and Physician-Assisted Suicide', *Annals of Internal Medicine*, vol. 133, no. 7, 2000, pp.1–39

Faber-Langendoen, K. and Karlawish, J.H.T. 'Should Assisted Suicide be Only Physician Assisted? *Annals of Internal Medicine*, vol. 132, no. 6, 2000, pp.482–7

Fallat, M.E., Caniano, D.A. and Fecteau, A.H. 'Ethics and the Paediatric Surgeon', *Journal of Paediatric Surgery*, vol. 42, no. 1, 207, pp.129–36

Ganzini, L. and Block, S. 'Physician-Assisted Death: A Last Resort?' *New England Journal of Medicine*, vol. 346, no. 21, 2002, pp.1663–5

Gedge, E., Giacomini, M. and Cook, D. 'Withholding and Withdrawing Life Support in Critical Care Settings: Ethical Issues Concerning Consent', *Journal of Medical Ethics*, vol. 33, no. 4, 2007, pp.215–18

General Medical Council, *Withholding and Withdrawing Life-Prolonging Treatments: Good Practice in Decision Making* (London: General Medical Council, 2002)

General Medical Council, *End-of-Life Treatment and Care. Good Practice in Decision Making: A Draft for Consultation* (London: General Medical Council, 2009)

Gillon, R. '"Futility": Too Ambiguous and Pejorative a Term?' *Journal of Medical Ethics*, vol. 23, no. 6, 1997, pp.339–40

Goh, A.Y. and Mok, Q. 'Identifying Futility in a Paediatric Critical Care Setting: A Prospective Observational Study', *Archives of Disease in Childhood*, vol. 84, no. 3, 2001, pp.265–8

Guild of Catholic Doctors, *A Response to the BMA Medical Ethics Committee's Consultation Paper: Withdrawing and Withholding Treatment* (London: Guild of Catholic Doctors, 1998)

Hollinger, D. 'Sanctity of Life', in S.G. Post (ed.), *Encyclopedia of Bioethics* (3rd ed., vol. 2) (New York: Macmillan, 2004)

In re a Ward of Court [1996] 2 IR 79

Irish Council for Bioethics, *Is it Time for Advance Healthcare Directives?* (Dublin: Irish Council for Bioethics, 2007)

Johnston, C. and Bradbury, P. *One Hundred Cases in Clinical Ethics and Law* (London: Hodder Arnold, 2008)

Joyce, T. and British Psychological Society Professional Practice Board, *Best Interests: Guidance on Determining the Best Interests of Adults who Lack Capacity to Make a Decision (or Decisions) for Themselves [England and Wales]* (Leicester: Professional Practice Board of the British Psychological Society, 2007)

Kelly, G. 'The Duty of Using Artificial Means of Preserving Life', *Theological Studies*, 11 June 1950, pp.203–20

Law Reform Commission, *Bioethics: Advance Care Directives [LRC 94 – 2009]* (Dublin: Law Reform Commission, 2009)

Lesage, P. and Portenoy, R.K. 'Ethical Challenges in the Care of Patients with Serious Illness', *Pain Medicine*, vol. 2, no. 2, 2001, pp.121–30

Madden, D. *Medicine, Ethics and the Law* (Dublin: Butterworths, 2002)

May, W.E. 'Tube Feeding and the "Vegetative" State', *Ethics and Medics*, 23 December 1998, pp.1–2

McCormick, R.A. *The Critical Calling* (Washington DC: Georgetown University Press, 1989)

McGinn, P.R. and Sheikh, A. 'Do Not Resuscitate! Who Decides?' *St Paul Medical Indemnity Scheme Newsletter*, Dublin, 2001, pp.1–8

Medical Council, *A Guide to Ethical Conduct and Behaviour* (6th ed.) (Dublin: Medical Council, 2004)

Medical Council, 'Good Medical Practice in Seeking Informed Consent to Treatment' (2008), http://www.medicalcouncil.ie/_fileupload/news/Informed_Consent.pdf [accessed 1 November 2009]

Medical Council, *Guide to Professional Conduct and Ethics for Registered Medical Practitioners* (7th ed.) (2009), http://www.medicalcouncil.ie [accessed 20 November 2009)]

Meidl, E.M.D. 'A Case Studies Approach to Assisted Nutrition and Hydration', *National Catholic Bioethics Quarterly*, Summer 2006, pp.319–36

Meisel, A. 'The Legal Consensus about Forgoing Life-Sustaining Treatment: Its Status and its Prospects', *Kennedy Institute of Ethics Journal*, vol. 2, no. 4, 1993, pp.309–45

Miller, F.G., Fins, J.J. and Snyder, L. 'Assisted Suicide Compared with Refusal Treatment: A Valid Distinction?' *Annals of Internal Medicine*, vol. 132, no. 6, 2000, pp.470–5

New South Wales (NSW) Department of Health, 'Guidelines for End-of-Life Care and Decision Making' (2005) http://www.health.nsw.gov.au/policies/gl/2005/pdf/GL2005_057.pdf [accessed 1 August 2009]

O'Keeffe, S.T. 'Development and Implementation of Resuscitation Guidelines: A Personal Experience', *Age & Ageing*, vol. 30, no. 1, 2001, pp.19–25

O'Brien, T., McQuillan, R. and Smullen, H. *Voluntary Euthanasia: A Position Paper by the Irish Association for Palliative Care* (Dublin: Irish Association for Palliative Care, 2000)

O'Rourke, K.D. 'The Catholic Tradition on Forgoing Life Support', *National Catholic Bioethics Quarterly*, vol. 5, no. 3, 2005, pp.537–53

O'Rourke , K.D. and Boyle, P. *Medical Ethics: Sources of Catholic Teachings* (2nd ed.) (Washington: Georgetown University, 1993)

O'Rourke, K.D. and Norris, P. 'Care of PVS Patients: Catholic Opinion in the United States', *Linacre Quarterly*, vol. 68, no. 3, 2001, pp.201–17

Panicola, M. 'Catholic Teaching on Prolonging Life', *The Hastings Center Report*, vol. 31, no. 6, 2001, pp.14–25

Peretti-Watel, P., Bendiane, M.-K., Galinier, A., Favre, R., Ribiere, C., Lapiana, J.-M. and Obadia, Y. 'District Nurses' Attitudes Toward Patient Consent: The Case of Mechanical Ventilation on Amyotrophic Lateral Sclerosis Patients. Results from a French National Survey', *Journal of Critical Care*, vol. 23, no. 3, 2008, pp.332–8

Pidd, H. 'Switzerland Considers Assisted Suicide Ban', *The Irish Times*, Thursday 29 October 2009, http://www.irishtimes.com/newspaper/world/2009/1029/1224257602232.html [accessed 8 December 2009]

President's Commission for the Study of Ethical Problems in Medicine and Biomedicine and Behavioural Research, *Deciding to Forego Life-Sustaining Treatment* (Washington DC: Government Printing Office, 1983)

Pretty v UK [2002] ECHR 2346/02

Quill, T.E. 'Legal Regulation of Physician-Assisted Death: The Latest Report Cards', *New England Journal of Medicine*, vol. 356, no. 19, 2007, pp.1911–13

Quill, T.E. and Battin, M.P. *Physician-Assisted Dying: The Case for Palliative Care and Patient Choice* (Baltimore: Johns Hopkins University Press, 2004)

Quill, T.E., Meier, D.E., Block, S.D. and Billings, J.A. 'The Debate over Physician-Assisted Suicide: Empirical Data and Convergent Views', *Annals of Internal Medicine*, vol. 128, no. 7, 1998, pp.552–8

Quinlan, C. and O'Neill, C. *Practitioners' Perspectives on Patient Autonomy at End of Life* (Dublin: Irish Hospice Foundation, 2009)

R v Cox (1992) 12 BMLR 38

Rachels, J. *The End of Life* (New Haven, CT: Yale University Press)

Rady, Mohamed Y. and Verheijde, Joseph L. 'Continuous Deep Sedation until Death: Palliation or Physician-Assisted Death?' *American Journal of Hospice and Palliative Medicine*, vol. 27, no. 3, 2010, pp.205–14

Raijmakers, N.J.H., van Zuylen, L., Costantini, M., Caraceni, A., Clark, J., Lundquist, G., Voltz, R., Ellershaw, J.E. and van der Heide, A. 'Artificial Nutrition and Hydration in the Last Week of Life in Cancer Patients: A Systematic Literature Review of Practices and Effects', *Annals of Oncology*, 2011, http://www.annonc.oxfordjournals.org [accessed 10 May 2011]

Ramsey, P. *The Patient as Person* (New Haven, CT: Yale University Press, 1970)

Royal College of Paediatrics and Child Health, *Withholding or Withdrawing Life-Sustaining Treatment in Children: A Framework for Practice* (London: Royal College of Paediatrics and Child Health, 2004)

Royal College of Physicians, *Concise Guidance to Good Practice: A Series of Evidence-Based Guidelines for Clinical Management. Number 12: Advance Care Planning: National Guidelines* (London: Royal College of Physicians, 2009)

Sacred Congregation for the Doctrine of the Faith, *Declaration on Euthanasia* (Rome: Vatican publications, 1980)

Sauer, P.J.J. 'Ethical Dilemmas in Neonatology: Recommendations of the Ethics Working Group of the CESP (Confederation of European Specialists in Paediatrics)', *European Journal of Paediatrics*, 160, 2001, pp.364–8

Schwartz, L., Preece, P. and Hendry, R.A. *Medical Ethics: A Case-Based Approach* (Edinburgh: Saunders, 2002)

McGinn, P.R. and Sheikh, A. 'Do Not Resuscitate! Who Decides?' *St Paul Medical Indemnity Scheme Newsletter*, Dublin, 2001, pp.1–8

Smith, D. 'Ethical Issues at the End of Life', unpublished study notes for MSc in pharmaceutical medicine at the Royal College of Surgeons of Ireland, Dublin, 2007, pp.1–29

Smith, D. *Key Guidelines on End-of-Life Care and Palliative Care* (Dublin: Royal College of Surgeons in Ireland, 2008), pp.1–62

Stanley, J. 'Developing Guidelines for Decisions to Forgo Life-Prolonging Medical Treatment', The Appleton International Conference (Appleton, WI: Lawrence University, 1991), pp.1–35

The, A.-M., Pasman, R., Onwuteaka-Philipsen, B., Ribbe, M. and van der Wal, G. 'Withholding the Artificial Administration of Fluids and Food from Elderly Patients with Dementia: Ethnographic Study', *British Medical Journal*, vol. 325, no. 7376, 2002, pp.1326–30

Tibballs, J. 'Legal Basis for Ethical Withholding and Withdrawing Life-Sustaining Medical Treatment from Infants and Children', *Journal of Paediatrics and Child Health*, vol. 43, no. 4, 2007, pp.230–6

Truog, R.D. 'Tackling Medical Futility in Texas', *New England Journal of Medicine*, vol. 357, no. 1, 2007, pp.1–3

Vanderpool, H.Y. 'Life-Sustaining Treatment and Euthanasia', in S.G. Post (ed.), *Encyclopedia of Bioethics* (3rd ed., vol. 2) (New York: Macmillan, 2004)

Veatch, R.M. 'Forgoing Life-Sustaining Treatment: Limits to the Consensus', *Kennedy Institute of Ethics Journal*, vol. 3, no. 1, 1993, pp.1–19

Verhagen, E. and Sauer, P.J.J. 'The Groningen Protocol: Euthanasia in Severely Ill Newborns', *New England Journal of Medicine*, vol. 352, no. 10, 2005, pp.959–62

Walter, J.J. 'Quality of Life in Clinical Decisions', in S.G. Post (ed.), *Encyclopedia of Bioethics* (3rd ed., vol. 2) (New York: Macmillan, 2004)

Warnock, M. and Macdonald, E. *Easeful Death: Is There a Case for Assisted Dying?* (Oxford and New York: Oxford University Press, 2008)

Watson, M., Lucas, C., Hoy, A. and Wells, J. *Oxford Handbook of Palliative Care* (2nd ed.) (Oxford and New York: Oxford University Press, 2009)

Way, J., Back, A.L. and Curtis, J.R. 'Withdrawing Life Support and Resolution of Conflict with Families', *British Medical Journal*, vol. 325, no. 7376, 2002, pp.1342–5

White, D.B., Braddock III, C.H., Bereknyei, S. and Curtis, J.R. 'Toward Shared Decision Making at the End of Life in Intensive Care Units', *Archives of Internal Medicine*, vol. 167, no. 5, 2007, pp.461–7

Woods, S. *Death's Dominion: Ethics at the End of Life* (Berkshire: McGraw-Hill, 2007)

Younger, S. 'Medical Futility', in S.G. Post (ed.), *Encyclopedia of Bioethics* (3rd ed., vol. 2) (New York: Macmillan, 2004)

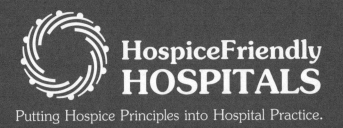

HospiceFriendly
HOSPITALS

Putting Hospice Principles into Hospital Practice.

Module 7

The Ethics of Confidentiality
and Privacy

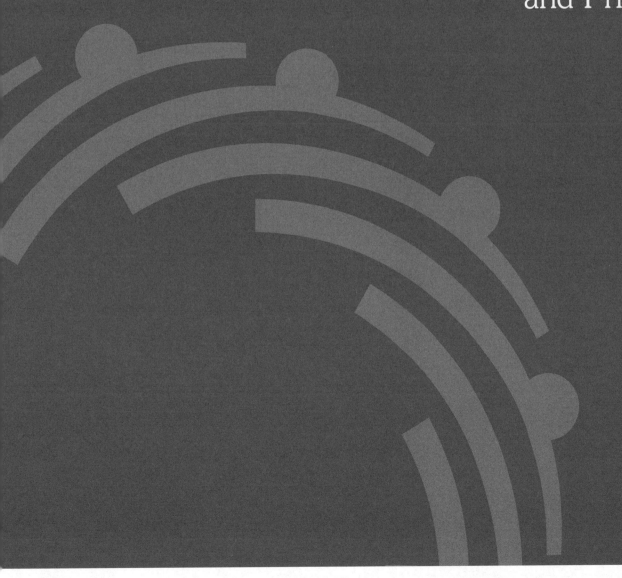

Module 7 Contents

Page

1. Module 7 Key Points

1.1 Confidential information is private information:

that a person shares with another on the understanding that it will not be disclosed to third parties. It includes identifiable patient information – written, computerised, visually or audio recorded – that health professionals have access to. Keeping patient confidentiality is important because it builds trust, respects patient autonomy and privacy and contributes to good patient outcomes.

1.2 Confidentiality is protected by professional codes and laws:

Ancient and modern medical and nursing codes stress the duty of confidentiality as a 'time honoured principle' that extends beyond death. Health professionals are also legally obliged to protect patient confidentiality under the Irish Constitution, the European Convention and the common law: legal sanctions are in place for breaches of patient confidence.

1.3 The principle of confidentiality is not absolute:

Exceptional circumstances where health professionals may ethically and legally qualify the principle of confidentiality centre on concerns about protecting the well-being of the patient themselves and protecting others from harm.

1.4 Health professionals should ask competent patients for permission to share information:

with third parties. In exceptional circumstances, such as abuse or threatened suicide, it may not be appropriate to seek permission on medical grounds. These circumstances have not been considered by the Irish courts but they are likely to look for very strong evidence regarding the medical grounds as to why it was not considered desirable to seek the patient's consent.

1.5 If patients lack the capacity to consent to sharing information, health professionals may need to share information:

with relatives, friends or carers in order to enable them to be involved in decisions about the patient's best interests. The sensitivity of the information and any known wishes of the patient in regard to it must be taken into account. The Irish law in relation to patients who lack capacity is currently unclear, though a forthcoming Mental Capacity Bill will help to clarify the position. Under the current Irish law, those close to the patient – spouses, partners, family members, friends – have no legal status in relation to healthcare decisions (and information in relation to decsion making) on behalf of people lacking capacity. While hospitals may routinely seek the consent of the 'next of kin' in relation to a healthcare decision, this consent has no legal basis. Ultimately, the lawfulness of sharing of information about a patient without capacity is likely to depend on whether it can be shown that it is in the patient's best interests that information about his or her condition should be shared with those close to them.

1.6 In exceptional circumstances,
health professionals may breach patient confidentiality in order to avoid serious risk of considerable harm to others (identifiable individuals and the public in general).
The decision to disclose patient information should not be made in haste or without due care and consideration of all concerned in the situation. Where disclosure is necessary, only information necessary to avoid harm should be provided.

1.7 The duty of confidentiality extends beyond death:
Guidelines that protect living patients equally apply after patients have died. Exceptions to confidentiality also equally apply. National and international guidelines governing the release of medical records of deceased patients generally consider: the known wishes of deceased patients in relation to their information; the impact of non-disclosure on the well-being and welfare of third parties – avoiding harming them or benefitting them; the impact of disclosure on the reputation of the deceased; the possibility of anonymising the information. The impact that posthumous breaches of confidentiality may have on the care of dying patients is also a concern.

1.8 Family members of deceased patients may ask for information and/or medical records:
because they may be anxious about a misdiagnosis, negligence or hereditary condition. Third parties may also request medical records because they are contesting a patient's will. Where disclosure is considered to be consistent with the wishes of the patient or to advance the best interests of the patient it is generally viewed as acceptable. Conflict arises where patients, while alive, did not consent to disclosure. In these circumstances, as with living patients, patients' rights to confidentiality are important but not absolute and the rights of others' well-being and welfare must also be taken into account. Recent legislation in relation to Freedom of Information confirms that access to information about deceased people may be obtained in some circumstances.

1.9 Privacy is valued in ethics and law:
(e.g. Irish Constitution and European Convention). Protecting someone's privacy involves protecting them from unwanted access or control by others. In this way it is linked with personal autonomy and it is also viewed as a key element of personal identity. Privacy can be thought of in terms of five dimensions: physical privacy, informational privacy, decisional privacy, personal property and expressive privacy.

2. Module 7 Definitions

2.1 Anonymised Data:

data from which the patient cannot be identified by the recipient of the information.
The name, address, and full post code must be removed together with any other information which, in conjunction with other data held by or disclosed to the recipient, could identify the patient. Unique numbers may be included only if recipients of the data do not have access to the 'key' to trace the identity of the patient.

2.2 Principle of Confidentiality:

obliges health professionals to respect the confidences that patients share with them.
By extension, health professionals are also obligated to keep confidential information that they might gain from sources other than the patient in their care, e.g. medical records or other health professionals.

2.3 Minimalist Principle:

where the interests of individuals or the general public require that patient confidentiality is qualified in some circumstances, the minimalist principle obliges health professionals to disclose to third parties only the patient information that is relevant to ensure their welfare or well-being.

2.4 Privacy:

refers to what belongs to individuals, e.g. bodily integrity, property, information, space. A right or claim to privacy is a right to control access to one's personal domain.

2.5 Right:

an entitlement that prohibits or obliges the actions of others. It is a justified claim that individuals or groups can make on other individuals or society generally. If a person is considered to have a right – to confidentiality, for example – they may be considered to be inviolable in some sense. In addition, a right may entitle a person to make certain claims on others for support or service – that their confidences will not be shared or that their medical records will be protected.

3. Module 7 Background

3.1 Confidential Information

Confidential information is usually understood to be private information that a person shares with another on the understanding that it will not be disclosed to third parties.

Keeping patient confidentiality is considered important because of its role in building patient trust and protecting patient privacy and autonomy. It is also considered important because the consequences of respecting patient confidentiality are generally seen as positive.

The British Medical Association (BMA) offers a useful list of what is considered confidential between health professionals and patients:

All identifiable patient information, whether written, computerised, visually or audio recorded or simply held in the memory of health professionals, is subject to the duty of confidentiality. It covers:

- any clinical information about an individual's diagnosis or treatment;
- a picture, photograph, video, audiotape or other images of the patient;
- who the patient's doctor is and what clinics patients attend and when;
- anything else that may be used to identify patients directly or indirectly so that any of the information above, combined with the patient's name or address or full postcode or the patient's date of birth, can identify them. Even where such obvious identifiers are missing, rare diseases, drug treatments or statistical analyses which have very small numbers within a small population may allow individuals to be identified. A combination of items increases the chance of patient identification.
- While demographic information such as name and address are not legally confidential, it is often given in the expectation of confidentiality. Health professionals should therefore usually seek patient consent prior to sharing this information with third parties.
(BMA, 2008, pp.5–6)

3.2 Confidentiality is Important

Confidentiality is a core element of all human relationships and so is basic to building trust between patients and health professionals. Keeping confidences is a form of keeping a promise or bond. In effect, the health professional promises the patient that they will keep a bond of trust – the patient trusts the health professional to keep confidence and the health professional trusts the patient to tell the truth (see Case 4).

Secondly, the assurance of confidentiality enables patients to be open about personal issues, concerns and questions and enhances their capacity to make decisions about their health care. Respecting a patient's choice to keep certain information about them confidential, e.g., deciding not to tell a family member about their illness, recognizes the patient's right to autonomy and privacy (see Privacy). It also acknowledges that it is the patient who must live with the consequences of their decision (not the health professional).

Finally, not only is the keeping of confidentiality considered worthwhile because it is viewed as an implicit part of the health professional/patient relationship, it is also seen as a means of ensuring other important benefits. For example, the trust engendered through confidentiality

- creates an open and supportive environment that encourages patients to disclose more of their symptoms and worries, fears and phobias
- ensures a better diagnosis and a higher quality of care – secures greater agreement and compliance with procedures and treatment
- encourages individuals, in particular vulnerable individuals, to seek help and increases their contact with the health services.

In sum, the keeping of patient confidentiality is considered important because it is basic to a relationship built on trust and respect. It is important also because the consequences of keeping confidentiality are generally beneficial to patients in that it ensures better outcomes for them.

3.3 Professional and Legal Accountability

3.3.1 Professional Codes

Because it has long been held as an honoured bond between health professionals and patients, the keeping of confidentiality has been enshrined in both professional and legal codes. It was first articulated in the Hippocratic Oath (*c.* fifth century BC):

What I may see or hear in the course of the treatment or even outside of the treatment in regard to the life of men, which on no account one must spread abroad, I will keep to myself, holding such things shameful to be spoken about. Translated by Ludwig Edelstein (1943), cited in University of Virginia Historical Collections (2007).

Florence Nightingale also set high standards for the nurse/patient relationship in relation to confidentiality. In 1859, she advised nurses in the following terms:

And remember every nurse should be one who is to be depended upon, in other words, capable of being a 'confidential' nurse. She does not know how soon she may find herself placed in such a situation; she must be no gossip, no vain talker, she should never answer questions about her sick except to those who have a right to ask them. **(Nightingale (1859), 1992, p.70)**

While the ancient oath points to shamefulness on the part of the health professional for breaking confidence, Nightingale draws attention to breaches of confidentiality that can happen through gossip and self-aggrandisement. Nightingale also indicates that anyone who asks for information about a patient must have a *right* to do so.

Modern codes of professional conduct for health professionals echo both Hippocrates' and Nightingale's stress on the professional/patient relationship and they also place emphasis on the notion of a presumed right on the patient's part to confidentiality. For example, the Irish Medical Council describes confidentiality as 'a fundamental principle of medical ethics [that] is central to the trust between patients and doctors'.
(Medical Council, 2009, p.26, section 24.1)

However, where contemporary codes differ from earlier ones is in the acknowledgement they make that some circumstances may give rise to the need for the principle of confidentiality to be qualified in some way. Such circumstances include situations where the well-being of the patient or the rights of those other than the patient may be at risk.
These codes are discussed in detail in the following sections.

3.3.2 Legislation

In addition to ethical obligations and professional codes, confidentiality is also protected by law, through legislation, in particular the Data Protection Acts 1988 and 2003, on the basis of court decisions and also on appeal to such mechanisms as the Irish Constitution and the European Convention on Human Rights. There is a legal duty on health professionals to respect the confidence of their patients. In the English case of Hunter v Mann (1974), the court set out the nature of the duty as follows: 'the doctor is under a duty not to [voluntarily] disclose, without the consent of the patient, information which he, the doctor, has gained in his professional capacity.'

Failure to respect the duty of confidentiality may lead to an action for breach of confidence and the award of damages to the patient. It may also cause a complaint to be made to the regulatory body responsible for the healthcare profession in question.

4. Qualifying the Principle of Confidentiality

While the principle of confidentiality holds an honoured place in professional codes and laws, serious extenuating circumstances occasionally call for the principle to be qualified in some way. The challenge for health professionals faced with such circumstances is to consider them carefully, to examine the implications of relevant codes and laws and to decide a course of action that they think best fulfils their various obligations as carers, professionals and citizens.

4.1 Disclosure with Consent

Health professionals do not breach the rule of confidentiality when they disclose information with the patient's permission. The least controversial circumstance that might arise is one where confidential information is shared between health professionals working in a multidisciplinary team (Medical Council, 2009, p.30). However, while many might presume that it is acceptable for members of a team to disclose confidential information about a patient to each other, even here care needs to be taken (BMA, 2008; Medical Council, 2009). The An Bord Altranais, *Code of Professional Conduct* (2000a), for example, advises nurses to use their professional judgement in relation to such disclosure:

> *Information regarding a patient's history, treatment and state of health is privileged and confidential. It is accepted nursing practice that nursing care is communicated and recorded as part of the patient's care and treatment. Professional judgement and responsibility should be exercised in the sharing of such information with professional colleagues.*
> (An Bord Altranais, 2000a, p.5)

The UK General Medical Council (2009) advises doctors to ensure that patients are aware that information might be shared:

> *You should make sure that information is readily available to patients explaining that, unless they object, their personal information may be disclosed for the sake of their own care and for local clinical audit* (p.6, section 7)

The Irish Medical Council advises that information shared among health professionals in relation to clinical audit, quality assurance systems and education and training should be anonymised as far as possible (2009, p.30). Where anonymisation is not possible, patients should be made aware of the possibility that identifiable information may be disclosed and that any patient's subsequent objections to such disclosure must be respected (2009, p.30).

In relation to end-of-life care, where a patient with the capacity to make healthcare decisions gives his or her consent to the sharing of information, then provided that the information sharing is done in accordance with the patient's instructions and does not exceed these, the health professional will not be in breach of her or his legal duties.

In other situations, patients are also likely to agree with disclosure to third parties when it is required to protect their interests, e.g. where insanity is a defence in a criminal action or for insurance purposes.

4.2 Disclosure without Consent

While these situations might be more contentious and troubling, there is considerable international consensus on what might be deemed grounds for qualifying the principle of confidentiality without the permission of a patient. Generally, codes delineate three circumstances where a health professional might, justifiably, share confidential information with people other than the patient or the multidisciplinary team. These circumstances relate to the interests of the law, the patient and other individuals and society. All three are explicitly detailed in the Irish Medical Council's *Guide to Professional Conduct and Ethics for Registered Medical Practitioners*:

1. Disclosure required by law

2. Disclosure in the interest of the patient or other people

3. Disclosure in the public interest (Medical Council, 2009, pp.27–9).

4.2.1 When Obligated Under the Law

Circumstances where the law can require a health professional to disclose confidential information include criminal investigations where the records of a suspected individual in a crime (e.g. road traffic offence, shooting offence) may be sought and legal actions where a professional might be asked to testify in a court or tribunal. They may also relate to Infectious Diseases Regulations which place an obligation on doctors and other health professionals to disclose information about 'notifiable' diseases to the public health authorities (Health Protection Surveillance Centre, 2009).

4.2.2 In the Interests of the Patient or Other People

Patients with Capacity

Ethical problems arise if the health professional and the patient disagree as to whether or not disclosing information is in their best interests. On such occasions, health professionals might find themselves torn between maintaining a patient's trust on the one hand and their duty to protect a patient from harm on the other. Circumstances where such conflicts arise might involve patients who share information in relation to abuse, neglect or suicidal intentions. In cases of abuse or neglect, the patient – young or old – may feel so dependent or fearful that they refuse to permit their doctor or nurse to disclose the abuse (Medical Council, 2009, p.7; Department of Health and Children, 2004). In cases of threatened suicide, the patient may be so severely depressed that they cannot rationally decide where their best interests lie.

Some commentators, for example Mason and Laurie (2006, p.259) suggest that, in some limited circumstances, it may also be legally permissible for a health professional to share information about a capable patient without the patient's consent where it is in the best interests of the patient that the information be shared and it is not desirable on medical grounds to seek the consent of the patient. Possible examples where this would arise would be sharing information between professionals responsible for the patient's care or sharing information with a close family member.

However, others, for example Brazier and Cave (2007, p.80), argue that paternalistic motives to protect the patient cannot justify the sharing of information about a patient with capacity without the patient's consent. The matter has not been considered by the Irish courts. However, even if the courts did adopt the first position, it is likely that they would take a strict view of the circumstances in which this exception would be allowed to arise and would look for very strong evidence regarding the medical grounds as to why it was not considered desirable to seek the patient's consent.

Temporary or Permanent Incapacity

If the patient lacks the capacity to consent to sharing information, health professionals may need to share information with relatives, friends or carers in order to enable them to be involved in decisions about the patient's best interests. In such circumstances, it is permissible for health professionals to provide information to those close to the patient. But caution is advised. According to the BMA (2008):

> *Where a patient is seriously ill and lacks capacity, it would be unreasonable to always refuse to provide any information to those close to the patient on the basis that the patient has not given explicit consent. This does not, however, mean that all information should be routinely shared,*

and where the information is sensitive, a judgement will be needed about how much information the patient is likely to want to be shared, and with whom. Where there is evidence that the patient did not want information shared, this must be respected. (BMA, 2008, p.28)

The Irish Medical Council advises the following:

While the concern of the patient's relatives and close friends is understandable, you must not disclose information to anyone without the patient's consent. If the patient does not consent to disclosure, you should respect this except where failure to disclose would put others at risk of serious harm.

If the patient is considered to be incapable of giving or withholding consent to disclosure, you should consider whether disclosing the information to family and carers is in the best interests of the patient. (Medical Council, 2009, p.26)

Unfortunately, Irish law in respect of patients who lack capacity is both unsatisfactory and unclear. The law is currently in the process of being reformed. A Mental Capacity Bill is due to be published but does not look like becoming law until well into 2012. Under the current law, a person who lacks capacity may be made a ward of court. If this happens, a committee of the ward (usually one person) is appointed to act on the person's behalf. The committee has the legal right to consent to some medical treatment for the ward provided that the treatment is not serious – the committee does not have the legal right to consent to serious treatment. Although the matter has not been considered by the Irish courts, where a person is a ward of court it would seem to be ethically appropriate and legally permissible for health professionals to share information with the ward's committee.

Wardship is still relatively uncommon in Ireland and most patients who lack capacity will not have a committee. Under the current Irish law, those close to the patient – spouses, partners, family members, friends – have no legal status in relation to healthcare decisions on behalf of people lacking capacity. While hospitals may routinely seek the consent of the 'next of kin' in relation to healthcare decisions, this consent has no legal basis. If a person is nominated by a patient as their next of kin, such a person may provide valuable insight to health professionals as to the patient's wishes. However they have no right to the patient's records nor can they consent to disclosing information about the patient to third parties.

Ultimately, the lawfulness of healthcare decisions about patients who are incapacitated depends on whether the decisions are in the best interests of the patient. It is likely that the best interests principle will also apply to the sharing of information about a patient without capacity. If it can be shown that it is in the patient's best interests that information about his or her condition should be shared with those close to them, then it is likely that the sharing of information will be legally permissible. The lack of clear legal guidance can create difficulties for health professionals especially in situations of family conflict. The new capacity legislation is likely to clarify the position considerably. It will allow for the appointment of adult guardians who will be the relevant people for all actions in respect of the person lacking capacity.

Healthcare surrogacy laws in many states in the US give decision-making authority for incapacitated patients to appointed surrogates where advance directives or living wills have not been executed. In these cases, surrogates are often granted access to patients' medical records. This might be ethically justified on the ground that it assists surrogates to make informed healthcare decisions which are consistent with the patient's own wishes and are also in their best interests.

The key test highlighted by Jansen and Friedman Ross (2000) is the degree to which the information that the patient does not want disclosed is relevant to the treatment decisions that the surrogate must make. Where it is not relevant, there is no justification for breaching confidentiality. Where adequate care requires information disclosure, then it would seem that the interests of the patient's welfare should be prioritised over his confidentiality. In cases where clinicians might reasonably disagree as to the relevance of certain information to treatment decisions, Jansen and Friedman Ross advise consultation with an ethics committee and tend to favour disclosure out of respect for the decision-making authority of the surrogate. However, we would urge caution in this regard on the grounds that it could be argued that, while the surrogate represents the patient, they are not themselves the patient and so their right to information is more limited. In any case, currently in Ireland there are no legal means of appointing surrogates and, if there were, the level of decision-making authority is uncertain.

In addition, the Freedom of Information Act 1997 (section 28(6) Regulations 2009 (SI 387/2009) allows access to information about people lacking capacity in some situations. Regulation 4 says that a request for personal information shall be granted where the requester is a parent or guardian of the individual to whom the information relates and the person has not reached the age of 18 or is a person with a mental condition or mental incapacity or severe physical disability provided that access to the information is in the person's best interests.

To Protect the Interests of Another Individual
These circumstances concern, not the public at large or society as a whole, but particular identifiable individuals who are at serious risk of harm which disclosure of information

might avert or minimise. The widely reported court case which first stipulated that health professionals had a legal obligation to breach confidentiality in circumstances where identifiable third parties were at risk is the Unites States case of Tarasoff v the Regents of the University of California (1976) (see Section 7. Further Discussion for details). The case was initially dismissed but, after several appeals, the California Supreme Court overturned the dismissal. In 1976 it stated:

> [O]nce a therapist does, in fact, determine, or under the applicable professional standards reasonably should have determined, that a patient poses a serious danger of violence to others, he bears a duty to exercise reasonable care to protect the foreseeable victim of that danger.
> (Tarasoff v the Regents of the University of California, 1976)

The court noted that the duty to protect might be fulfilled in different ways, such as issuing a warning to the presumed intended victim or others likely to tell the potential victim of the danger, notifying the police, or initiating steps reasonably necessary under the circumstances.

The duty or obligation on the part of health professionals to warn an identifiable person who is at risk of serious harm that was articulated by the Californian Supreme Court in the Tarasoff case has also been expressed in many contemporary codes. The Irish Medical Council, for example, puts it in the following way.

> Disclosure of patient information without their consent may be justifiable in exceptional circumstances when it is necessary to protect the patient or others from serious risk of death or serious harm. You should obtain consent of the patient to the disclosure if possible.
> If you consider that disclosing patient information is justifiable, you should carefully consider whether anonymisation of the information (sharing it without revealing the patient's identity) would achieve the same potential benefits. You must also be careful to disclose the information to an appropriate person (or body) who understands that the information must be kept confidential. You should only disclose the minimum information that is necessary in the circumstances.
> In the preceding instances, you should inform patients of the disclosure unless this would cause them serious harm. (Medical Council, 2009, p.28)

The position of the Medical Council in relation to disclosure in these circumstances is supported by the Irish Data Protection Acts 1988 and 2003 and the EU Data Protection Directive 1995 (Council of Europe 1995). Specifically, the Irish Acts permit disclosure of otherwise confidential information where 'required urgently to prevent injury or other damage to the health of a person' (Data Protection Acts 1988 and 2003, Section 8 [d]).

A duty to warn: Who? When? How? What?

While the law (legislation and court decisions) and professional regulations clearly stipulate a duty on the part of health professionals to warn those at risk, there remains some uncertainty in relation to the precise circumstances that would prompt the disclosure of information (who to warn) and also in relation to the process of carrying out such a duty (when, how and what). However, some guidelines exist.

In relation to whom to warn:

The Californian Supreme Court stipulates that the person at risk must be identifiable and that the risk to them must be one of a serious danger of violence (Tarasoff v Regents of the University of California, 1976).

In relation to when and how:

The Data Protection Act 1988 permits disclosure in urgent circumstances to prevent injury or other damage.

The Irish Medical Council cites 'serious risk of death or serious harm' as a condition of disclosure (2009, p. 29, section 28.1).

The Californian Supreme Court advises taking steps that are reasonably necessary under the circumstances (Tarasoff v Regents of the University of California, 1976).

In relation to what:

If a health professional decides to disclose confidential information to a third party, either in the interests of the patient or to protect other individuals from harm, they might ask themselves a further question: what should they tell them? This question is based on a rule of thumb, the minimalist principle of disclosure. The principle can be formulated in the following way: 'Only tell a relevant third party the minimum that is necessary to achieve the end of disclosure.' This can afford protection of patient confidence as much as possible, while recognising an obligation to disclose pertinent information to protect patients, or others, from harm.

What these provisos indicate is a general concern that confidentiality is not breached lightly: that the decision to disclose is not made in haste without due care and consideration of all concerned in the situation.

4.2.3 In the Interests of Society

As Module 4, 3.4 indicated, the right of an individual to exercise autonomy is limited by the similar rights of others to live autonomously. So also, in the case of confidentiality, the interest of a patient in having their confidences protected is limited by the legitimate interests of others. Those interests may be deemed to outweigh an individual's right to confidentiality in circumstances where nondisclosure threatens the well-being and welfare of others. The discussion in the previous section relates to the interests of identifiable other individuals but a health professional also has obligations in relation to society in general. For example, a health professional might be justifiably concerned if she or he becomes aware that an airline pilot or bus driver suffers from epilepsy or that a patient has murderous intentions and seems capable of carrying them out. In these circumstances, the health and even lives of members of the public are at risk if the health professional does not disclose what she or he knows to other relevant parties.

4.3 Deceased Patients

The status of deceased patients in uncertain in ethics and law, but there is general consensus that the obligation to respect patients' confidentiality extends beyond death.

4.3.1 US Guidelines

Opinion 5.051 – Confidentiality of Medical Information Postmortem

All medically related confidences disclosed by a patient to a physician and information contained within a deceased patient's medical record, including information entered postmortem, should be kept confidential to the greatest possible degree. However, the obligation to safeguard patient confidences is subject to certain exceptions that are ethically and legally justifiable because of overriding societal considerations (Opinion 5.05, 'Confidentiality'). At their strongest, confidentiality protections after death would be equal to those in force during a patient's life. Thus, if information about a patient may be ethically disclosed during life, it likewise may be disclosed after the patient has died.

Disclosure of medical information postmortem for research and educational purposes is appropriate as long as confidentiality is maintained to the greatest possible degree by removing any individual identifiers. Otherwise, in determining whether to disclose identified information after the death of a patient, physicians should consider the following factors:

(1) The imminence of harm to identifiable individuals or the public health

(2) The potential benefit to at-risk individuals or the public health (e.g. if a communicable or inherited disease is preventable or treatable)

(3) Any statement or directive made by the patient regarding postmortem disclosure

(4) The impact disclosure may have on the reputation of the deceased patient

(5) Personal gain for the physician that may unduly influence professional obligations of confidentiality.

When a family member or other decision maker has given consent to an autopsy, physicians may

disclose the results of the autopsy to the individual(s) that granted consent to the procedure.
(American Medical Association Council on Ethical and Judicial Affairs, 2000, p.5)

4.3.2 UK Guidelines

Your duty of confidentiality continues after a patient has died. Whether and what personal information may be disclosed after a patient's death will depend on the circumstances. If the patient had asked for information to remain confidential, you should usually respect their wishes. If you are unaware of any instructions from the patient, when you are considering requests for information you should take into account:

(a) whether the disclosure of information is likely to cause distress to, or be of benefit to, the patient's partner or family

(b) whether the disclosure will also disclose information about the patient's family or anyone else

(c) whether the information is already public knowledge or can be anonymised or coded, and

(d) the purpose of the disclosure. (General Medical Council, 2009, p.28, section 70)

You are personally accountable for your professional practice and must always be prepared to justify your decisions and actions. (General Medical Council, 2009, p.2)

4.3.3 Irish Guidelines

The Irish Medical Council also addresses the issue briefly and confirms that the ethical duty of confidentiality extends beyond death:

Patient information remains confidential even after death. If it is unclear whether the patient consented to disclosure of information after their death, you should consider how disclosure of the information might benefit or cause distress to the deceased's family or carers. You should also consider the effect of disclosure on the reputation of the deceased and the purpose of the disclosure. Individual discretion in this area might be limited by law. (Medical Council, 2009, p.27, section 24.2)

What is at the heart of these guidelines is concern for the wishes of the patient, worry about harm to others and the need to anonymise information where possible.

Other good reasons for protecting confidentiality after death centre on the impact that posthumous breaches of confidentiality may have on the care that the dying patient receives. Robinson and O'Neill (2007) frame the problem in the following way:

Although certain ethicists may argue that the dead have no interests to protect, some individuals' fear of disclosure of information posthumously may be as great as contemporaneous disclosure.

Such fears affect patient behaviour and candor, which may result in suboptimal care during life. Individuals frequently withhold information from loved ones to protect them, and there is no reason to assume that this should be different after a person's death. An expectation among the living that their private medical information may be released after death may inhibit the patient–clinician relationship. (Robinson and O'Neill, 2007, p.634)

This obligation is particularly weighty if the patient requested confidentiality when they were alive. The usual exceptions remain, however, that the patient's right to confidentiality is not absolute, and confidentiality may be breached in certain circumstances. Of these, the possibility that non-disclosure of confidential information may cause serious harm to other individuals or the general public are the most pressing.

The legal position is less clear. There is some authority from the European Court of Human Rights that a duty of confidentiality survives after death: see European Court of Human Rights Plon v France (2004). However, in Rotunda Hospital v Information Commissioner (2009), McCarthy J held that there was no right of privacy in deceased people. This decision is currently on appeal to the Supreme Court.

Access to information about deceased people may be obtained in some circumstances. The Freedom of Information Act 1997 and the Freedom of Information Act 1997 (Section 28(6)) Regulations 2009 (SI 387/2009) allow access to information about deceased people to certain classes of requesters. These are: a personal representative of the deceased person acting in due course of the administration of the estate of the deceased person; a person upon whom a function is conferred by law in relation to the estate of the deceased person; the spouse or next of kin of the deceased person where in the opinion of the head of the body from whom the information is sought, having regard to all circumstances, the public interest, including the public interest in the confidentiality of personal information would, on balance, be better served by granting than by refusing to grant the request.

The Regulations also define a 'spouse' and a 'next of kin'. A 'spouse' includes a party to a marriage which has been dissolved or who is living apart from the deceased person under a deed of separation and a man or woman who is not married to the deceased but who has cohabited as husband or wife with the deceased person. A 'next of kin' is 'the person or persons standing nearest in blood relationship' to the deceased person in accordance with the order set out in the Succession Act 1965.

5. Privacy – A Space to Call One's Own

5.1 Scope and Limits

'Privacy' is a rich concept that plays an important role in the assessment of healthcare policies and practices. The question of how to define privacy is a controversial one. Some say that privacy should be defined as a moral claim while others argue that privacy should be construed as a legal right. For a society to value individual privacy, it needs to specify and clarify what might be considered to be in the private domain and, therefore, worthy of protection. Bok offers a definition of privacy that is helpful when considering privacy in relation to end-of-life care:

> *the condition of being protected from unwanted access by others – either physical access, personal information, or attention. Claims to privacy are claims to control access to what one takes – however grandiosely – to be one's personal domain.* (Bok 1989, pp.10–11)

The law also fleshes out the meaning of privacy and links it with dignity and autonomy. For example, the Irish courts recognise a right to privacy (and by implication, a right to confidentiality) which is loosely derived from the Irish Constitution:

> *Though not specifically guaranteed by the Constitution, the right to privacy is one of the fundamental personal rights of the citizen which flow from the Christian and democratic nature of the State [...] The nature of the right to privacy must be such as to ensure the dignity and freedom of an individual in the type of society envisaged by the Constitution, namely, a sovereign, independent and democratic society.* (Hamilton P. in Kennedy and Arnold v Ireland [1987] cited in Madden, 2002)

The European Convention on Human Rights also protects privacy under Article 8: 'Everyone has the right to respect for his private and family life, his home and his correspondence' (Council of Europe, 1998, Art. 8.1, p.9).

However, just as professional codes consider exceptional circumstances where the principle of confidentiality might be qualified, so also legal rights to privacy are not considered absolute.

The European Convention, for example, also stipulates under Article 8 that:

There shall be no interference by a public authority with the exercise of this right except such as is in accordance with the law and is necessary in a democratic society in the interests of national security, public safety or the economic well-being of the country, for the prevention of disorder or crime, for the protection of health or morals, or for the protection of the rights and freedoms of others. (Council of Europe, 1998, Art. 8.2, p.9)

What is at the heart of qualification of the right to privacy in Article 8 is a concern for the interests of others and the public interest generally.

While private matters are often kept secret, there is an important difference between privacy and secrecy. What is kept private does not have to be secret, and what is kept secret does not have to be private. For example, a private house or a private life is not always a secret house or life. In turn, a secret ballot for government elections is not a private concern, nor is a secret plan to assassinate a president.

Control over secrecy provides a safety valve for individuals in the midst of communal life – some influence over transactions between the world of personal experience and the world shared with others. With no control over such exchanges, human beings would be unable to exercise choice about their lives. To restrain some secrets and to allow others freer play; to keep some hidden and to let others be known; to offer knowledge to some but not to all comers; to give and receive confidences and to guess at far more: these efforts at control permeate all human contact. Those who lose all control over these relations cannot flourish in either the personal or the shared world, nor retain their sanity. If experience in the shared world becomes too overwhelming, the sense of identity suffers. (Bok, 1989, p.20)

Why should we have some control over our secrets? One reason is that having control over our secrets protects a key element of personal autonomy: identity.

[Secrecy] [p]rotects identity, the sacred, unique and unfathomable nature of human beings: [Secrecy] protects vulnerable beliefs or feelings, inwardness, and the sense of being set apart; of having or belonging to regions not fully penetrable to scrutiny, including those of memory and dream; of being someone who is more, has become more, has more possibilities for the future than can ever meet the eyes of observers. [...] Human beings can be subjected to every scrutiny, and reveal much about themselves; but they can never be entirely understood, simultaneously exposed from every perspective, completely transparent either to themselves or to other persons. They are not only unique but unfathomable. (Bok, 1989, pp.20–1)

Bok emphasises the importance of individual rights to privacy and, linking them with autonomy, argues that conflicts about concealing or revealing personal information should be understood as conflicts of power. She claims:

Conflicts over secrecy – between state and citizen … or parent and child [or between health professional and patient] or in journalism or business or law – are conflicts over power: the power that comes through controlling the flow of information. To be able to hold back some information about oneself or to channel it and thus influence how one is seen by others gives power; so does the capacity to penetrate similar defenses and strategies when used by others. [...] To have no capacity for secrecy is to be out of control over how others see one; it leaves one open to coercion. To have no insight into what others conceal is to lack power as well.

(Bok, 1989, p.19)

5.2 Dimensions of Privacy

Judith DeCew (1997) analyses a range of privacy theories and privacy claims and believes that, rather than think of privacy as a single concept, we should look at it as an umbrella term or broad and multifaceted cluster concept for a wide variety of interests. Drawing on DeCew's and Bok's (1989) work on privacy, we suggest that there are five dimensions of privacy that health professionals might consider:

1. physical privacy
2. informational privacy
3. decisional privacy
4. personal property
5. expressive privacy

5.2.1 Physical Privacy

Physical privacy is a popular usage of the concept of privacy and it means freedom from unwanted contact with other people. This sense of privacy recognises the need for bodily privacy and environmental privacy and protects a desire for limited accessibility from others.

Complete physical privacy is inconsistent with the requirements of modern healthcare. Patients know that medical and nursing care may involve touching, invasive probing, nudity, and observation as necessary aspects of many examinations, treatments and surgeries. This is the privacy price of hopefully gaining better health. Nevertheless, patients can rightfully expect doctors, nurses and other carers to take special care against unnecessary or insensitive bodily exposure or contact. When it is necessary to have physical examinations, it is important and courteous to offer a brief explanation of what is being done, why it is necessary and some indication of the time duration of the physical contact.

These are minimal markers of respect for bodily privacy.

Because healthcare workers get accustomed to nudity and body exposure in various examinations and caring tasks, they might too readily become inured to the customary embarrassment that patient modesty causes. Respect for physical privacy should alert health professionals to try and keep 'alive' their awareness of patients' discomfort under examinations.

Physical privacy can also respect desires for seclusion and solitude that allow for peace of mind and intimacy. However, it does not imply that all patients would want to be in a room by themselves. While privacy is a most important value for patients, being in a room with two or three other patients can often help pass the time with friendly banter. People vary on what they would consider intrusive but individuals might consider some of the following as invasions of their physical privacy: unexpected and unexplained physical touch, telephone calls, other patients and their visitors coming in at will, their own visitors, chaplaincy visits, photography.

A commitment to the goal of protecting patients' physical privacy will also alert staff to:

- Introduce physical touch with request and explanation
- Minimise the duration and the extent of exposure
- Minimise or get permission for the bedside presence of medical/nursing students, spectators, or cameras producing photographs for study purposes
- Provide explanations to patients of what happens during times when they are unconscious
- The importance of expanding the number of single over shared hospital rooms
- The sensitivity of many patients to rooms of mixed sexes
- The possible preference of some patients for doctors or nurses of their own sex.

It may not always be possible to fulfil these aims but one can develop sharper sensitivity to these potential intrusions on patient privacy.

5.2.2 Informational Privacy

Secrecy, confidentiality, anonymity and protection of patient data would come under this meaning of privacy. Informational privacy calls for access to personal information to be limited and this is especially true with respect to health information, present and past. Limiting access to medical and insurance records are fundamental protections required under the principle of confidentiality in the professional–patient relationship.

5.2.3 Decisional Privacy

Decisional privacy can be understood as having control over intimate aspects of personal identity. Under decisional privacy a person can expect to be allowed, if not encouraged, to make their own decisions and act on their decisions if they so choose free from state, governmental or health professional interference. There is, however, at least one important constraint on decisional privacy. A person cannot make a decision that causes harm to a third party and expect that the decision will have no interference or opposition. Obviously, what is covered by 'harming third parties' would need to be clarified if individuals are to observe care and consideration when making decisions (see Module 4, 3.4).

This area of decisional privacy in healthcare contexts is a central issue in ethics, medical and nursing codes and hospital administration guidelines. In the healthcare context, decisional privacy concerns responsibility for very important choices about treatment, termination of treatment, and involvement in clinical trials. Who has the authority to decide about treatment, commencement and termination is often a point of contention. Patients may not wish to have decisional authority in these matters and give permission to health professionals to make those decisions for them (paternalism with permission). Health professionals have expertise to advise patients in decisions about treatment or life supports and most patients appreciate such advice (see Module 3, Module 4 and Module 6 for more on patient authority over decision making).

5.2.4 Personal Property

Respect for personal property includes all of a patient's personal belongings and, especially, those items that are considered by them to be most important, e.g. personal diaries, letters, handbags and wallets.

5.2.5 Expressive Privacy

This dimension of privacy protects a realm for expressing one's self-identity or personhood through activity or speech. Self expression is critical for lifestyle choices that contribute greatly to defining oneself and one's values. If expressive privacy is a value that facilitates or supports self-expression and self-identity, then as an element of expressive privacy we add a concept of personal space.

Iris Marion Young thinks privacy theories have given inadequate attention to material support for privacy in guaranteeing personal space. An essential element of privacy, for Young, is:

[…] having a dwelling space of one's own to which a person is able to control access and in which one lives among things that help support the narrative of one's life […] Services and institutions giving shelter and care to needy persons fail to appreciate what is required for individuals not simply to stay alive, physically well and nourished but to have the life of a person (**Young, 2005, pp.155–6**).

Studies of older people's feelings of at-homeness emphasise the embodied understanding of security in oneself as surrounded by familiar things – especially those that form a connection with a life lived. The sense of personal integrity and sense of self is linked to control. Older people, like people of all ages, resist attempts of organisers and managers to direct their routines and activities. The same can be applied to patients, residents of long-stay units or residents suffering from dementia.

6. Cases: Respecting Confidentiality of the Dying and Deceased

6.1 Case 1: The Rights of Relatives to Medical Records

Particular circumstances may arise where relatives of deceased persons may ask for information. The British Medical Association (BMA) cites a common example: 'when the family requests details of the terminal illness because of anxiety that the patient might have been misdiagnosed or there might have been negligence' (BMA, 2008, p.47). Because such disclosure is likely to be what the deceased person would have wanted, and because it might also be a matter of justice, disclosure is usually justified in such cases.

Medical records may also be requested in circumstances where a will is contested on the basis of doubts raised as to the capacity of an individual to execute it. Again, disclosure in this case is generally viewed as acceptable because it is considered to advance the interests of the patient. Robinson and O'Neill (2007) note that the situation is less clear in cases where the disclosure of a hereditary or infectious condition might benefit those close to the patient.

Freedom of information (FOI) legislation in many countries, including Ireland, governs access to personal information. In line with existing legislation protecting confidentiality, freedom of information laws protect private information but also allow for exceptions. The following case illustrates the balance that is sometimes struck between protecting patient confidentiality and the rights of interested others to access patient information.

The Rights of Relatives to Medical Records

Ms X requested access to her deceased brother's records held by Cork University Hospital but was refused by the Irish Southern Health Board. In refusing access to the patient's records the Board Submission made the following general observations:

- *that the doctor–patient relationship is inherently private and based on confidence;*
- *following the death of a patient, it is reasonable to assume that his/her privacy rights will continue to be respected;*
- *any public perception that medical records may be released to others, following the death of the patient, may inhibit the provision of relevant medical information by patients generally;*
- *once records are released under FOI there are no restrictions on the manner in which they may be used.'* (5th December, 2002)

On appeal to the Office of the Information Commissioner, the rights of Ms X to access the medical records were upheld. Specifically, the Commissioner took the following into account:

- *all of his siblings, who were his nearest next of kin, agreed to the records being released to Ms X (Ms X had provided evidence that her two sisters agreed to the release of the records to her);*

- *the fact that Ms X's sister was named as his next of kin and personal carer in his hospital admission records suggests that he had confidence in her judgement in relation to matters concerning him;*

- *the fact that the patient had good relations with his siblings and that there was no evidence of estrangement between them – all three sisters visited him in hospital and were with him when he died;*

- *there was no evidence that the patient would have objected to the release of the records;*

- *there was nothing of unusual sensitivity in the patient's records; and nothing that Ms X was not aware of in general terms;*

- *the patient's GP saw fit to release the records to Ms X.*

(Office of the Information Commissioner, 2003, Case 020561)

6.1.1 Discussion

On the one hand, in this case, the Southern Health Board was concerned about patient privacy, the lack of restriction on how the records might be used and the worry that it might change the public's trust that confidentiality is protected. On the other hand, the Information Commissioner focussed on the wishes of the patient, the non-sensitive nature of the information requested and evidence of the (good) relationship between the requester and the patient.

In Case 1, the family of the patient had concerns about the patient's will. Considering the decision of the Commissioner in light of situations where patients' relatives seek information because they are anxious about hereditary risks to themselves, Robinson and O'Neill propose that a more cautious approach to the release of information might serve to protect confidentiality and reassure relatives. They suggest 'an expert review of the likelihood of genetic risk or of inadequate care' rather than, necessarily, the release of full medical records (Robinson and O'Neill, 2007, p.635). Moreover, these authors suggest that such a review could form 'part of a bereavement care program following death, ideally involving the patient's personal physician' who would have cared for the patient in the terminal phase of their illness (Robinson and O'Neill, 2007, p.635). They argue that such support could be supplemented by providing the advice of expert clinicians who are independent of the institutions and individuals at the centre of the situation.

However, while Robinson and O'Neill's proposal goes some way towards balancing the obligation to protect patient confidentiality with the needs of those who might benefit from disclosure, critics of their position might see the reliance on 'expert opinion' to decide what should and should not be disclosed as overly paternalistic. Glen (1997) distinguishes between confidentiality understood as respect for privacy and confidentiality understood as a means of control. She worries that the duty of confidentiality may be misused by health professionals and organisations in order to maintain control over information.

> *'Confidentiality' can become a somewhat embellishing signboard for paternalistic caring. In essence, one needs to distinguish between confidentiality as a respectful attitude to a patient/ client, where it becomes credible that the caring professional will not misuse the information she or he obtains about the patient/client, and between confidentiality misused as an instrument of power to keep the patient/client outside the processes in which it might be important or advantageous for him or her to participate.'* (Glen, 1997, p.403)

In a similar vein, Bok draws attention to the way in which maintaining confidentiality might not serve vulnerable populations well. She notes:

> *The sick, the poor, the mentally ill, the aged, and the very young are in a paradoxical situation in this respect. While their right to confidentiality is often breached and their most intimate problems bandied about, the poor care they may receive is just as often covered up under the same name of confidentiality. That is the shield held forth to prevent outsiders from finding out about negligence, overcharging, unnecessary surgery, or institutionalization. And far more than individual mistakes and misdeeds are thus covered up, for confidentiality is also the shield that professionals invoke to protect incompetent colleagues and negligence and unexpected accidents in, for instance, hospitals, factories, or entire industries.* (Bok, 1983, p.30)

6.1.2 Suggested Professional Responsibilities

- Health professionals have an obligation to respect patient confidentiality which extends beyond the patient's death.

- Consideration should be given to the wishes of the patient prior to their death in relation to the confidentiality of information relating to them if these are known or can be otherwise determined.

- The sensitivity of the information sought should be taken into account.

- Health professionals also have a duty of care in relation the well-being and welfare of those who are bereaved.

- Access to patient information should not be considered as an automatic right. In deciding access to patient information professionals should be aware of legislation pertaining to Freedom of Information.

- Health professionals should consider carefully the particular circumstances that give rise to the relatives' request for access to the patient's records.

6.2 Case 2: The Patient with HIV – Silence of the Tomb

Consider the following case where the patient, Peter, has not made known whether or not information about his illness should be disclosed to anyone:

Silence of the Tomb

Peter died suddenly following a short illness. HIV was diagnosed post mortem. There had been no indication from Peter of his wishes with regards to telling his friends and family. Similarly, he had denied any risk factors for HIV. A week following his death, Peter's sister Ann visited from Australia and asked to see a doctor to discuss the cause of her brother's death. She also wanted to know specifically if he had been infected with HIV. Ann was subsequently informed only of his heart failure and not of his HIV status [...]. Before seeing her, the treating physicians were told by a representative legal body that: 'the duty of confidentiality of Peter persists after his death – we may talk to her about the cause of death only as it appeared on the death certificate (which did not mention HIV)'. **(adapted from Wildfire, Stebbing and Gazzard, 2007, p.474)**

6.2.1 Discussion

According to Wildfire et al. (2007), the advice to Peter's doctors implies that only publicly available information may be shared and that Peter's HIV status was no-one else's business as it had no bearing on the health or welfare of anyone else.

Wildfire et al. pose a number of questions in relation to this scenario that might be considered here:

1. Do dead patients have a right to confidentiality?

-   if so, health professionals are obliged to respect their confidentiality but they must consider this duty in the light of their other duties to protect the health and well-being of others (individuals and society).

-   if dead patients are not considered to have a right to confidentiality, then health professionals 'can primarily consider the mental and physical welfare' of any other relatives or persons who might benefit from the information shared (Wildfire et al., 2007).

2. Do health professionals have a right to tell the truth or avoid deception?

If we accept that the duty of confidentiality persists beyond death, Wildfire et al. (2007) present one argument for maintaining Peter's confidentiality in the following way:

> *Patient P's right to confidentiality has moral supremacy, as he is the patient with the problem and the vulnerable should be protected. His trust in the doctor, that was inherent in their professional relationship, is preserved by maintaining privacy and discretion. His right as the patient overrides the wishes of his sister, or the doctor's right to tell the truth.* (Wildfire et al., 2007, p.475)

6.2.2 Suggested Professional Responsibilities

- Health professionals have a duty of care towards the living as well as the dead. In response to requests for information about deceased persons, health professionals need to determine whether or not the disclosure of that information has any implications for the health and well-being of others.

- In order to avoid situations where health professionals are torn between the duty of confidentiality and the duty to warn or protect others, those who treat HIV-positive patients should discuss with them as early as possible the limits of patient confidentiality.

- Such a discussion could include making a plan for what might happen should the patient lose their capacity to make decisions about their care and who might be involved (and perhaps informed) about their status in order that their best interests are preserved.

- A balance has to be struck between respect for confidentiality and the legitimate interests of others.

6.3 Case 3: Refusing to Disclose – Don't tell anyone until I'm gone

Consider a slightly different scenario for Peter. The following case relates to the duty to warn and illustrates some of the complex ethical tensions that arise when a health professional must contemplate breaching confidentiality in these circumstances.

Don't Tell Anyone Until I'm Gone

Peter is imminently dying and staff are aware that he has HIV/AIDS. Peter is in a coma and, prior to lapsing into the coma, Peter specifically asked that the fact that he has AIDS not be shared with anyone until after his death. Peter's partner Salma and his sister have been regular visitors to the ICU unit where Peter is being cared for. They are not aware of Peter's condition. One morning, Salma asks the nurse who seems to be Peter's main carer to tell her more about Peter's condition.

6.3.1 Discussion

One morally significant difference between Case 2 and Case 3 is that, in Case 3, there is an identifiable person who is at risk of harm (and of harming others) if the information is not disclosed. As Peter has given his permission to disclose that he has HIV/AIDS after his death, disclosure post-mortem would be ethically acceptable. The question that arises here relates, primarily, to the 'when?' of disclosure.

In Case 3, the nurse must decide whether he should inform Salma about Peter's condition or whether he should protect the confidentiality of the therapeutic relationship. It seems that he must choose between two competing moral obligations, the obligation to keep patient confidentiality and the obligation to protect another person whose life may be at risk if he fails to disclose. To help him in making the decision, he must ask himself the following questions about the situation.

1. Is it within the scope of his practice to give this kind of information to anyone?
2. What values are protected by the principle of confidentiality and are they relevant in this case?
3. Does he have an obligation to protect a third party who is not his patient?
4. If there is both a duty to a patient and a duty to a third party, which is the most compelling duty?
5. If he is considering telling Salma, how much should be told?

As indicated earlier, the principle of confidentiality is basic to all human relationships, is essential to the promotion of trust between health professional and patient and is an expression of respect for patient autonomy and privacy. The positive consequences to the patient of keeping confidentiality are also considered important. In Case 3, Peter has asked that no-one is told until after his death. In considering his situation, the nurse is obliged to maintain his trust in him as much as possible, he is also obliged to respect his autonomy, i.e. the decisions he makes in relation to his own life (see Module 4. 3.2, 3.3).

In addition to these duties, the nurse must also consider the consequences of disclosure. Not everyone agrees that making exceptions to the principle of confidentiality is helpful in the longer run. Utilitarian ethicists such as Helga Kuhse are concerned that allowing exceptions to the rule of confidentiality with the intention of protecting third-party interests will not achieve their intended effect in the long term (Kuhse, 1999, pp.493–6). Kuhse's basic concern is that a more relaxed confidentiality requirement on the part of health professionals will inhibit people who are most in need of health services from availing of them:

> *The point is that if known breaches of confidentiality are likely to prevent individuals from seeking treatment or to hinder them from seeking treatment in a timely fashion, then a rule requiring disclosure is likely to do more harm than good.* (**Kuhse, 1999, p.495**)

The cost of breaches of confidentiality is the loss of patient trust and (though this doesn't apply to Peter's case) the subsequent inability to support patients to modify behaviour that is harmful to others. In brief, on Kuhse's view, while harm might be prevented on some occasions, in the longer term the overall harm to society will not be reduced.

On the other hand, even though Peter's partner is not his patient, it could be argued that the nurse also has a moral obligation to protect her. Not just Peter's, but also Salma's autonomy is very much at risk in this situation. While the consequences of disclosure might be serious for Peter, the consequences of nondisclosure are also serious for Salma.

The most compelling argument for disclosure is a health-related one based on general agreement that early access to anti-retroviral therapy and healthcare management are likely to prolong the health and welfare of individuals with HIV (Woodman, 2003, p.7).
The nurse might also consult relevant professional and legal regulations. For example, the guidelines of the UK Society of Sexual Health Advisers (SSHA) (2004) acknowledge that sexual health advisers have a professional duty to protect third parties and an important function of GUM clinics in Ireland and elsewhere is the process of partner notification. Partner notification, or contact tracing, describes the process whereby individuals who may have been in contact with a sexually transmitted infection (STI) are contacted (by the partner

or by the health professional) in order to prevent the spread of the infection.

From a legal point of view, the Tarasoff case and other legislation indicate that there is a duty to warn an identifiable third party of serious danger. In this case, the third party is identifiable – the nurse needs to consider if she (and others) are also in serious danger: Salma may already be HIV positive and is in need of treatment. Additionally, the nurse needs to determine if she or other visitors need to take precautions against contracting the disease.

The ethical dilemma that the nurse is faced with then is very real; he has a duty to the patient and he has a duty to protect the patient's partner. It seems that he cannot fulfil both duties at once; if he fulfils his duty to Salma, he must neglect his duty to Peter and vice versa. Case 3 seems to evolve into a 'win–lose' situation, where Peter wins and Salma loses or vice versa.

6.3.2 Suggested Professional Responsibilities

- Health professionals must balance a duty to respect patient confidentiality with a duty to warn identifiable others at risk of serious harm.

- The health professionals involved must consider whether or not Peter will regain consciousness.

- In general, those who treat HIV-positive patients should discuss with them as early as possible the limits of patient confidentiality.

- The health professionals in this case need to distinguish between the weight of two possible requests for information; from Salma and from Peter's sister Ann. They must consider the health-related argument in favour of disclosing information to Salma because she may benefit from access to anti-retroviral therapy and healthcare management.

- The nurse must consider who is best placed to talk to Salma about Peter's situation.

6.4 Case 4: Trust and Confidentiality – Privacy, a Bond of Trust

Consider the following case which illustrates the links between trust, confidentiality, privacy and identity and demonstrates how health professionals can nurture and protect all of these.

Privacy, a Bond of Trust

Julie, an otherwise healthy 66-year-old woman, presents to her doctor with a three-month history of weight loss, sleep disturbance, and loss of appetite. The exchange with the busy physician is brief:

'Do you live alone?'

'Yes.'

'What about your husband?'

'He died twenty years ago.'

The physician diagnoses depression and prescribes an antidepressant with follow-up in two weeks. When Julie returns, a different doctor is covering that day.

'Who do you live with?'

'No-one – I'm alone.'

'Is that a change for you?'

'Yes.'

'Tell me about what has happened recently.'

'Sheila died.'

'Sheila … did she live with you?'

'Yes.'

'How long did the two of you live together?'

'Eighteen years.'

'Were the two of you close?'

'Yes. Very.' (patient in tears …)

In addition to the antidepressant, the physician offers Julie bereavement counselling. In future follow-up, Julie reveals a relationship with Sheila that the two women had hidden from their children and community, all of whom assumed they were 'just roommates.'

(Peterkin and Risdon, 2003, p.25)

6.4.1 Discussion

Peterkin and Risdon (2003) draw attention to the need for health professionals to be especially sensitive and open to Lesbian, Gay, Bisexual and Transgender (LGBT) patients – this case illustrates the impact that a conversation that does not assume that all patients are heterosexual can have on the outcome for the patient.

The need for health professionals to be more sensitive to the lives and health of LGBT patients, family members and health professionals is supported by international research on the physical and mental dangers that many LGBT individuals must face in every part of the world. One recent and sobering example of this is found in a very comprehensive report on levels of discrimination and homophobia across the European member states, which includes very large surveys of individuals' experiences at the hands of health professionals (European Union Agency for Fundamental Rights, 2009).

Recent Irish research indicates that LGBT people living in Ireland face particular challenges in relation to the recognition of partners in healthcare contexts. This is especially true in relation to decision making around end-of-life care, for example withholding and withdrawing treatment, last rites and hospital visits (Higgins and Glacken, 2009). In addition, as the Health Service Executive (HSE) Report on LGBT Health (2009a) and the Equality Authority (2002) indicate, 'the invisibility of older LGBT people may lead to a reluctance to disclose a same-sex relationship. This may impact on the ability to express grief when a partner dies or to be involved in the funeral arrangements' (HSE, 2009a, p.38).

6.4.2 Suggested Professional Responsibilities

- Don't assume everyone is heterosexual (e.g. service users, carers, parents, colleagues).
- Respond positively when people disclose their sexual orientation and/or gender identity.
- Ensure respect, confidentiality and privacy is shown to all LGBT people.
- Address issues of same-sex partners and next-of-kin in care settings in a sensitive manner.
- Be informed about the health issues of LGBT people.
- Ensure all relevant paperwork uses language which is inclusive of LGBT people and their families (e.g. information leaflets, questions used in history taking).
- Address unacceptable, offensive or discriminatory comments and/or actions relating to LGBT people. (Drawn from HSE, 2009b)

7. Module 7 Further Discussion

7.1 The Tarasoff Case (1976)

In that case, the California Supreme Court imposed on a psychotherapist a limited duty to warn a presumed intended victim of a patient's aggression. The case came about when the parents of a murdered student, Tatiana Tarasoff, sued the University of California and the professionals involved for their failure to notify them that their daughter was in grave danger. Her killer, Prosenjit Poddar, had been undergoing outpatient psychotherapy with the student health services during which he had admitted to having violent fantasies in relation to Tarasoff. The therapist, who learned from Poddar's friend that he had purchased a gun, took steps to hospitalise him for further evaluation, against his will if necessary. However, Californian law makes involuntary hospitalisation difficult and, while Poddar was still at large, he shot and killed Tarasoff and was subsequently convicted of second-degree homicide.

The parents claimed that the defendant (University of California, therapist and campus police) failed to notify them or their daughter that she was in danger. The providers involved claimed that they could not warn Tatiana Tarasoff because it would violate patient confidentiality.

(Unites States case of Tarasoff v the Regents of the University of California, 1976)

8. Module 7 Summary Learning Guides

8.1 Confidential Information

Confidential information

- is private information that a person shares with another on the understanding that it will not be disclosed to third parties.

Keeping patient confidentiality is important because it

- builds patient trust
- protects patient autonomy and privacy
- contributes to good treatment and care outcomes.

8.2 Professional Codes and Laws

- Professional codes stipulate that patients have a right to confidentiality.
- Confidentiality is also protected by law: court decisions, the Irish Constitution and the European Convention on Human Rights.

Qualifying the principle of confidentiality

The principle of confidentiality is not considered absolute. Exceptional circumstances where the principle may be qualified include:

- Disclosure required by law
- Disclosure in the interest of the patient or other people
- Disclosure in the public interest.

8.3 Privacy

Privacy can be defined as the condition of being protected from unwanted access by others.

There are five dimensions of privacy that health professionals might consider:

1. physical privacy
2. informational privacy
3. decisional privacy
4. personal property
5. expressive privacy

9. Module 7 Activities

9.1 Consider again the principle of confidentiality:

a. Can you give one example from your professional experience where the breaching of a patient's confidentiality undermined their trust in the health professions?

b. Re-read Bok's argument that conflicts about disclosing or not disclosing personal information are about power. Can you think of any example from your professional experience that might support Bok's view?

c. Nightingale suggests that confidentiality may be breached through 'gossip' and 'vain talk'. Can you think of contemporary examples where such breaches might arise?

d. Can you think of any other circumstances where in the process of ordinary, everyday routine activities in a clinic or hospital, patient confidentiality might be breached?

9.2 Reflect back on the particulars of Case 1:

a. Jot down your own unanalysed response to the position of the HSE and the position of the Information Commissioner. Which position is closest to your own?

b. Give reasons for your answer.

c. Critically consider the more cautious approach towards information sharing with relatives that Robinson and O'Neill advise. Do you think that they are being overly cautious and/or paternalistic? Or do they have the balance right between protecting patients and their families?

9.3 Reflect back on the particulars of Cases 2 and 3:

Consider the following questions that clinicians and nurses might ask themselves:

a. How do I treat the information that a patient shares with me?

b. How do I treat what I know about the patient from other colleagues or from the patient's records?

c. How much of a say does the patient have in what I do with this information?

d. Where do my loyalties lie: to the patient or the patient's family? To my profession, my colleagues, my employer, other affected parties?

e. If I were given a piece of information about a patient in the strictest confidence, would I be able to keep that confidence?

f. If I thought that not disclosing the confidential information of a patient might cause harm to another individual or individuals, what would I do? What level of harm is enough harm?

9.4 Reflect back on the particulars of Case 4:

a. Consider each of the HSE Good Practice Guidelines (2009). Decide the ways in which these guidelines might be applied to LGBT patients who are terminally ill and LGBT families of dying or deceased patients.

b. Check if the contact details, posters and literature of local and national LGBT services are displayed in the waiting areas of your place of work.

c. Consider what you might need to do to become familiar with local LGBT groups and services in order to develop working relationships with them.

10. Module 7 References and Further Reading

Ainslie, D.C. 'Questioning Bioethics, AIDS, Sexual Ethics, and the Duty to Warn', *The Hastings Center Report*, vol. 29, no. 5, 1999, pp.26–35

Allen, A. 'Privacy in Health Care', in S.G. Post (ed.), *Encyclopedia of Bioethics* (3rd ed., vol. 2) (New York: Macmillan, 2004)

American Medical Association Council on Ethical and Judicial Affairs, 'Confidentiality of Health Information Postmortem (Rep. No.5-A-00)', http://www.ama-assn.org/ama1/pub/upload/mm/code-medical-ethics/5051a.pdf [accessed 16 June 2009]

Beauchamp, T. and Childress, J. *Principles of Biomedical Ethics* (5th ed.) (Oxford and New York: Oxford University Press, 2001)

Bok, S. 'The Limits of Confidentiality', *The Hastings Center Report*, vol. 13, no. 1, 1983, pp.24–31

Bok, S. *Secrets* (New York: Vintage Books, 1989)

An Bord Altranais, *Code of Professional Conduct for Each Nurse and Midwife* (Dublin: An Bord Altranais, 2000a)

An Bord Altranais, *Scope of Nursing and Midwifery Practice Framework* (Dublin: An Bord Altranais, 2000b)

Brazier, M. and Cave, E. *Medicine, Patients and the Law* (4th ed.) (London: Penguin Books, 2007)

British Medical Association (BMA), 'Confidentiality and Disclosure of Health Information Toolkit' (2008), http://www.bma.org.uk/ethics/confidentiality/ConfToolKit08.jsp [accessed 10 June 2009]

Constitution of Ireland (Bunreacht na hÉireann), 1937

Council of Europe, *The European Convention for the Protection of Human Rights and Fundamental Freedoms as Amended by Protocol No. 11 (ETS No. 155)* (Rome: Council of Europe, 1950)

Council of Europe, *Data Protection Directive 95/46/EC* (1995) http://europa.eu.int/ISPO/legal/en/dataprot/directiv/directiv.html [accessed 1 May 2004]

Council of Europe, Article 8. 'Right to Respect for Private and Family Life', *The European Convention on Human Rights and Fundamental Freedoms as Amended by Protocol No. 11 (ETS No. 155)* (Strasbourg: Council of Europe, 1998)

Data Protection Act No. 25/1988,

http://www.irishstatutebook.ie/1988/en/act/pub/0025/index.html [accessed 1 May 2004]

Data Protection (Amendment) Act No. 6/2003, http://www.justice.ie/802569B20047F907/vWeb/wpMJDE5NKDM9 [accessed 1 May 2004]

DeCew, J. *In Pursuit of Privacy: Law, Ethics and the Rise of Technology* (Ithaca and London: Cornell University Press, 1997)

Department of Health and Children, *Children First: National Guidelines for the Protection and Welfare of Children*, http://www.dohc.ie/publications/pdf/children_first.pdf?direct=1 [accessed 12 December 2009]

Donnelly, M. and McDonagh, M. Personal communication, 2009

Edelstein, L. *The Hippocratic Oath: Text, Translation, and Interpretation* (Baltimore: Johns Hopkins University Press, 1943)

Equality Authority, *Implementing Equality for Lesbians, Gays and Bisexuals* (Dublin: Equality Authority, 2002)

European Court of Human Rights (Second Section), Case of Plon (Société) v France Application No. 56148/00 of 18 May 2004

European Union Agency for Fundamental Rights, *Homophobia and Discrimination Grounds of Sexual Orientation and Gender Identity in the EU Member States. Summary Report*, http://fra.europa.eu [accessed 12 September 2009]

Freedom of Information Act 1997 (Section 28(6)) Regulations 2009, http://www.foi.gov.ie/legislation [accessed 12 September 2009]

Freedom of Information Act. No. 13/1997, http://www.irishstatutebook.ie/1997/en/act/pub/0013/index.html [accessed 12 September 2009]

Garro, L.C. 'Culture, Pain and Cancer', *Journal of Palliative Care*, vol. 6, no. 3, 1990, pp.34–44

General Medical Council (GMC), *Confidentiality: Guidance for Doctors* (London: General Medical Council, 2009)

Glackin, M. and Higgins, A. 'The Grief Experience of Same-Sex Couples Within an Irish Context: Tacit Acknowledgement', *International Journal of Palliative Nursing*, vol. 14, no. 6, 2008, pp.297–302

Glen, S. 'Confidentiality: A Critique of the Traditional View', *Nursing Ethics*, vol. 4, no. 5, 1997, pp.403–6

Greenhalgh, T. and Hurwitz, B. *Narrative-Based Medicine: Dialogue and Discourse in Clinical Practice* (London: British Medical Journal Books, 1998)

Health Protection Surveillance Centre, *Notifiable Infectious Diseases* (22 January 2009), http://www.ndsc.ie/hpsc/NotifiableDiseases/NotificationLegislationandProcess [accessed 12 December 2009]

Health Service Executive (HSE), *LGBT Health: Towards Meeting the Health Care Needs of Lesbian, Gay, Bisexual and Transgender People* (2009a), http://www.hse.ie/eng/services/news/2009_Archive/May_2009/LGBT_HEALTH_Towards_meeting_the_Health_care_Needs_of_Lesbian,_Gay,_Bisexual_and_Transgender_People.html [accessed 12 December 2009]

Health Service Executive (HSE), *Good Practice Guidelines for Health Service Providers Working with Lesbian, Gay, Bisexual and Transgender People* (Dublin: HSE, 2009b), http://www.hse.ie/eng/newsmedia/Archive/LGBT_HEALTH_Towards_meeting_the_Health_care_Needs_of_Lesbian,_Gay,_Bisexual_and_Transgender_People.html [accessed 1 June 2009]

Higgins, A. and Glacken, M. 'Sculpting the Distress: Easing or Exacerbating the Grief Experience of Same-Sex Couples', *International Journal of Palliative Nursing*, vol. 15, no. 4, 2009, pp.170–6

Hunter v. Mann [1974] 2 All ER 414 QBD England

Jansen, L.A. and Friedman Ross, L. 'Patient Confidentiality and the Surrogate's Right to Know', *The Journal of Law, Medicine & Ethics*, vol. 28, no. 2, 2000, pp.137–43

Kennedy & Arnold v Ireland [1987] IR1 per Hamilton P

Kuhse, H. 'Confidentiality and the AMA's New Code of Ethics: An Imprudent Formulation?' in Kuhse, H. and Singer, P. (eds), *Bioethics: An Anthology* (London: Blackwell, 1999), pp.493–6

Madden, D. *Medicine, Ethics and the Law* (Dublin: Butterworths, 2002)

Mason, J.K. and Laurie, G.T. 'The Principle of Confidentiality: Relaxation of the Rule', in *Mason and McCall Smith's Law and Medical Ethics* (Oxford and New York: Oxford University Press, 2006), pp.253–79

Mason, T. 'Tarasoff Liability: Its Impact for Working with Patients who Threaten Others', *International Journal of Nursing Studies*, vol. 35, nos 1–2, 1998, pp.109–14

McDonald, L. (ed.), *Florence Nightingale: The Nightingale School. The Collected Works of Florence Nightingale* (vol. 12) (Waterloo, ON: Wilfrid Laurier University Press, 2008)

Medical Council, *Guide to Professional Conduct and Ethics for Registered Medical Practitioners* (7th ed.) (2009), http://www.medicalcouncil.ie [accessed 20 November 2009)]

Mills, S. *Clinical Practice and the Law* (Dublin: Butterworths, 2002)

Murray, T. and Jennings, B. *The Quest to Reform End-of-Life Care: Rethinking Assumptions and Setting New Directions. A Hastings Center Special Report, 'Improving End-of-Life Care'*, pp.S52–S59

Nightingale, F. 'Notes on Nursing: What It Is, and What It Is Not' (1859), http://www.nursingcenter.com/library/JournalArticle.asp?Article_ID=270233#13 [accessed 1 May 2004]

Nightingale, F. *Notes on Nursing: What It Is, and What It Is Not* (commemorative edition) (Philadelphia: J.B. Lippincott, 1992)

Office of the Information Commissioner, 'Case 020561 – Ms X and the Southern Health Board' (2003), http://www.oic.gov.ie/en/DecisionsoftheCommissioner/ LetterDecisions/Name,1287,en.htm [accessed 9 June 2009]

Perez-Carceles, M.D., Perniguez, J.E., Osuna, E. and Luna, A. 'Balancing Confidentiality and the Information Provided to Families of Patients in Primary Care', *Journal of Medical Ethics*, vol. 31, no. 9, 2005, pp.531–5

Peterkin, A. and Risdon, C. *Caring for Lesbian and Gay People: A Clinical Guide* (Toronto: University of Toronto Press, 2003)

Phukan, J.F.M., Cunney, A., Getty, S. and O'Neill, D. 'How is My Mother, Doctor? *Irish Journal of Medical Science*, no. 173 (Supplement 1), 2004, p.47

Rotunda Hospital v Information Commissioner [2009], IEHC 315, http://www.bailii.org/ie/ cases/IEHC/2009/H315.html [accessed 12 May 2010]

Robinson, D.J. and O'Neil, D. 'Access to Health Care Records after Death', *JAMA: Journal of the American Medical Association*, 2007, pp.634–6

Schwartz, L., Preece, P. and Hendry, R.A. *Medical Ethics: A Case-Based Approach* (Edinburgh: Saunders, 2002)

Society of Sexual Health Advisers (UK), 'Code of Professional Conduct', http://www.ssha.info/ member/code.htm [accessed 1 May 2004]

Succession Act 1965 No. 27/1965

Tarasoff v. the Regents of the University of California et al., 551 P.2d 334 131 Cal Rptr 14 (1976) [Tarasoff II]

Torrance, I. 'Confidentiality and its Limits: Some Contributions from Christianity', *Journal of Medical Ethics*, vol. 29, 2003, pp.8–9

University of Virginia Historical Collections, 'Vaulted Treasures. Hippocrates (460 BCE-ca. 370 BCE) (2007), http://historical.hsl.virginia.edu/treasures/hippocrates.html [accessed 12 December 2009]

Werth, J.L., Burke, C. and Bardash, R.J. 'Confidentiality in End of Life and after Death Situations', *Ethics & Behavior*, vol. 12, no. 3, 2002, pp.205–22

Whipple, V. *Lesbian Widows: Invisible Grief* (New York: Harwood Press, 2006)

Wildfire, A., Stebbing, J. and Gazzard, B. 'Rights Theory in a Specific Healthcare Context: "Speaking Ill of the Dead"', *Postgraduate Medical Journal*, vol. 83, no. 981, 2007, pp.473–7

Woodman, M.A. 'Partner Notification for Sexually Transmitted Infections in the Republic of Ireland', unpublished MComm., University College Cork, 2003

Young, I.M. 'A Room of One's Own: Old Age, Extended Care and Privacy', in *On Female Body Experience: 'Throwing Like a Girl' and Other Essays* (Oxford and New York: Oxford University Press, 2005), pp.155–6; 160–3

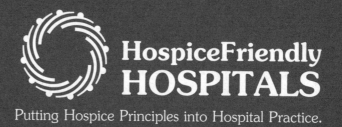

HospiceFriendly HOSPITALS

Putting Hospice Principles into Hospital Practice.

Module 8

Ethical Governance in Clinical Care and Research

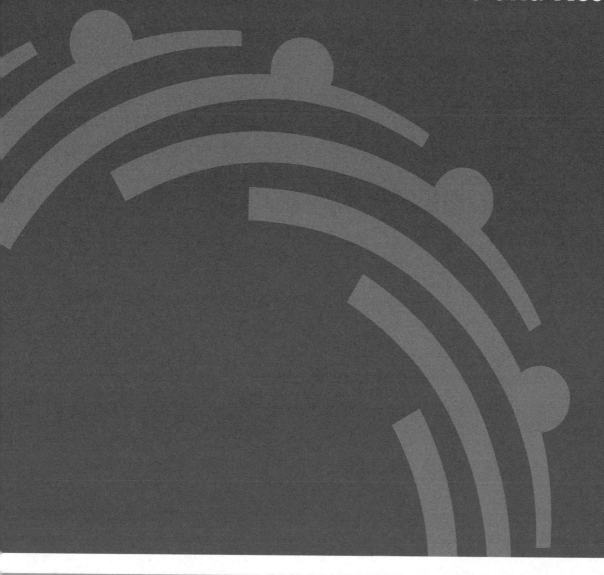

Module 8 Contents

1. Module 8 Key Points

1.1. There is a need for formal ethics support in clinical practice:

Recent advances in biomedical technology and the identification of an increased range of values and needs in the patient population have led to a growing awareness of the complexity of healthcare provision and the need for formal ethics support for health professionals in the day-to-day treatment of patients. In the US and UK, this support most commonly takes the form of a healthcare or clinical ethics committee, although it can also be provided by an individual ethicist trained in the skills necessary for ethics consultation.

1.2. Constitution and terms of reference of ethics committees:

Unlike research ethics committees, healthcare or clinical ethics committees have no legal standing, and there are different interpretations of their mandate. However, central to the effective functioning of such committees is their multidisciplinary constitution, with members drawn from nursing, medicine, psychology, law, ethics, theology, social work and administration. This diverse range of expertise allows the members of these committees to explore more comprehensively the different aspects of an ethically challenging case or situation.

1.3. The role of healthcare or clinical ethics committees:

In the US, Europe and Australia, healthcare ethics committees (HECs) or clinical ethics committees (CECs) perform a threefold function: they provide ethics education for health professionals, hospital staff, patients and families; they contribute to the formulation and revision of hospital policy, and they provide a consultation service to support practitioners in resolving difficult or demanding clinical cases. While the first two of these functions are relatively uncontroversial, the third is more contentious.

1.4. Defining clinical ethics consultation:

Ethics consultation may take a number of forms. There are different models of consultation, as well as different methods for conducting consultations. Because the practice of ethics consultation is still evolving, there is no universally accepted definition of its nature or purpose. However, commentators agree that the following tasks are central to the process of ethics consultation: the identification and clarification of values, the exploration of diverse perspectives, the creation of an open environment for discussion, the determination and analysis of available options, the facilitation of communication between involved parties, and the building of consensus.

1.5. Reasons for ethics consultation:

Historically, HECs or CECs were consulted primarily for guidance in relation to issues such as the withholding or withdrawing of treatment, competent refusal of treatment, advance directives and DNR (do not resuscitate) orders, or in relation to problems involving capacity, consent and confidentiality. In recent years, however, the focus has shifted to questions of communication, negotiation and mediation. Requests for ethics consultations may arise as a result of conflict between the healthcare team and the patient or member of the patient's family during the course of the routine provision of care, or from disagreements between members of the healthcare team concerning the nature of the treatment provided or the manner in which it is provided. They may also issue indirectly from flawed or short-sighted management practices, or they may arise as a response to the culture of the organisation, in the form of unease with decisions taken at the executive level and their implications for the quality of patient care.

1.6. Clinical ethics committees: concerns and challenges:

As the provision of clinical ethics consultation services becomes more widespread in the US and Europe, the role of HECs and CECs is subject to increasing scrutiny. Issues raised include concerns about the moral authority, expertise and qualification of members of CECs, in addition to concerns about the legitimacy of their recommendations and concerns about the lack of standardisation in relation to the objectives and terms of reference of HECs and CECs. Some commentators have drawn attention to the need for more information about the efficacy of the HEC or CEC in improving the moral quality of decision making within a healthcare institution, and to the need for the provision of ethics education and further training for committee members. Liability and lack of regulation pose further challenges for clinical ethics services.

1.7. Research ethics governance and research ethics committees:

Abuses perpetuated on vulnerable populations in the name of research during the twentieth century have led, over the course of the past forty years, to the creation of a number of mechanisms for the regulation of research and the protection of research participants. Guidelines for the ethical conduct of research include the Nuremburg Code (1947), the Declaration of Helsinki (World Medical Association, 1964, 1975, 1883, 1989, 1996, 2000, 2002, 2004, 2008), the Belmont Report (National Commission for the Protection of Human Subjects of Biomedical and Behavioral Research, 1979) and the guidelines of the Council of International Organisations for Medical Science (CIOMS) (1982 and revisions 1993, 2002). In the US, research is subject to stringent regulations which are enforceable by federal law (United States Department of Health and Human Services, 2005: Code of Federal Regulations 45, section 46). The European equivalent of the 45CFR 46 is the EC Clinical Trials Directive of

2001 (European Parliament and Council of the European Union, 2001). Both sets of legislation mandate the establishment of research ethics committees (RECs), whose function it is to review research protocols for any ethical issues which may arise in the process of conducting the research in question. While in jurisdictions such as the US, Canada and the UK, the system of research ethics review is highly regulated and systematic, there is no central coordination of research review in Ireland and this has given rise to a certain amount of concern.

2. Module 8 Definitions

2.1 Accreditation:

a process of self-assessment and external peer assessment for evaluating the performance of healthcare organisations against a set of pre-determined standards, with the aim of improving the quality and safety of patient care and implementing strategies for continuous improvement.

2.2 Clinical Ethics:

an approach to resolving conflicts arising in the context of clinical care which relies on a fusion of clinical and ethical expertise and employs frameworks for clarifying, analysing and mediating value differences.

2.3 Clinical Ethics Committee (CEC):

a multidisciplinary committee which functions within a healthcare organisation on three levels: to educate health professionals and staff in relation to ethical issues, to create and revise institutional policies related to ethical issues, and to provide an ethics consultation service to staff and patients. In this module, the terms 'clinical ethics committee' and 'healthcare ethics committee' will be treated as synonymous. In what follows, the term 'healthcare ethics committees' (HECs) will be used when discussing the situation in the US, and 'clinical ethics committees' (CECs) will be used in the European context. In some contexts, both in the US and in the Netherlands, these committees may also be referred to as 'institutional ethics committees' (IECs). Although clinical ethics committees are not yet a common feature of healthcare provision in the Republic of Ireland, the past ten years have seen the establishment of a number of clinical ethics committees in major hospitals around the country.

2.4 Clinical Ethicist (sometimes referred to as a 'bioethicist' or 'ethics consultant'):

a trained consultant with a professional qualification in clinical ethics employed by a healthcare organisation to oversee all aspects of the delivery of clinical ethics services, namely education, policy development and ethics consultation. In-house clinical ethicists are not a feature of the Irish healthcare landscape, although they are increasingly prevalent in the North American context.

2.5 Clinical Ethics Consultation:

a service provided by an individual ethics consultant, team or committee to enable managers or health professionals to address the ethical issues involved in a specific clinical case. Its central purpose is to improve the process and outcomes of patient care by helping to identify, analyse and resolve ethical problems and by providing health professionals with decision-making support.

2.6 Decision-making Framework:

a method used for the analysis of ethical issues arising in the context of the provision of clinical care, which focuses on the identification and clarification of the values and perspectives of the parties involved.

2.7 Ethical Leadership:

activities carried out by an organisation's leaders to foster an environment and culture which supports ethical practices throughout the organisation.

2.8 Governance:

derived from the Greek word gubernator, meaning 'helmsman', the term 'governance' refers to the overseeing of processes designed to improve the quality of an institution's or entity's performance. In this module 'governance' refers to the regulation and standardisation of clinical and research ethics activities, in addition to attempts at the organisational level to promote ethical conduct throughout the organisation.

2.9 Organisational Ethics:

is concerned with the ethical issues faces by managers and governors of healthcare organisations, and the ethical implications of organisational decisions and practices on patients, staff and the community.

2.10 Research Ethics Committee:

a multidisciplinary committee which functions to review research proposals ('protocols') in any organisation in which research involving human subjects is carried out; this includes research involving biological samples and human tissue, as well as behavioural and observational studies.

2.11 Value System:

a set of beliefs – personal, social or institutional – about what is valuable, or good, or desirable or worth pursuing.

2.12 Value Pluralism:

the – sometimes uneasy – coexistence in a given society of a number of different value systems, some of which may be in conflict although none has authority over the others.

3. Module 8 Background

3.1. The Need for Formal Ethics Support

During the course of the past three decades, advances in medical technology and a growing awareness of the range of diverse needs and values in the patient population have led to an acknowledgement of the ethical complexity of healthcare provision (Shelton and Bjarnadottir, 2008, p.49) and the need for formal ethics support in healthcare institutions. Awareness of the ethical obligations inherent in healthcare provision may be said to date at least as far back as the time of Hippocrates, yet developments in modern biomedical science have created possibilities undreamt of by Hippocrates. New diagnostic techniques and therapeutic interventions, coupled with advances in life-prolonging technologies and rapid expansion in the field of clinical research, provide healthcare teams with an ever-increasing array of options in their treatment of patients. These advances have important ramifications for the day-to-day provision of care; for example, health professionals now have to make choices in situations whose outcome would previously have been determined by the progression of the patient's illness. Moreover, not only may the availability of these technologies create unrealistic expectations amongst patients and families, so too do they confront health professionals and hospital governors with an increased variety of choices about how best to allocate expensive and scarce resources. More often than not, clinical education does not provide doctors and nurses with the resources needed to make these difficult decisions. The establishment of healthcare ethics committees (HECs) in the US and clinical ethics committees (CECs) in Europe has been driven by the recognition that health professionals require additional decision-making support in the day-to-day provision of treatment to patients.

Historically, the call for the establishment of ethics committees in healthcare institutions arose in the US as a response to several specific developments in medical technology and the new ethical dilemmas engendered by them. The first successful heart transplant in 1967 led to a determination of the criteria for brain death, for use in pronouncing death in patients who were being maintained on ventilators so that their organs could be used for transplantation without physicians incurring the risk of prosecution (Wilson Ross, Bayley, Michel et al., 1986, p.4). Debates about the acceptability of these criteria for brain death and about the acquisition of donated organs formed the foundation for the emerging bioethics movement. Similarly, the introduction of haemodialysis in the 1960s led to a wide-ranging public discussion about the criteria employed in selecting patients for dialysis. These discussions resulted in the consolidation of bioethics as a discipline, with its own dedicated scholars, institutes and publications. By the early 1970s, professional organisations had begun to establish committees to examine ethical issues in healthcare, and hospitals too had started to consider how bioethical concerns influenced the care provided to patients (Wilson Ross et al., 1986, p.5).

Around the same time, the revelation of research abuses involving vulnerable populations – such as the infamous Tuskegee study of untreated syphilis carried out between the 1930s and the 1970s – gave rise to public outrage and mandated the formation in 1974 of the National Commission for the Protection of Human Subjects of Biomedical and Behavioural Research (the Research Commission). This Commission was responsible for the publication in 1979 of the Belmont Report (National Commission for the Protection of Human Subjects of Biomedical and Behavioral Research, 1979) which remains a seminal achievement in articulating the need to protect research participants from exploitation. In a parallel development, the founding of the Research Commission was followed in 1978 by the establishment of the President's Commission for the Study of Ethical Problems in Medicine and Biomedical and Behavioural Research (the President's Commission). Between 1978 and 1983, the Commission published several high-profile reports which underpinned the 'organised and socially-sanctioned' study of the ethical implications of high-technology medical care and drew attention to the need for ethical regulation of the healthcare industry (Wilson Ross et al., 1986, p.5).

The first HECs were created to deal with the ethical issues which emerged around the provision of dialysis to patients with chronic kidney disease. Insufficient numbers of dialysis machines during the 1960s and early 1970s necessitated selecting patients for treatment on the basis of specific criteria. Critics of the selection process argued that the standards guiding these life-or-death decisions were based on partial or biased judgements concerning the value of certain people's lives (Murphy, 2008, p.215). Controversy surrounding the selection process employed by these 'dialysis treatment committees' – sometimes referred to as 'God committees' – was quelled in 1972 when the federal government opted to fund all life-prolonging treatment for end-stage renal disease. But the role of the HECs was revisited in 1976 in the Quinlan case, when the US Supreme Court ruled that Karen-Ann Quinlan's respirator could be withdrawn at the behest of her family if the HEC agreed with her attending physician that she would never be restored to a 'cognitive sapient state' (Wilson Ross et al., 1986, p.6). Subsequent to this ruling, small groups began to form in hospital settings to discuss the ethical issues inherent in the clinical application of advanced technologies. During the late 1970s and early 1980s, some of these groups came to take on a more formal role than others, providing institution-wide education programmes, developing decision-making guidelines and, in some cases, providing a forum in which specific cases could be discussed.

Why the Need for Clinical Ethics Support?

- The provision of healthcare involves achieving a balance between promoting the well-being and best interests of patients and respecting their right to be partners in decisions made about their treatment. This balance requires accommodating a number of different value systems, some of which may be in conflict with one another. Clinical ethics support contributes to the clarification and resolution of these valuen conflicts.

- Excellence in the delivery of care requires ongoing education of staff in relation to patient rights, issues of consent and confidentiality, communication methods and mediation techniques.

- Mechanisms and frameworks for ethical decision making are needed to assist practitioners in making difficult decisions.

- There is a need for a fair and reasonable process for the resolution of conflicts arising in the context of the provision of care.

- There is a need for past mistakes to be acknowledged and skilfully converted into learning opportunities for health professionals and staff, in order to prevent re-occurrence.

- There is a need for advocacy on behalf of those who do not have a voice because they lack power in the medical hierarchy (patients, members of minority populations, staff in vulnerable positions, low-paid contract employees).

3.2 The Formation of HECs and CECs

3.2.1 HECs in the US

In the early 1980s, a number of controversial cases involving treatment decisions made on behalf of patients lacking decision-making capacity, particularly neonates – specifically the cases of Baby Doe and Baby Jane Doe – focused public attention on the ethical difficulties inherent in such cases and the need for guidelines and policies to assist health professionals, with special reference to the withholding or withdrawing of treatment. Recommendations were made for the establishment of 'infant care review committees' which would assume the role of reviewing decisions to withhold life-prolonging treatment from severely handicapped neonates. In 1983, a report by the President's Commission suggested that HECs might provide a reasonable means of promoting effective decision making through education, policy recommendations and case review (Wilson Ross et al., 1986, p.7) – the three principal responsibilities of the present-day HEC. With this endorsement, the interest of the healthcare industry was finally awakened, and a rapid increase in the number of ethics committees in the US followed. By the mid-1980s, an estimated 50% of American hospitals had an ethics committee, and by 1987 this figure had risen to 67% (Edwards and Street, 2007, p.254). In 1992, the Joint Commission for the Accreditation of Healthcare Organisations (JCAHO) made it a requirement that healthcare organisations 'have in place a defined mechanism for the consideration of ethical issues arising in the care of patients, and to provide education to caregivers and patients on ethical issues in health care' (JCAHO, 1992, p.104). Currently 95% of US hospitals have an ethics committee, although there is considerable variation in the size, function and effectiveness of these committees (Hackler and Hester, 2008, p4; Fox et al., 2007, p15).

3.2.2 CECs in the UK

In the UK and mainland Europe, the establishment of clinical ethics committees (CECs) took place in a more piecemeal fashion and at a slower rate than in the US (Slowther, Johnston, Goodall and Hope, 2004a; Doyal, 2001). Reasons for the more rapid pace of development in the US may include a longer tradition of federal and state regulation of ethico-legal aspects of clinical activity in the US, a more accessible legal system and less tolerance of overt paternalism in medicine (Doyal, 2001, p.i44). During the early 1990s, a small number of isolated CECs existed in the UK, with an impetus to the establishment of further committees provided in the mid-1990s by the need expressed by some health professionals for support in the decision-making process (Edwards and Street, 2007, p.255). In 2001, the UK Clinical Ethics Network, an unofficial network of CECs, was established under the auspices of the Oxford Centre for Ethics and Communication in Health Care Practice (ETHOX). At that time, there were 20 CECs in the UK. By 2002, this figure had risen to 47, with 85 CECs currently registered with the Clinical Ethics Network. The aims of the Clinical Ethics Network are to promote the development of clinical ethics support in the UK, to encourage a high level of ethical debate in relation to clinical practice, and to facilitate the sharing of best practice between CECs (Slowther, Johnston, Goodall and Hope, 2004b, p.950). Recently, both the Royal College of Physicians and the Nuffield Trust have endorsed the role played by CECs in healthcare provision in the UK. In its report on *Critical Care Decisions in Foetal and Neonatal Medicine* (2006), the Nuffield Council on Bioethics explicitly recommended that difficult decisions in neonatal medicine should be reviewed by CECs, particularly those relating to the withholding or withdrawing of treatment.

While the number of CECs in the UK has increased steadily since 2000, not every trust within the NHS has a CEC to date. Nor is there a uniform mandate shared by the diverse CECs within the NHS as a whole. Most of these committees function within the working context of a particular NHS Trust and have evolved in response to the particular needs and resources of the institution they serve; they are linked to the functioning of a particular organisational system and have no 'absolute' authority (Edwards and Street, 2007, p.256). A 2001 survey of UK CECs found that some of the committees surveyed were not yet clear about the exact nature of their role within the institution (Slowther, Bunch, Woolnough and Hope, 2001). Despite their increase in status in the intervening years, another survey conducted in 2007 concluded that the functioning of CECs in the UK remains unregulated and under-researched (Williamson, McLean and O'Connell, 2007, p.4).

3.2.3 CECs in Europe

The role played by CECs in Europe varies from country to country, with some countries having legislation in place recommending the establishment of CECs, and others – including Ireland – still lacking a formally recognised ethics support structure. In most European countries – with the exceptions of Belgium and Italy – clinical and research ethics are regarded as separate jurisdictions and are dealt with by different committees (Meulenbergs, Vermylen and Schotsmans, 2005, p.319). In Belgium it is a legal requirement that every hospital should have an ethics committee which addresses both research and clinical issues (Slowther, Johnston, Goodall and Hope, 2004a, p.7). All 86 Norwegian hospital trusts have at least one clinical ethics committee, coordinated at a national level by the Section for Medical Ethics at the University of Oslo. Although they have existed in various forms in the Netherlands since the 1980s, institutional ethics committees (IECs) have become an accepted part of the healthcare landscape over the course of the past decade. In most Dutch healthcare institutions, an institutional ethics committee may serve a number of functions: it may provide the opportunity for consultation in relation to complicated cases, it may provide advice on institutional policy, or it may simply raise moral awareness among the institution's employees (van der Kloot Meijburg and ter Meulen, 2001, p.i36). Most healthcare organisations in the Netherlands – not only acute care hospitals but also nursing homes and psychiatric hospitals – have institutional ethics committees, many of which combine the provision of a clinical ethics service with research ethics oversight (van der Kloot Meijburg, 2001, p.i36). In larger hospitals, these institutional ethics committees are distinct from research ethics committees (RECs) but function alongside them.

3.2.4 CECs in Australia

A survey of 79 CECs conducted in Australian hospitals between 1991 and 1994 revealed that CECs in Australia function primarily as policy formation bodies, although some have an educational function in the hospitals they serve, with very few performing any advisory role (McNeill, 2001, p.443-4). Those few committees which do provide patient care advice, do so within a very limited remit, and generally only in relation to those issues dealt with by the policies under consideration by the committees. McNeill concludes that, while CECs do have a valuable role to play, the range of issues they deal with is very narrow and excludes broader considerations such as the functioning of the hospital as an ethical enterprise (2001, p.459).

3.3 Differences between CECs and RECs

Research ethics, like clinical ethics, is an emerging field whose roots can be traced back to the early 1970s. However, although both research ethics committees (RECs) and clinical ethics committees (CECs) may serve as overseeing mechanisms in the healthcare setting, the ethical governance of research differs in a number of ways from clinical ethics governance. Most significantly, while the operation of RECs is mandated by law in the US and Europe, CECs have no legal standing. Second, whereas CECs perform a purely advisory function, RECs make decisions about whether or not to approve a given research protocol, and they are held to account for these decisions. The ethical governance of research will be discussed below at 3.7.

3.4 CECs: Constitution and Terms of Reference

3.4.1 Clinical Ethics

Clinical ethics emerged in the late 1980s as a response to the increasingly abstract orientation of medical ethics. Less an academic sub-discipline within bioethics than a form of practice in its own right, the aim of clinical ethics is to make the concepts and principles of medical ethics more clinically relevant by bridging the gap between ethical theory and the concrete reality of clinical practice. As a practice oriented towards the resolution of concrete clinical problems, clinical ethics 'takes place' in the healthcare setting, not in the university environment, and what is most distinctive about it is its fusion of clinical and ethical perspectives and skills. Clinical ethics is reducible neither to theoretical disciplines such as philosophy or ethics nor to clinical knowledge and expertise; rather, it must genuinely integrate both. The legitimacy of clinical or healthcare ethics committees rests on their ability to provide a genuinely multidisciplinary approach to the analysis and resolution of ethical problems.

Although the HEC has now become a fixture of the US hospital system and is gaining ground in the UK, such committees are still in the process of defining themselves, their role and their mandate. In the US – as in the UK – the general idea of a HEC must in each case be adapted to the structure, mission and size of the institution to which the committee belongs, and to the resources available to it (Hackler and Hester, 2008, p.18). The Joint Commission for the Accreditation of Healthcare Organisations (JCAHO) makes no recommendations for the constitution or development of a 'mechanism' for addressing ethical concerns, nor does it specify the role it should play (Hackler and Hester, 2008, p.12). Since HECs have no legal standing, they have no fixed terms of reference, nor have set rules been established to regulate membership or composition. For this reason, a number of different approaches to clinical ethics consultation and a variety of models of consultation have developed over the course of the past twenty years.

Where such committees have been effective, however, multidisciplinary and diverse membership has been regarded as a key factor in their success (Schick and Moore, 1998, p.78), with members drawn from a number of different areas of specialisation, including medicine, nursing, psychology, law, theology, ethics, social work and hospital administration. While not a requirement, the inclusion of community and patient representatives is recommended as a means of achieving a more balanced composition. Patient and community perspectives are often seen as providing a valuable external viewpoint and a check on the institutional interests of the committee (Hackler and Hester, 2008, p.14). The multidisciplinary composition of the HEC or CEC reflects the shift in the culture of healthcare delivery which has taken place over the course of the past twenty years, from an authoritarian approach to decision making to a more inclusive and participatory model. Central to the efficacy of such a committee is professional respect for the contribution of each individual member (van der Kloot Meijburg and ter Meulen, 2001, p.i39) and a willingness to disregard differences in status within the organisation. Ultimately, the functioning of the committee rests on the variety of expertise and the range of professional perspectives on clinical care – and on the broader social context of healthcare provision – brought to bear by its members on the issues under consideration (Hackler and Hester, 2008, p.14). Ethical issues in healthcare are multifactorial and stem from a variety of sources, and a wide range of expertise is required to address them. However, while the combined expertise of each CEC is unique to that committee, strong leadership, clarity of purpose, the support of management and some level of formal training in ethics are indispensable to its effectiveness within the institution in which it functions (Schick and Moore, 1998).

4. The Role of Ethics Committees: What do they do?

Broadly speaking, the function of the healthcare or clinical ethics committee is threefold (Fletcher and Siegler, 1996; Slowther et al., 2001):

1. it provides ethics education to health professionals and administrative staff,

2. it provides institution-wide guidance on matters of policy development and revision, and

3. it provides support to individual health professionals in the form of a clinical ethics consultation service, which may take a number of forms.

While the first two functions are relatively uncontroversial, the third is more contentious and has given rise to considerable debate (Fletcher and Siegler, 1996). What is clear, however, is that virtually all healthcare or clinical ethics committees understand their role as advisory, not as authoritative: even in cases in which healthcare or ethics committees intervene, the making of the clinical decision is the responsibility of the health professionals involved, and the committee's primary role is to provide support during the decision-making process.

During the course of the past twenty years, the evolution of clinical ethics has been marked by a 'shift in emphasis from issues of content to issues of process: from what the ethicist [or CEC] does to what the ethicist enables' (Walker, 1993, p.33). Slowther et al. (2002) emphasise that a central role played by the CEC is to bring into being a fair and reasonable process for the resolution of ethical issues, and argue that the existence of a CEC testifies to the seriousness which the organisation attaches to the discussion of ethical issues arising in the course of the delivery of care (2002, p.6). Rather than perceiving themselves as ethics 'experts', ethics committees and individual ethicists are 'architects of the moral space within the healthcare setting as well as mediators of the conversations which take place within that space' (Walker, 1993, p.33).

In other words, in addition to meeting health professionals' need for decision-making support in difficult cases, these committees also perform the more general role of raising – and maintaining – awareness of ethical issues in the institution (Slowther et al., 2004a, p.6). Part of their mandate is to provide a 'reflective space' within the institution where healthcare providers feel comfortable discussing ethical issues (Walker, 1993). Similarly, Gillon argues that, despite the lack of agreement in the US concerning the function of HECs, such committees represent the values and practices that 'define the healthcare institution as a "moral community" and reinforce its moral mandate' (Gillon, 1997, p.204).

4.1 Education

Some commentators view the educational function of the healthcare or clinical ethics committee as its most fundamental function, and as indispensable to the performance of its other functions (Kinlaw, 2008, p.204). Healthcare or clinical ethics committees have an explicit mandate to educate health professionals and administrative staff with regard to ethical and legal principles and guidelines, but they also have a responsibility to identify areas in which they themselves may require further education (Hackler and Hester, 2008, p.7).

Because not every member of a clinical ethics committee will have formal training in ethics, the education of the staff of the organisation is necessarily intertwined with the education of the members of the committee themselves (Kinlaw, 2008, p.203). Every HEC or CEC should include members with ethics expertise or should have an ethics resource readily available to it. It should also be able to identify effective mechanisms for self-education, which would provide its members with a basic knowledge of the field of bioethics and furnish them with the competencies required to carry out ethics consultation and policy formulation, such as the competencies specified by the American Society for Bioethics and Humanities (ASBH) Task Force report of 1998. An effective HEC or CEC will use every consultation and every policy review as an opportunity to educate its own members, health professionals and hospital staff, and patients.

One of the first tasks of any HEC or CEC as educator is to recognise the potential suspicion with which it may be viewed in the organisation, and to address this proactively. The willingness of members of the committee to participate in educational sessions on the various hospital units provides an opportunity to 'demythologise' the role of the HEC or CEC and emphasise the relevance of ethics to the everyday life of staff, patients and families (Kinlaw, 2008, p.210). In addition to existing weekly divisional or unit meetings, clinical staff meetings or Grand Rounds may also provide collaborative opportunities for institution-wide education.

4.2 Policy Guidance and Revision

While there is general agreement about the moral and legal principles associated with the duty of care, there is often serious disagreement about how these principles are to be implemented in practice (Doyal, 2001, p.i45). The formulation of each aspect of the duty of care contains variables which are open-ended and subject to interpretation. When health professionals interpret the same duties of care in different ways or cannot agree about the resolution of conflict between such duties, they are thrown into a state of moral and legal indeterminacy (Doyal, 2001, p.i46).

One of the functions of the HEC or CEC is to provide a practical resolution of this indeterminacy. Good clinical practice requires a procedural means of generating the most rational course of action in such circumstances. An effective HEC or CEC can resolve indeterminacy and optimise opportunities for rational deliberation by facilitating wider debate and discussion about the formation of clinical policies, in which contesting parties have an equal opportunity to put forward their views. The proactive involvement of a HEC or CEC in formulating policies concerning good clinical practice also creates a feeling of 'institutional ownership of moral and legal principles which have been agreed nationally' (Doyal, 2001, p.i46).

In addition to the formulation of clinical policy, HECs or CECs are also responsible for the review of existing policies. Providing an effective policy review service entails getting policies which could benefit from an ethics review to the committee (Ells, 2006, p.268). In some institutions in the US, a process is in place which requires that certain policies be submitted to the HEC for review. Another option is to recommend the policy review service to policy-makers themselves, and encourage voluntary referral. An ethics review of an existing policy may be triggered by a number of factors, including the negative impact of that policy on patient autonomy, privacy or well-being, or an inconsistency between the policy and the institution's stated mission or values (Ells, 2006, p.271). In the US and Canada, accreditation standards may serve as a checklist of items to be addressed by the institution in a particular policy, for example the elements to be included in a policy on informed consent. Finally, in reviewing a policy, the HEC or CEC should try to anticipate the moral significance of its implementation and its impact on patient care and organisational systems (Ells, 2006, p.272).

4.3 Clinical Ethics Consultation

In the US and Canada, clinical ethics consultation has become a standard way for hospitals to meet the accreditation requirement that they address the ethical issues arising in healthcare provision (American Society for Bioethics and the Humanities, 2009). In the UK and in Europe, ethics consultation is increasingly becoming an accepted part of the landscape of healthcare provision. However, while there has been much talk about the provision of a consultation service, little guidance has been provided as to how to design such a service and what its responsibilities might be (Fletcher and Siegler, 1996, p.122). As clinical ethics consultation becomes more widespread, a number of commentators have drawn attention to the need for greater clarity in defining its nature and goals. Tulsky and Fox define ethics consultation as

a service provided by a committee, team or individual to address the ethical issues involved in a specific, active clinical case (1996, p.112).

The Task Force report produced by the American Society for Bioethics and the Humanities (ASBH) defines ethics consultation as

> *a service provided by an individual or group to help patients, families, surrogates, health care providers or other involved parties to address uncertainty or conflict regarding value-laden issues that emerge in health care* (1998, p.3).

Elsewhere, the report defines the goal of clinical ethics consultation as that of 'assist[ing] the interested parties in addressing an ethical issue in patient care' (ASBH, 2009, p.15). This assistance may take the form of helping the parties involved to understand the moral problem and the relevant facts at issue, and to reflect on alternative courses of action and their probable consequences, or it may serve to enable more effective communication between the parties involved.

Fletcher and Siegler summarise the objectives of ethics consultation as the clarification of ethical issues, the facilitation of discussion of particular cases and the resolution of ethical disputes (1996, p.122). Hester suggests that the common goals of ethics consultations are 'clarification, conflict resolution or mediation, and treatment recommendation' (Hester, 2008, p.10). Conversely, Zaner argues that the job of an ethics consultation service is not to recommend a course of action, but

> *to help individuals whose situation it is to think through their circumstances as thoroughly as possible, then help them understand what must be decided and what aftermath can be expected* (Zaner, 2007, p.29).

While there is considerable debate concerning the legitimacy of any treatment recommendations which might be made by CECs, what is uncontroversial is that the ultimate goal of all clinical ethics services is to improve the outcome of healthcare provision and the quality of patient care (ASBH, 1998, p.8). In their 2009 report, the ASBH Task Force points out the importance of differentiating clinical ethics consultation from other practices carried out in the hospital context with which it might be confused, such as medical consultation, risk management, compliance and organisational ethics consultation. The goals of these various practices are different:

*[W]hile the objective of clinical ethics consultation is to provide defensible solutions to clinical moral problems, medical consultations provide medical information, risk management protects the institution from liability, compliance programmes promote institutional adherence to legal standards and organisational ethics consultations offer guidance on moral issues arising in the management of health care institutions. (*ASBH, 2009, pp.12–13)

4.4 Value Clarification in a Pluralistic Society

In their summary of the 1998 ASBH Task Force report, Aulisio et al. point out that contemporary Western healthcare provision takes place in a pluralistic society, governed by the idea that each individual has the right to pursue her own conception of the good life, and to live by her own values, provided that this does not prevent others from doing the same. In this context, the delivery of clinical care is fraught with ethical difficulty, much of it generated by inadequate communication and the confrontation between conflicting value systems. Yet, while the differences between the value systems of the parties involved in an ethics consultation may be irreducible, good communication, inclusiveness and attention to process often help to reduce or resolve conflict (Harrison, 2008).

Essential to all three of its functions, but particularly to its consultative function, is the pivotal role played by the HEC or CEC in clarifying the value differences which underpin most conflicts arising from medical decisions. Resolution of value conflict in the clinical setting requires not only attention to societal and cultural differences but also sensitivity to the communication needs of the various parties involved, as well as awareness of the barriers to communication which may thwart the process. In order to achieve this aim, the HEC or CEC must have in place a transparent process for the systematic review and analysis of information relevant to the decision at hand.

One of the most important contributions made by ethics committees or consultants is to ensure that the decision-making process is

inclusive, educational, respectful of cultural values and supportive of institutional efforts at quality improvement and appropriate resource utilisation (Schneiderman, 2005, p.601).

Although in fraught clinical environments it may not always be possible to meet all of these requirements, health professionals and practitioners must acknowledge them as a goal to aim for in the process of improving the quality of care.

Clinical ethics consultation can be structured in a variety of different ways, and can involve the use of a number of different procedures and tools (ASBH, 2009, p.16). Consultations can be provided by individuals, by small teams, or by entire ethics committees (Shelton and Bjarnadottir, 2008, p.72). The dominant model in the UK and Europe is the multidisciplinary committee, whereas individual consultants with specialist training are more common in the larger hospitals in the US and Canada, which have more frequent need for ethics consultations, often on an urgent basis.

Multidisciplinary collaboration and the ability to accommodate a plurality of perspectives are essential to the effective functioning of any ethics service, regardless of whether the service is provided by an individual or by a team. Although to date no one method for conducting ethics consultation has been universally adopted, there is widespread agreement that ethics facilitation is the most appropriate general approach for ethics consultation (Sheldon and Bjarnadottir, 2008, p.56; Zaner, 2007).

The two goals of ethics facilitation are:

1. the identification and analysis of the nature of value uncertainty and
2. the facilitation of consensus between the parties involved
(Aulisio, Arnold and Younger, 2000, pp.60–1).

In contrast to a more authoritarian form of decision making by ethical 'experts', ethics facilitation rests on an open-ended approach which requires that the building of consensus be an inclusive process, in which all parties have a voice. This approach is based on the recognition that societal values, law and institutional policy all have a bearing on what can count as a morally acceptable consensus (Aulisio et al., 2000, p.61).

The American Society for Bioethics and Humanities describe the tasks associated with ethics consultation as (2009, pp.77–8):

- *Effective navigation of the clinical setting in order to perform the various tasks demanded by ethics consultation*
- *Collection of information (a multi-part task utilizing the medical records and carrying out appropriate interviews) and assessing the appropriateness of the case for ethics consultation*
- *Determination of whether the case falls within the scope of the ethics consultation service (the case must be referred to an appropriate resource if deemed outside the scope of ethics consultation)*
- *Evaluation, interpretation and analysis of the information*
- *Fostering communication between the parties to the consultation or facilitating a meeting of the principal parties and an understanding of each perspective; assessing options for moral acceptability; and assisting the parties to identify and think through ethically acceptable options*
- *Promoting implementation of an ethically acceptable plan of action by identifying responsibilities, documenting agreements and points of consensus the principals achieve in the meeting and/or documenting recommendations or ethically acceptable options.*

4.5 Competencies for Clinical Ethics Consultation

The principal goal of the American Society for Bioethics and Humanities Task Force report of 1998 was the improvement of the quality of clinical ethics resources in the US. The report documented the minimum training requirements and skills for those providing clinical ethics advice, drawing a distinction between the knowledge required for ethics consultation and the skills needed to conduct ethics consultation. The knowledge required for ethics consultation includes a broad familiarity with the concepts and issues of bioethics as a discipline, familiarity with the clinical context as it relates to ethics consultation, familiarity with the systems, policies and practices of the healthcare institution in which the consultation takes place, knowledge of relevant codes of ethics and professional practice guidelines and, finally, familiarity with local health law (1998, p.20).

The report lists three categories of skill needed for ethics consultation: 'ethical assessment skills', 'process skills' and 'interpersonal skills', and distinguishes between 'basic' and 'advanced' skills in each of these categories.

- Ethical assessment skills form the basis for identifying the value uncertainty or conflict which underlies the request for consultation. These skills include the ability to distinguish the properly ethical aspects of the situation from other aspects (legal, medical, psychiatric), the ability to identify the assumptions underlying the positions of the various parties involved (e.g. assumptions about value or quality of life), and the ability to clarify concepts and issues relevant to the case discussion (ASBH, 1998, p.13).

- Process skills are needed in order to resolve the value uncertainty or conflict, and these include the ability to identify key decision makers and include them in discussions, to create an atmosphere of trust in which participants feel free to express their concerns, to help individuals analyse the values underlying their positions, and to negotiate between competing moral perspectives (ASBH, 1998, p.14).

- Interpersonal skills are crucial for every aspect of ethics consultation and include the ability to listen well and to communicate interest, respect, support and empathy to the involved parties, the ability to elicit the moral views of the respective parties, the ability to enable the involved parties to communicate effectively and be heard by other parties, and the ability to recognise and transcend barriers to communication.

Individuals from a variety of academic and health-related backgrounds can be trained to develop the competencies necessary to become ethics consultants (Sheldon and Bjarnadottir, 2008, p.55). What primarily differentiates the approach of a qualified ethics consultant from that of an untrained lay person is the understanding and use of a method or framework for the systematic collection and analysis of information in the resolution of difficult ethical cases (Sheldon and Bjarnadottir, 2008, p.56).

4.6 Tools for Collection and Analysis

Examples of such frameworks include the following Case Analysis Tool developed by Christine Harrison, Clinical Bioethics Service, Hospital for Sick Children, Toronto:

4.6.1 Harrison's Case Analysis Tool

1. Clearly articulate what the problem is.

2. Gather and consider all relevant information, both medical and non-medical (see 'Four-Box' method below).

3. Identify the various courses of action possible, collaborating with colleagues where possible.

4. Identify the appropriate decision makers and those who should participate in the decision-making process.

5. Identify the various values and ethical principles associated with each alternative. Remember that individuals' value systems may vary radically.

6. Consider the consequences of each alternative – including probable harms and benefits and who will be affected.

7. Select the best – or the 'least bad' – course of action.

8. Implement the action, and review the outcome.

4.6.2 Dubler and Liebman's Guidelines

Dubler and Liebman have formulated a related set of guidelines for ethics mediation in the clinical setting (Shelton and Bjarnadottir, 2008, p.72):

1. Understand the stated and latent interests of the participants.

2. Level the playing field to minimise disparities in power, knowledge, skill and experience.

3. Help the parties define their interests, search for common ground and maximise options for conflict resolution.

4. Ensure that the consensus is justifiable as a principled resolution compatible with ethical principles and legal rights.

4.6.3 Jonson, Siegler and Winsdale's 'Four-Box' Method

Jonson, Siegler and Winsdale (2010), the 'pioneers' of clinical ethics, have developed a comprehensive method for gathering information prior to conducting clinical ethics consultation. These four categories of question have become known as the 'four-box' method:

Medical Indications

The Principles of Beneficence and Nonmaleficence

1. What is the patient's medical problem? Is the problem acute? chronic? critical? reversible? emergent? terminal?

2. What are the goals of treatment?

3. In what circumstances are medical treatments not indicated?

4. What are the probabilities of success of various treatment options?

5. In sum, how can this patient be benefited by medical and nursing care, and how can harm be avoided?

Patient Preferences

The Principle of Respect for Autonomy

1. Has the patient been informed of benefits and risks, understood this information, and given consent?

2. Is the patient mentally capable and legally competent, and is there evidence of incapacity?

3. If mentally capable, what preferences about treatment is the patient stating?

4. If incapacitated, has the patient expressed prior preferences?

5. Who is the appropriate surrogate to make decisions for the incapacitated patient?

6. Is the patient unwilling or unable to cooperate with medical treatment? If so, why?

Quality of Life

The Principles of Beneficence and Nonmaleficence and Respect for Autonomy

1. What are the prospects, with or without treatment, for a return to normal life, and what physical, mental, and social deficits might the patient experience even if treatment succeeds?

2. On what grounds can anyone judge that some quality of life would be undesirable for a patient who cannot make or express such a judgment?

3. Are there biases that might prejudice the provider's evaluation of the patient's quality of life?

4. What ethical issues arise concerning improving or enhancing a patient's quality of life?

5. Do quality-of-life assessments raise any questions regarding changes in treatment plans, such as forgoing life-sustaining treatment?

6. What are plans and rationale to forgo life-sustaining treatment?

7. What is the legal and ethical status of suicide?

Contextual Features

The Principles of Justice and Fairness

1. Are there professional, interprofessional, or business interests that might create conflicts of interest in the clinical treatment of patients?

2. Are there parties other than clinicians and patients, such as family members, who have an interest in clinical decisions?

3. What are the limits imposed on patient confidentiality by the legitimate interests of third parties?

4. Are there financial factors that create conflicts of interest in clinical decisions?

5. Are there problems of allocation of scarce health resources that might affect clinical decisions?

6. Are there religious issues that might influence clinical decisions?

7. What are the legal issues that might affect clinical decisions?

8. Are there considerations of clinical research and education that might affect clinical decisions?

9. Are there issues of public health and safety that affect clinical decisions?

10. Are there conflicts of interest within institutions and organizations (e.g., hospitals) that may affect clinical decisions and patient welfare?

Reproduced with the permission of The McGraw-Hill Companies, Clinical Ethics, 2010, Seventh Edition, Albert R. Jonsen, Mark Siegler, William J. Winslade, McGraw Hill, New York.

4.7 Reasons for Consultation

Healthcare provision is fraught with ethical difficulty and requests for ethics consultations are 'triggered' by a wide variety of situations. In the course of meeting the day-to-day needs of patients, health professionals encounter numerous situations which may prove ethically challenging or troubling and which, if unacknowledged, may result in moral distress, burnout or compassion fatigue on the part of the individual health professional. The need for formal clinical ethics support may express itself in a number of different ways, including the following:

1. It may emerge as a result of conflict between the healthcare team and the patient or member of the patient's family during the course of the routine provision of care.

2. It may arise from disagreements between members of the healthcare team concerning the nature of the treatment provided or the manner in which it is provided.

3. It may issue indirectly from flawed or short-sighted management strategies, which can leave individual health professionals feeling unsupported or unheard, resulting in symptoms associated with moral distress, burnout and compassion fatigue.

4. It may arise as a response to the culture of the organisation, in the form of unease with decisions taken at the executive level and their implications for the quality of patient care.

4.7.1 Kinds of Issues

Historically, healthcare or clinical ethics committees were consulted primarily in relation to issues such as the withholding or withdrawing of treatment, competent refusal of treatment, advance directives and DNR (Do Not Resuscitate) orders, in addition to problems involving capacity, consent and confidentiality. In recent years, however, the focus of these committees has shifted to issues of communication, negotiation and mediation.

A number of recent surveys have examined the need for ethics support in the clinical context and the kinds of situation in which ethics consultations are requested. In 2001, a survey of 344 physicians across the US found that the most common factors underlying physician requests for ethics consultation were: the need for help in resolving conflicts, the need for assistance in dealing with difficult family members, the need for support in making treatment decisions and, finally, 'emotional triggers' (Du Val, Sartorius, Clarridge, Gensler and Danis, 2001, p.i28).

To the 'traditional' list of skills expected of an ethics consultant – the ability to identify and analyse ethical problems, the use of reasonable clinical judgement, communication and educational skills and the ability to facilitate negotiation – Du Val and colleagues added the skill of conflict 'or even crisis' resolution in emotionally charged situations (Du Val et al., 2001, p.i29). If ethicists are to earn the respect of health professionals, according to Du Val et al.

(2001) they must also be 'adept' at identifying the particular needs of the individual health professional.

> *The ethicist must do more than grasp the clinical situation and analyse it from an ethical standpoint. The factors that trigger a consultation request must be clearly identified so that they can be properly addressed.* (Du Val et al., 2001, p.i29)

Du Val et al. concluded that the increasing frequency with which physicians appeal to ethics consultants to mediate conflict suggests that the earlier intervention of ethicists in difficult situations might serve to reduce conflict (2001, p.i29). Similarly, Arnold and Wilson Silver argue that an understanding of the process by which conflicts arise and are resolved – basic knowledge about group process, mediation and conflict resolution – should form part of the training of every ethics consultant (2003, p.73).

Goals of Ethics Consultation

In the first major study to explore how ethics consultation is conducted in hospitals across the US, the following were ranked in order of prevalence as the primary goals of ethics consultation (Fox, Myers and Pearlman, 2007, p.16):

- Intervening to protect patient rights
- Resolving real or imagined conflicts
- Changing patient care to improve quality
- Increasing patient or family satisfaction
- Educating staff about ethical issues
- Preventing ethical problems in the future
- Meeting a perceived need of a staff member
- Providing moral support to a staff member
- Suspending unwanted or wasteful treatments
- Reducing the risk of legal liability.

4.8 Evaluation of Ethics Consultation

The ASBH Task Force report emphasises the need for evaluation of ethics consultation at three levels: the competencies of those who conduct consultations, the process of consultation itself and the outcomes of consultation (ASBH, 1998, p.27). The report acknowledges that a major impediment to the evaluation of the outcome of ethics consultation has been the lack of specification of the goals of consultation, but suggests that the success of the consultation can be determined by answering the following questions:

- Was there a consensus?
- Was the consensus within the boundaries set by societal values, law and institutional policy?
- Was the consensus implemented?
- What was the level of satisfaction among participants?

4.9 Ethics Committees: Concerns and Challenges

As clinical ethics services become more prominent in healthcare provision, the role played by HECs or CECs has come under increasing scrutiny.

Concerns include:

- Concerns about the legitimacy of the recommendations made by clinical ethics consultation services
- Concerns about the qualifications and expertise which give the CEC authority to issue recommendations (Fiester, 2007, p.31)
- Concerns about a lack of standardisation in relation to the objectives and terms of reference of HECs and CECs
- Concerns about the need for ethics education and further training of CEC members
- Need for more information about the efficacy of the CEC in improving the moral quality of decision making within healthcare institutions (van der Kloot Meijburg and ter Meulen, 2001, p.i39)
- Concerns about the lack of regulation and the need for accreditation of CECs
- Concerns about committee liability
- Demand for patient representation on HECs and CECs.

While empirical research observing or measuring the efficacy of clinical ethics committees' discussion of difficult cases is rare (Pedersen, Akre and Forde, 2009, p.147), a series of recent studies conducted by Schneiderman and colleagues claim to show that clinical ethics consultation is effective in reducing hospital days, hospital costs and ventilator days in the ICU (Schneiderman, Gilmer and Teetzel, 2000; Schneiderman, Gilmer, Teetzel et al., 2003;

Schneiderman, 2005). However, as Slowther et al. point out, there is little published evidence of the effectiveness of HECs in changing behaviour in the North American context (Slowther, Hill and McMillan, 2002). Fletcher and Hoffmann (1994) argue that, before granting ethics committees additional authority,

> there is a need for more research on their performance and a period of experimentation with quality standards governing their membership and operations (p.335).

In their 2002 study, Slowther et al. note a concern among health professionals that an interest in ethics on the part of its members does not provide the HEC with sufficient qualification to wield the ethical authority it has within the institution in which it functions, despite a perceived need for some form of clinical ethics support (2002, p.5). This is linked to a doubt that committee members who themselves lack formal training in ethics can provide a credible education for health professionals. However, Slowther et al. point out that the existence of a HEC within a healthcare institution does not imply that health professionals themselves lack the expertise to make ethical decisions, but rather that the principal function of a HEC is to provide a forum to assist health professionals in thinking through and reflecting upon the decisions they make (2002, p.5).

What health professionals lack is not ethical expertise but decision-making support. Any moral credibility or authority wielded by a HEC within a healthcare institution would be derived from its balanced consideration of a variety of points of view and the fairness and transparency of its processes (2002, p.6). Similarly, Williamson et al. concur that the results of studies designed to determine the 'success' of ethics consultation are 'mostly moot', but point out that the use of resources by healthcare organisations to address ethical conflicts within the institution

> plays an important role in increasing public and institutional confidence in clinical decisions (Williamson et al., 2007, p.3).

Further, even though the question of the effectiveness of HECs in the US has not been definitively answered, the establishment of a HEC can lead to a reduction in the acute stress often experienced by health professionals involved in difficult treatment decisions, by giving them the opportunity to share the load (Slowther et al., 2002, p.7).

Repeated again and again in the literature on ethics committees is the necessity of the support of institutional leadership for the work of the committees (van der Kloot Meijburg and ter Meulen, 2001, pp.i38–9; Pearson, Sabin and Emanuel, 2003; Gibson, 2007, p.33). Given

its lack of legal standing,

if management does not endorse the initiative, it becomes extremely difficult for the committee to become firmly grounded in the organisation

(van der Kloot Meijburg and ter Meulen, 2001, pp.i38–9).

Similarly, Moreno argues that mechanisms must be put in place to define and promote the moral climate of the healthcare organisation, with the ethics committee as 'one action arm':

> *[I]f the organisation as a whole isn't committed to this effort, no ethics entity can rise above benign neglect.* (Moreno, 2006, p.369)

Management helps to legitimise the role of ethical consultation and awareness-building within the hospital by providing for it and integrating it with hospital policy and services, and this support from management should be made visible by its providing the committee with training programmes and promoting the continuing education of its members (van der Kloot Meijburg and ter Meulen, 2001, p.i39).

Slowther et al. point out that if an ethics committee is to change practice within an institution, it needs to be seen as having authority within that institution, yet if it is seen as too close to the management structure of the institution, health professionals may see it as a regulatory or monitoring body and be reluctant to approach it. For this reason, a 'delicate balance' needs to be struck between being aligned closely enough with management to be respected and being distant enough from management to remain autonomous within the institution (Slowther et al., 2002, p.9).

In some cases, the complexity of the role played by the ethics committee may result in the allegiance of the committee becoming divided: confusion may arise as to whether its primary objective is to facilitate and promote high-quality moral standards in the delivery of care or to provide policy advice which will minimise the risk of litigation or adverse publicity to the institution (2002, p.8). What is crucial is that the organisational climate must be such that the committee can perform its work with authority in an environment free of concerns about job security, reprisals and undue political pressure.

Senior administrative personnel should anticipate that ethics consultation is inherently a controversial, potentially divisive and sometimes personally uncomfortable activity, and should ensure that the ethics committee can function without compromising its integrity (Miles and Purtillo, 2003, p.125). To demonstrate this support, the ethics service should be written into the institution's governance documents, and the chair of the committee should be accountable in that role to a senior-ranking administrator, such as a vice-president or director of nursing or medical staff (Miles and Purtilo, 2003, p.122).

The prevailing consensus among members of healthcare or clinical ethics committees and commentators that institutional support is central to the success of ethics consultation services points to a further aspect of the concept of ethical governance: the internal ethical climate of the healthcare organisation itself. The attempt to create organisations which are ethical in character is known as organisational ethics (see Further Discussion section).

4.10 CECs in Ireland: The Current Situation

At the time of writing, there are at least ten functioning CECs in the Republic of Ireland. In Dublin, Beaumont Hospital has a clinical ethics forum and Our Lady's Hospital for Sick Children, Crumlin, and the Mater Hospital have clinical ethics committees. The Bon Secours Hospital, the Daughters of Charity and the Sisters of Charity of Jesus and Mary all have clinical ethics committees. Wexford General Hospital has a newly established ethics advisory committee, while the Mid-Western Regional Hospital in Limerick has an ethics committee which provides both research ethics and clinical ethics oversight. In Cork, the Mercy University Hospital has an ethics committee and Cork University Hospital has an ethics forum. Most of these committees meet on a quarterly basis and have an average membership of between nine and thirteen members from a range of backgrounds. Most committees have been in existence for approximately four years, although the establishment of the Bon Secours clinical ethics committee dates back to 1989.

The composition and terms of reference of these clinical ethics committees vary from institution to institution, although they have much in common. Generally speaking, these committees see their role as advisory. The Cork University Hospital Ethics Forum was established in 2002 to provide support, consultation and clarification in relation to ethical issues arising from healthcare practice. It also provides education on issues in healthcare and guidance in the development of protocols and procedures. Likewise, the ethics committee of the Daughters of Charity, founded in 2006, provides education, policy advice and guidance on ethical issues arising in the course of providing patient care. The clinical ethics committee of the Mercy University Hospital, founded in 2006, serves as a referral facility and an ethics information resource for hospital staff. Its members facilitate ethics education within the hospital, assist in the development of ethical guidelines and provide a consultation service where appropriate. Established in 2006, the Beaumont Clinical Ethics Forum functions as an advisory body in relation to ethical issues arising in the course of providing care, and it also produces educational pamphlets dealing with ethical matters.

5. Research Ethics Committees (RECs)

5.1 Aims of Research Ethics

The initial purpose of identifying ethical principles to govern the conduct of biomedical research was to ensure that research participants or subjects are protected from exploitation. One of the earliest sets of guidelines for the ethical conduct of research was the Nuremberg Code of 1947, developed to prevent the reoccurrence of atrocities committed in the name of medical research by Nazi physicians during the Second World War (Anon., 1996). Like the Nuremberg Code, the Declaration of Helsinki (World Medical Association, 1964, 1975, 1983, 1989, 1996, 2000, 2002, 2004, 2008) emphasised the protection of subjects and the importance of obtaining informed consent for research. The Council for International Organizations of Medical Sciences (CIOMS) guidelines (1982) and later revisions of the Declaration of Helsinki stressed the need to extend this protection to research participants in developing countries.

Biomedical research on human subjects requires ethical regulation

- because of its inherent potential for the exploitation of vulnerable persons
- because the frequency of past abuses necessitates the ongoing oversight of research involving human subjects
- because conducting research with human participants is a privilege grounded in trust, and for this reason investigators have ethical obligations to research participants, however low-risk the research study may seem
- because the increasing prominence of, and expenditure on, research in the biosciences imposes stricter demands for responsibility and transparency in the conduct of research
- because advances in the field of new biotechnologies such as stem cell research, human germline genetic modification and nanotechnology have generated novel ethical challenges which must be addressed.

5.1.1 Belmont Report (1979)

The publication of the US Belmont Report in 1979 by the National Commission for the Protection of Human Subjects of Biomedical and Behavioural Research drew attention to the need for the regulation of research involving human participants, and listed three principles which should form the basis for all such research:

1. respect for persons
2. beneficence
3. justice.

The Belmont Report called for the creation of local oversight bodies charged with reviewing the ethical issues arising in research involving human subjects. In the US, Institutional Research Boards (IRBs) came into existence to satisfy federal sponsors that human beings were not inappropriately subjected to harm or exploited during the course of their involvement in research (Murphy, 2008, p. 217).

The fact that guidelines such as the Belmont Report and the Declaration of Helsinki lacked legal authority, although they possessed significant moral authority, led to the creation of legislation designed to protect subjects participating in clinical trials, such as

1. Title 45 of the US Department of Health and Human Services' Code of Federal Regulations (United States Department of Health and Human Services, 2005) and
2. The EC Clinical Trials Directive (2001).

Both pieces of legislation mandate the independent review of all clinical research protocols by committees whose members have no affiliation with the research. This legislation also reflects an awareness at both national and international level of the need for regulation to keep pace with advances in biomedical and biotechnological research.

5.1.2 Clinical Trials Directive (2001)

The main aim of the Clinical Trials Directive (2001) is to standardise and streamline the research ethics application process, while enshrining in law the subject protections codified in the Declaration of Helsinki and the Belmont Report. The Directive has recently been transposed into law in all EC member states, including Ireland. Under European law, each member state must have in place a system of research ethics committees (RECs) charged with ensuring that any clinical research carried out in that state meets the requirements set out in the Clinical Trials Directive. The primary purpose of RECs is to review research protocols in order to determine their ethical acceptability. In its Operational Guidelines for Ethics Committees, the World Health Organisation (WHO) defines the role of research ethics committees as contributing to

safeguarding the dignity, rights, safety, and well-being of all actual or potential research participants (WHO, 2000, p.1).

5.2 Research Ethics in the UK

RECs were set up across the UK to review the ethical issues arising from research conducted within the National Health Service. The Department of Health has mandated that all research involving NHS patients or NHS resources must receive REC approval prior to commencement of the research. The role and conduct of RECs in the UK is closely regulated, and is the responsibility of the relevant Strategic Health Authority. A central co-ordinating office for RECs was established to issue guidance and facilitate the provision of training for REC members (Slowther et al., 2004a, p.9).

5.3 Research Ethics in Ireland

Approximately 72 RECs have been identified in the Republic of Ireland. There is considerable variation in the size, function and level of activity of the different RECs. According to a recent study of research ethics committees in Ireland commissioned by the Health Service Executive (HSE), the number of submissions received in 2006 by the committees surveyed ranged from 0 to 278, with a median of 36.5 applications (HSE, 2008, p.42). Most RECs reviewed between 11 and 50 applications in 2006, with an average time period of 21.7 days between protocol submission and committee response (HSE, 2008, p.48). Only 60% of RECs had drawn up standard operating procedures for the review of research protocols, and only 13.3% had a dedicated budget for the education and training of members (HSE, 2008, p.42).

According to the Irish Council for Bioethics, RECs should comprise members who are drawn from a broad range of disciplinary backgrounds in order to maximise the breadth of their expertise. They advise that REC membership should include (2004, p.10):

- Member(s) with knowledge of and current experience in the areas of research which are regularly considered by the REC (e.g. scientist)
- Members with knowledge of and current experience in the professional care, counselling or treatment of people (e.g. nurse, medical practitioner, clinical psychologist, as appropriate)
- Member(s) with training in ethics (e.g. ethicist, philosopher, theologian)
- Member(s) with training in law
- Member(s) with training in statistics
- Lay member(s).

However, the HSE study found that, whereas the vast majority of RECs in Ireland have a legal representative, a medical doctor, a nurse and a lay person on the committee, few committees have a statistician or an ethicist available to them (HSE, 2008, p.38).

Activities requiring REC review include the following (Irish Council for Bioethics, 2004, p.8):

1. Clinical trials involving human participants

2. Trials of new treatment or interventions

3. Research involving human remains, cadavers, tissues, discarded tissue (e.g. placenta) or biological fluids

4. Physiological studies

5. Comparison of an established procedure – whether therapeutic, non-therapeutic or diagnostic – with other procedures which are not recognised as established

6. Innovative practices in health and disability services

7. Research conducted by students, including all activities which meet the definition of research with human participants

8. Observational clinical research

9. Research requiring access to personal information by means of questionnaires, interviews or other techniques of information gathering

10. Research involving the secondary use of data (use of data not collected for that research purpose), if any form of identifier is involved and/or if health information pertaining to individuals is involved

11. Case studies, when a series of subject observations 'allow possible extrapolation or generalisation of the results from the reported cases and when there is an intent to publish or disseminate the data'.

The HSE report concluded that (2008, p.49):

- Overall, there is great commitment to, and participation in, RECs in Ireland.

- What was found to work well, where they existed, were standardised application forms, standard operating procedures (SOPs), reliance on available expertise, feedback mechanisms and adequate resources.

- Those areas in need of improvement include the development of standardised national application forms and SOPs.

- There is a need for a resource of expert opinion which can be accessed by RECs when the need arises.

- Training and administrative resources are inadequate.

- There is a need for improved communication on several levels.

- There is a need for the development of a knowledge network for research ethics.

- Participants strongly suggested the need for a central national resource to coordinate and support some of the suggested improvements.

5.4 Principles for the Ethical Conduct of Research

While the Clinical Trials Directive provides general guidance in relation to the constitution, role and function of RECs, it provides little detail in relation to the complex ethical concerns generated by clinical research. Emanuel, Wendler and Grady (2000) have proposed a checklist of seven requirements which all clinical research must meet if it is to be considered ethically sound:

1. **Social or scientific value.** The proposed research must have social, scientific or clinical value, i.e. the intervention or study must have the potential to lead to improvements in human health or well-being or to increase knowledge through the dissemination of results (2000, p.2703).

2. **Scientific validity.** In order to avoid exploiting subjects and wasting resources, the research must be carried out in a methodologically rigourous manner; the study must be soundly designed, feasible and unbiased, with a valid hypothesis, a clear scientific objective and a plausible data analysis plan (2000, p.2704). In clinical research which compares different therapies, there must be at the outset a genuine lack of consensus within the scientific community as to whether or not the new intervention is more effective than the standard therapy. This is known as 'clinical equipoise' (2000, p.2704).

3. **Fair subject selection.** The determination of inclusion and exclusion criteria and recruitment strategies for the study must be based on the scientific goals of the study, not on arbitrary factors such as social status (vulnerability or privilege) or convenience.

- Subjects should be selected in a way which minimises risk and enhances benefit both to individual subjects and to society (2000, p.2704).

- Participants who are at greater risk of harm through participating in the study should be excluded, although no groups or individuals who could benefit from participation should be excluded without good scientific reason.

- Those who accept the risks and burdens of research should be in a position to avail of its benefits, and subjects who will not benefit should not assume the burdens of participation so that others may avail of the benefits.

- Both the benefits and the burdens generated by participation in the study should be distributed as fairly as possible.

4. **Favourable risk–benefit ratio.** Because clinical research tests interventions about which only limited knowledge is available, there is often great uncertainty about the degree of risk or benefit associated with participation. In these circumstances, clinical research is justifiable only if

- the potential risks to individual participants are minimised;

- the potential health-related benefits to individual participants are maximised;

- the potential benefits to both individual subjects and to society outweigh the risks; and,

- the probability and severity of the risk must be proportionate to the benefit involved.

- Assessments of risk and benefit should rely on explicit standards based on existing data. Where there is little probability of the individual subject receiving any direct benefit from the research, an evaluation of whether the benefit to society justifies the risk to the subject must be carried out (2000, p.2706).

Research in which the risks outweigh the benefits cannot be justified because it contravenes the principles of nonmaleficence and beneficence by imposing harm on the subject.

5. **Independent review.** Independent review of research protocols by persons unaffiliated with the research (generally research ethics committees or research ethics boards) helps to ensure the quality of the study and to rule out any potential conflicts of interest which could arise in the course of carrying out the study. Independent review promotes social accountability and assures members of the public that research participants will be treated ethically (2000, p.2706).

6. **Informed consent.** The purpose of the requirement that investigators obtain informed consent from subjects prior to enrolment in a study is to give the subject control over the decision to become involved in the research. Informed consent is closely linked to the idea of autonomy and indicates respect for the subject's capacity to determine his or her own values, interests and preferences and to act on the basis of these values and interests.

Informed consent presupposes that the subject has received accurate and adequate information about the nature, purpose and methods of the study and its risks, benefits and alternatives, has understood the relevance of this information and has made a voluntary and uncoerced decision to participate in the research (2000, p.2706). Persons with diminished decisional capacity have interests of their own and should not automatically be excluded from research which may benefit them directly or indirectly. Where a person is unable to provide informed consent, a proxy or surrogate may agree or refuse to participate in the research on the subject's behalf, by trying to determine what the subject would have wanted had he or she not lacked capacity to decide.

7. **Respect for subjects.** Research participants are not mere means to the ends of the investigator, but are owed respect as persons in their own right. Respecting participants involves ensuring that a number of conditions are met:

- the subject's personal health information must be kept confidential;

- subjects must be permitted to change their minds and withdraw from the study at any point;

- subjects should be provided with any additional information about the intervention or its effects which comes to light during the course of the study; and

- subjects should be continuously monitored for adverse reactions or changes in clinical status (2000, p.2707).

6. Cases: CECs, RECs and Ethical Decision Making

6.1 Case 1: Ethics Consultation – Premature Neonate

Premature Neonate

A child lies in the neonatal intensive care unit of a local hospital, having been born twelve weeks premature. During delivery, the child suffered severe respiratory distress and had to be intubated and ventilated. An ultrasound scan performed shortly afterwards showed massive bilateral intracranial haemorrhage, with cortical extension. For three weeks, she has been on a ventilator, assisted by pulmonologists, cardiologists, neurologists and other specialists. She has dedicated nursing care, and her neonatologist visits the bedside daily.

The doctors agree that there is no realistic hope that the child will survive intensive care. While avoiding absolute pronouncements, they try to explain to her parents that their daughter is not responding to treatment, that in all likelihood she will not live to leave the hospital, and that the treatment she is receiving involves considerable discomfort and pain. Her parents are young and distraught, and, believing that their child will recover, request that staff continue all aggressive treatment.

Some of the nurses find this difficult, because they consider that the treatment is medically futile and simply prolongs the child's suffering. When they ask their supervisor about the hospital policy on this issue, they are informed that there is no such policy. The doctors are confused about what 'futility' might mean in this situation, and are unsure whether or not they are legally and ethically bound to provide the treatment the parents demand. When they approach the parents about shifting to 'comfort care', the parents become confused and angry and accuse the clinical team of abandoning their child's only means of survival. They insist that all aggressive measures continue. A team meeting is called and the hospital's recently appointed in-house ethicist is asked to provide an opinion about how to proceed.

(Adapted from Hackler and Hester, 2008, p.1)

6.1.1 Discussion

A case like this one, although not uncommon, is extremely difficult to resolve satisfactorily, and great care must be taken to be as inclusive as possible in the process of determining what should be done. A delicate balancing act is required if the ethicist is to ensure that all parties to the conflict are heard and validated. In clinical contexts, there is often a great variance of opinion about what constitutes 'futile' treatment: patients and families may often disagree strongly with health professionals on this issue. The bottom line is that there is no consensus in our society on this question, and intense negotiation is often the only way to resolve situations of this kind. Negotiation is not possible, however, if the confidence and trust of the parents are lost or if the health professionals caring for the child end up feeling alienated. There should also be an awareness that concepts such as 'value of life' and 'best interests' may be defined in a number of different ways.

To prepare for the meeting, the ethicist needs to study the patient's chart and gather as much information as possible about the child's medical condition and about her family from the doctors and nurses who have been looking after her for the past three weeks. She then needs to assess this information systematically, and recommend a process for arriving at a decision, for example the process for decision making identified at 4.6.1 above:

Harrison's Case Analysis Tool:

1. Clearly articulate what the problem is.
2. Gather and consider all relevant information (both medical facts and non-medical factors).
3. Identify the various courses of action possible, collaborating with colleagues where possible.
4. Identify the appropriate decision makers and those who should participate in the decision-making process.
5. Identify the various values and ethical principles associated with each alternative. Remember that individuals' value systems may vary radically.
6. Consider the consequences of each alternative – including probable harms and benefits and who will be affected.
7. Select the best – or the 'least bad' – course of action.
8. Implement the action and review the outcome, including the effects of the decision on the decision makers.

1. Articulate the problem. What is the issue which needs to be resolved? What decision has to be made? Where is the conflict?

2. Gather all relevant information: 'Relevant information' refers to any information which is needed to inform or enrich the decision-making process, including both medical and non-medical facts. Medical facts include diagnosis, prognosis (and the estimated certainty of outcomes), health professionals' past experience with the condition, and information about the organisation, such as relevant institutional policies and relevant professional guidelines. Non-medical facts include information about the parents, family relationships, language barriers, cultural and religious beliefs, and the family's past experiences with the healthcare system. In gathering information, it is vital to ascertain the parents' understanding of the facts, their expectations of the technology involved, and the nature of the communication between the parents themselves.

3. Explore the available courses of action: This entails an explicit discussion of the range of treatment options available for the infant. This range of options is limited in two ways:

a. parents may not refuse life-sustaining measures which would be beneficial for their child, and

b. health professionals are not obliged to provide medical interventions that would be non-beneficial and harmful for the child.

4. Identify decision makers and participants: The decision lies primarily with the clinician but the opinion of parents should be included in all medical decisions. The lead clinician is responsible for surveying the available treatment options and proposing the options that are appropriate for that infant in her specific circumstances, for explaining the options to the parents and for supporting the parents in a shared decision-making process. Those who should participate in the process are those who bear the greatest burden of care and conscience (the parents), those with special knowledge (the responsible clinician, relevant sub-specialists), and those with the most continuous, committed and trusting relationship with the patient and parents (members of the healthcare team directly involved in the care of the infant, extended family, religious leaders identified by the parents).

5. Identify the values and principles associated with each alternative:
All participants in the decision-making process need to take into account the professional and personal beliefs, values and preferences of the decision makers.

Because the neonate's perspective on the treatment she is receiving is unascertainable, the concept of her 'best interests' comes into play. Best interests are usually decided by considering the balance of burdens and benefits of treatment, within the context of the longer-range goals for the child.

The nurses' distress is caused by the fact that they perceive a conflict between the treatment the child is receiving and their obligation to promote the welfare of the child, while minimising harmful effects. This discomfort is significant in light of the fact that many health professionals who care for seriously ill patients over a protracted period of time are prone to developing burnout or compassion fatigue.

As her surrogate or proxy decision makers, the child's parents may not in this instance be impartial judges of what her best interests might be. However, what the parents are hoping for needs to be established and explicitly acknowledged by the health professionals caring for their child.

The attending doctors must accept that no prognosis, however 'certain', is infallible, and that circumstances can influence the way patients or family members interpret the medical information they are given. As long as a patient can be seen to be breathing, family members can often remain in denial about the true nature of the patient's condition.

In situations of this kind, it is often the case that the parents are simply not ready, emotionally or psychologically, to accept the truth about their child's condition. In this particular case, understandably, the distraught parents are unwilling to believe that there is 'no hope' for their daughter, and the reasons for this must be explored. If the basis for their belief that she will survive – or their unwillingness to discuss discontinuing treatment – is rooted in religion or in a religious interpretation of the principle of the sanctity of life, a chaplain should be invited to attend the case conference. If the basis for their belief is not religious, then the child's medical condition and prognosis must again be discussed with them in a gentle and sensitive manner.

Ensuring full parental comprehension may require a formal interdisciplinary case conference in order to identify and clarify what information has been and needs to be provided to the parents. This is best achieved without the parents present, but they should be aware of the meeting taking place and appraised of its conclusions. It should be made clear to the parents that, when guided by the best interests of the baby, withholding or withdrawing treatment does not mean to withhold or withdraw care; rather, it is to substitute another form of care for one which is judged not to benefit the child (Nuffield Council on Bioethics, 2006, [2.33], p.18).

6. Identify the consequences: This requires a projection of the known and potential short- and long-term benefits and harms for each treatment option, including not just the medical consequences for the child but also the psychological and emotional implications of each course of action for the principal decision makers.

7. Select the best course of action. Once the values and perspectives of the various parties have been explored in a respectful and sensitive manner, and the available options and their implications investigated, the 'least bad' course of action should emerge from the decision-making process. If the process has resulted in a consensus, this option may be implemented.

(For discussion of a similar case, see Module 6, 6.4 Case 4: Withholding LPT in a Neonatal Unit – A Low Birth Weight Baby)

6.1.2 Suggested Professional Responsibilities 8

- A consensual decision-making process must be employed throughout. All participants should be invited to contribute to this process, with the common objective of achieving what is in the child's best interests. A decision which respects parental authority and honours the clinicians' commitment to promoting the child's best interests can usually be achieved through a process of explanation, dialogue, and negotiation between the participants. Ultimately, all decision makers must be in agreement with the plan of action proposed at the time, even though on occasion the agreement may be only temporary.

- The creation of an environment in which ethical issues and values can be thoroughly explored requires not only finding the appropriate physical environment for a formal meeting with the parents and whomever else they may choose to have present, but also an environment in which the responsible clinician creates an opportunity for open discussion. Additional, more private conversations between parents and the responsible clinician should be accommodated whenever possible. It is important not to overwhelm parents and family with the size of the group.

- The participation and views of decision makers should be documented. Documentation should also include who was present at the discussion, what was discussed, what was decided, which issues remain outstanding, and any plans for future meetings.

- If, even after this process has taken place, consensus has still not been achieved, time should be allocated for further clinical observation, provided the child is not in discernible pain or otherwise compromised by the continuation of current treatment. The process should move as fast as the slowest participant in the decision-making group.

- Health professionals should continue to discuss and explore with parents the underlying reasons for their disagreement. Early expressions of preference by parents, such as 'do everything possible' or 'stop everything', need to be carefully and sensitively re-examined over time.

- The cultural complexity of the decision-making process should be further explored. Practitioners must recognise that ethnic and cultural traditions, customs, and institutions inform parents' beliefs and values, and that these influences may diverge from the practitioners' own value systems.

- Efforts to negotiate towards consensus should continue. The consensual nature of the decision-making process and the shared 'burden' of the decision must be reinforced.

- The attention of senior management should be drawn to the need for a comprehensive institutional policy to provide guidance on end-of-life care in the Neonatal intensive care unit (NICU).

(Drawn from Clinical Bioethics Service, Hospital for Sick Children, Toronto [Harrison, 2008])

6.2 Case 2: Respecting the Dead – The Lost Baby

This is an unusual case, in which ethical concerns arise at a number of different levels. At issue is not harm done to a living being, but, rather, the question of the respect owed to a deceased neonate; given that no harm was done to the neonate while alive, what exactly is the responsibility of the hospital in this situation? In addition to the question of respect for the neonate, there is the more pragmatic question of how to disclose the error to the fragile and already distraught mother, and a further ethical concern relating to the DNA test, which was conducted without obtaining maternal consent.

The Lost Baby

A neonate of 37 weeks' gestation was delivered stillborn at a large community hospital and an autopsy was scheduled to determine the cause of death. Customary practices in such situations included shrouding and tagging the neonate's body. The distraught mother, who had had two previous miscarriages, requested that the neonate be dressed in the clothes she had provided for the cremation once the autopsy had been completed. Admissions were notified of the death and the neonate's body was transported to the morgue in a bag by a porter, accompanied by security, again customary practice. Given that an autopsy was to take place, the neonate was not dressed and his clothes were sent to the morgue in a separate tagged bag. After the autopsy had taken place, the bags containing the neonate and his clothes were returned to the morgue, in identical bags of the same size, both bearing the same name and date.

When the transport company contracted by the crematorium later came to collect the neonate's body, they picked up the first bag bearing the correct name and date. The bag containing the neonate's clothes was logged out and brought to the crematorium, where it was cremated, on the assumption that it contained the body. The bag containing the neonate's body remained in the morgue for a further four weeks, until somebody finally noticed it during an inventory audit. When staff checked the name on the tag and consulted the records, it turned out that a body under that name had been logged out four weeks previously. A complete check of records had then to take place to determine what had happened.

A lengthy investigation led to a stored sample of the placenta, on which a DNA test was performed, and the results were matched against a snip of the neonate's hair, which was covered in fluid from the mother's birth canal. The lab analysis yielded a 'highly probable' match between the two samples. The crematorium was then contacted by the hospital and the director became livid when the mistake was explained. Instead of waiting for the hospital to approach the family, the crematorium director disclosed the error directly to the mother's sister, who had made the cremation arrangements. The sister insisted that the mother, a single parent with no local family support, be shielded from this new information. The memorial service for the neonate had not yet taken place and was scheduled for the following week. Nursing staff from the neonatal unit felt strongly that the mother deserved to be told the truth about what had happened to her child.

The hospital CEO approaches the in-house ethicist and wonders how the hospital should respond to the situation.

6.2.1 Discussion 8

The situation is a difficult one to classify, since the usual categories pertaining to disclosure of unanticipated outcomes – adverse event, medication error, system error, 'patient protection event', 'environmental event' – fail to capture what happened. The event is probably best defined simply as an error – the 'failure of a planned action to be completed as intended' (College of Nurses of Ontario, 2006).

Professional guidelines stipulate that, in all of the above kinds of situation, the patient or family must be informed of harm caused by negligence or human error. In this case, however, there was no 'subject' to whom harm was caused. Rather, expectations developed and articulated in the context of a highly sensitive and distressing situation were not met and procedures for the respectful disposal of human remains were not properly followed. The neonate's remains 'slipped through the net' and there was no system of checks in place to ensure that the body was actually cremated. Neither the hospital nor the crematorium showed sufficient respect for either the neonate or the mother, and neither followed through on their obligations to ensure that the neonate was properly prepared for cremation. There was no continuity of care. The harm in this instance was symbolic, involving a violation of convention and a distortion of what we feel is the 'right' way to dispose of the dead. What complicates this case further is the fragility of the mother and the risk of adding to her distress by disclosing the error.

Prior to arranging a meeting between the neonate's family and representatives of the hospital, the ethicist must consider ethical issues that arise in relation to the patient and family as well as the organisation.

Ethical issues that arise in relation to the patient and family include respect, fidelity, truthfulness, nonmaleficence and consent.

Respect for persons: How should we think about the way in which persons are dealt with after death? Does the hospital owe anything to the neonate? What are its obligations towards the neonate's mother? How desensitised do persons dealing with the dead become in their work environments?

Fidelity (promise-keeping) and the ideal of patient-centred care: The mother was promised that the neonate would be dressed in his own clothes prior to cremation. She relied on the hospital to fulfil this promise and to ensure that the neonate's body would be delivered intact to the crematorium. In a situation as sensitive as this, the failure to meet these expectations could cause enormous distress. Why were the mother's wishes not respected?

Truthfulness: Are we obligated to be truthful even in cases where the truth may be more harmful than continuing to maintain the illusion that nothing out of the ordinary has happened? From what does this obligation arise? Truth-telling is tied to the need to respect people as autonomous beings and observe their right not to be manipulated (this issue has been extensively discussed in Module 2).

Nonmaleficence: Can it be claimed that the hospital is obligated to respect the aunt's request and shield the mother from further suffering? How will the news that her child lay in a plastic bag on the morgue floor for four weeks affect the mother? Is this desire to protect the mother motivated by paternalism or by a genuine concern for her well-being – or simply by an interest in defending the reputation of the hospital?

DNA testing without consent: Can the DNA test be justified, even though prior maternal consent was not obtained? Should any unexpected results have come to light in the course of conducting the analysis – e.g. information about a genetic disorder – was there a mechanism in place to disclose these new results to the mother, or to provide her with counselling?

Ethical issues that arise in relation to the organisation can be considered in terms of the benefits versus the risks of disclosure:

Benefits:

- From an organisational perspective, public confidence and trust in healthcare organisations is enormously important. It is widely acknowledged that transparency strengthens this covenant of trust between the healthcare organisation and the public, whereas the relationship would be seriously undermined if the organisation were seen to be acting in secret or attempting to cover up an error.

- Surveys have shown that handling disclosure properly minimises damage to the patient–provider relationship.

- Patients are often more disappointed that an error has been concealed from them than they are angry about the initial error.

- Cases involving disclosure are less likely to involve litigation than cases involving non-disclosure.

- Disclosure provides an opportunity to re-examine practices and processes which may not have been recently reviewed and to implement policies which may lead to an overall improvement in care.

- An emphasis on transparency and disclosure can lead to a more open institutional culture and away from a culture of blame.

Risks:

- Even greater distress and grief will be caused to the mother and family.

- Disclosure might lead to bad publicity, which in turn might lead to a loss of public confidence in the institution.

- The hospital might be sued.

Organisation's responsibilities:

- To strive for transparency in all aspects of its operation.

- To comply with the duty to disclose errors and unanticipated outcomes, since this is a key element of the patient safety movement.

- To ensure that the organisation as a whole has a progressive attitude towards disclosure, and that senior leaders take responsibility for ensuring that health professionals and staff receive education in relation to disclosure.

- To improve processes and procedures by creating a policy, or revising an existing policy, with the aim of preventing the recurrence of such incidents.

What Should be Done?

The ethicist needs to set up a meeting between the crematorium director and representatives from hospital governance, nursing staff, the hospital morgue, risk management, patient safety and ethics services. It is important that the meeting does not turn into a finger-pointing exercise and that the morgue staff are not made to feel responsible for the incident: equal responsibility should be accepted by both institutions.

The central question to resolve is the issue of whether and how to approach the neonate's mother, and what mechanisms would need to be put in place to counter the damaging effect that the disclosure may have. Ultimately, if the hospital decides to disclose the incident to the mother, the necessity of providing support and counselling for her is as pressing as the question of whether or not to disclose (Ouellet, 2009). In addition to the organisational benefits of disclosure, in this case disclosing the truth to the mother might allow her to make alternative arrangements for the disposal of the neonate's remains, and to hold a funeral service rather than a memorial service, which might provide her with closure.

What this and other cases of disclosure of unintended outcomes have in common is that truthfulness, respect and compassion must play a role in the way the situation is managed. More important than trying to explain the event itself, ascribe blame or defend the hospital's position is empathising with the mother and enabling her to understand and come to terms with what happened.

- In organising the initial meeting, a great effort should be made to create an appropriate environment for discussion, and all perspectives must be explored in an open-ended, non-confrontational way, avoiding the impulse to ascribe blame and employing mediation techniques if necessary.

- It is important that the clinical ethics component in this case does not disappear behind the organisational ethics component. The ethicist should point out in unambiguous terms that, aside from its responsibility to society to pursue transparency (organisational ethics), the hospital has a responsibility to the mother – rooted in the duty of care (clinical ethics) – to disclose both the error itself and the fact that a DNA test has been performed without her consent. What remains to be determined is the timing and manner of the disclosure, and this requires a detailed discussion about the benefits and risks of disclosing information of this nature to someone in such a vulnerable condition.

- The neonate's mother, or her sister, should receive a genuine apology from the hospital and a guarantee that every effort will be made to prevent a similar incident from happening in the future.

- Counselling should be offered to the mother to provide support in the aftermath of the disclosure.

- The hospital should commit itself to establishing a policy describing and clarifying procedures for the transferral of the bodies of patients who have died while in hospital.

Postscript

In this complex case, the hospital decided to respect the wishes of the mother's sister and did not disclose the incident to the mother. Hospital management made a commitment to creating a policy specifying procedures for care of the dead in the hospital and in the hospital morgue. The mother's sister promised to disclose the event to the mother when she was strong enough to accept the news, and requested that the new policy be named after the neonate ('_____'s Policy'). The hospital agreed to this, and, during the course of ratifying the policy, the neonate's story was retold several times. Each occasion was poignant and it was felt that the incident, although regrettable, had provided an opportunity for the hospital to review and improve the quality of care it provided.

6.3 Case 3: Research with Young People – Risking Suicide

Since many members of research ethics committees (RECs) receive little or no formal ethics education, they are increasingly turning to ethics consultants to help them to think about difficult ethical issues. Just as clinical ethics consultation fuses the expertise of the ethicist with that of the medical team, research ethics consultation requires a collaboration which unites the experience of the ethicist with the various kinds of medical or scientific expertise represented by the members of the research ethics committee. This collaboration is illustrated in the analysis of the following case:

Risking Suicide

Suicide among youths is a growing problem, with suicide the third leading cause of death among 10 to 24-year olds in the US (National Institutes of Health (NIH), 2009). Ireland has the highest youth suicide rate in the EU. Depression is a major risk factor for suicide in both youth and the general population. Standard clinical practice has been to treat depressed teens with antidepressants, even though most antidepressants on the market have not been approved for use in populations under 18. Whether the use of antidepressants in teens is associated with increased or decreased risk of suicide continues to be a matter of debate.

A clinical trial is now being proposed to determine the safety of a commonly prescribed antidepressant in children and young people aged 12–17. Because there has been controversy regarding the relationship between the use of antidepressants and the risk of suicide, the investigators will treat suicidality as an outcome measure. The investigators define suicidality to include suicidal ideation, attempted suicide or death by suicide. Whereas most pharmaceutical clinical trials exclude patients who are at high risk for suicidality from participation, this trial proposes to include them. Investigators will randomise participants to one of four treatment arms: the drug under investigation (approved for adult use only), cognitive behavioural therapy (CBT), the experimental drug combined with CBT, and a competitor drug – also approved for use in adults only which is widely used but has greater side-effects.

The hospital REC is uncertain about whether to recommend that the study be undertaken. Its members approach the hospital ethicist to help them resolve the issue. Should the study be approved with suicide as an outcome measure? If not, why not? If it is to be approved, what additional special protections should be put in place? (Adapted from James Dubois, 2008, pp.115–16)

6.3.1 Discussion 8

In this case, given that the hospital has an in-house ethicist (as do many Canadian and some major US hospitals), she would also be a member of the hospital REC. As such, she would be in a position to educate the other members of the REC about the principles for the ethical conduct of research (5.4 above) and to supply information about the current legislative context, while the scientific and medical members of the REC would be responsible for interrogating the scientific evidence in favour of the study. It is then up to the committee as a whole to work together to think through the question of whether the proposed study is ethically acceptable, or whether it runs the risk of exploiting a doubly vulnerable patient population.

The committee should devote special attention to the following ethical issues:

1. **Social and Scientific Validity**

   A research study is valid if the research hypothesis has value for members of a particular group or for society at large, provided that the risks imposed on the participants are proportionate and do not outweigh the benefits of participation. It is an ethical requirement that those who bear the burdens and inconveniences of a given research study should be in a position to benefit from the research. It has also been argued that persons whose decision-making capacity may be impaired should not be summarily excluded from participation in research. Subject to certain restrictions, then, persons suffering from psychiatric disorders or lacking decisional capacity due to age or illness may be enrolled in research studies, provided that the risks are proportionate and that there is no other way of answering the research question than by studying the particular group in question.

Despite the public health and personal burdens associated with suicide,

> *the empirically-validated knowledge base is limited and clinical wisdom and empirical evidence have minimal overlap when it comes to interventions with persons at high risk for suicidality*
> (Pearson, Stanley, King and Fisher, 2001).

This is because, among other factors, suicidal behaviours are relatively rare and often difficult to predict, making it difficult to conduct studies with statistically significant samples. Further, persons at high risk for suicide are frequently excluded from participation in clinical trials, and few trials are specifically designed to target people at high risk for suicide (Dubois, 2008, p.116). Because pharmaceutical companies tend to be reluctant to fund 'risky' studies involving vulnerable populations, particularly if these studies promise low market returns, this ultimately means that a group which could benefit greatly from research of this nature is being denied this benefit.

2. **Relationship of Risk to Benefit**

The EC Clinical Trials Directive permits research involving minors, provided that a certain 'risk threshold' is not exceeded (Article 4). However, the US Code of Federal Regulations (United States Department of Health and Human Services, 2005: Title 45, Part 46, Subpart D) is more stringent, distinguishing between four categories of risk in research involving minors:

i. research involving minimal risk,

ii. research involving risk which is greater than minimal risk but offers the prospect of direct benefit to the subject,

iii. research involving risk which is greater than minimal and has no prospect of benefiting the individual subject, but is likely to yield generalizable knowledge about the subject's condition,

iv. research not otherwise approvable but which provides an opportunity to 'understand, alleviate or prevent a serious medical problem affecting the health or welfare of children'. (The same system of risk classification also protects prisoners and foetuses from exploitation.)

In the absence of a further set of conditions, parents may not consent to the enrolment of their children in research which promises no direct benefit to the child, unless the research is classified as presenting a 'minor increase over minimal risk'. These standards are highly protective, and many commentators regard them as overprotective, serving ultimately to deny many children with chronic conditions – particularly psychiatric illnesses – the fruits of much-needed research.

The reluctance on the part of pharmaceutical companies to conduct clinical trials involving minors with chronic illnesses has led to a practice known as 'off-label' prescribing: the prescribing for children of medicinal products licensed only for use on adult populations, since children were excluded from the clinical trials which tested the product. There are serious concerns about the safety and legitimacy of this practice. Tan and Koelch argue that the need to protect vulnerable participants from exploitation in research 'has had the consequence of generating a lower standard of routine care for those very patients', and they point to the need for research and clinical studies to reduce the high rate of 'off-label' medication use in minors (Tan and Koelch, 2008, p.2).

In light of this, and given that the population involved in the above study is underrepresented in research, the trial in question is justified, provided that the risk–benefit ratio is favourable and additional protections are implemented in acknowledgement of the vulnerability of the study group as a whole. In this study, no-one is being denied a known effective treatment, and everyone is receiving some form of treatment. The experimental drug is already being prescribed off-label for children. If the research proved the drug safer than its competitor, or established the efficacy of the drug when combined with CBT, the benefits of the study would be significant. If the study has the support of the participants' families, and if participants are carefully monitored, the risk of participation should not outweigh the benefits. This attempt to obtain the necessary knowledge while minimising the risk to participants is known as the principle of least infringement.

3. **The Informed Consent Process**

   Great care needs to be taken when designing the informed consent form. Under the Mental Health Act (2001), young people suffering from psychiatric illnesses are regarded as minors until they reach 18 years of age. Although their decisional capacity may well be fully developed, these young people – like younger children who are not yet capable of making mature decisions for themselves – require written parental consent if they are to participate in research.

In order to make the decision-making process as inclusive as possible, a separate assent form should be designed for these young people which explains in clear and non-patronising language the nature, purpose and potential risks and benefits of the study and stresses the participants' freedom to withdraw from the study at any time. Ideally, the decision to participate should be a joint decision made by the young person in conjunction with his or her parents. To ensure medication adherence, the consent form should emphasise the importance of parental support for the young person participating in the study. The need for close monitoring for indications of increased risk during the course of the study should also be emphasised. Participants should be supplied with contact numbers and encouraged to contact the investigators if they have further questions.

6.3.2 Suggested Professional Responsibilities 8

- The study should be allowed to proceed, subject to the implementation of the following safeguards, which are based on the principle of least infringement (Dubois, 2008, pp.118–19).
- All participants should be monitored closely for signs of increased suicidal ideation.
- Clear criteria – such as the experience of severe side-effects – should be established for the withdrawal of participants from the trial.
- Criteria should be established for 'rescue treatment', including the provision of emergency coverage and a protocol for hospitalisation.
- Family involvement should be sought in monitoring for suicidality and in promoting compliance.
- The informed consent process should be modified to include additional efforts to foster decision-making capacity among participants, including younger participants.
- 'Cross-over' and stopping rules should be established (provision should be made for participants to switch from one treatment arm to another, depending on their response to the intervention).
- Appropriate community consultation should shape the development and review of the protocol.
- Suicidality should replace suicide as an outcome measure.

7. Module 8 Further Discussion

7.1 Organisational Ethics and the Governance of Healthcare Organisations

During the course of the past decade, increased attention has been paid to the organisational or institutional backdrop against which ethical issues arise in healthcare. Ethical issues do not arise within a 'vacuum', yet hospital ethics programmes – where they exist – often tend to focus exclusively on specific decisions and behaviours, while the underlying 'root cause organisational factors' which influence these actions are frequently overlooked. Given that individual behaviours are particularly influenced by an organisation's systems, processes, environment and culture, these larger contextual factors must also be taken into consideration (MacRae, Fox and Slowther, 2008, p.319).

As Chen, Werhane and Mills (2007) observe, it is the healthcare organisation and its various subunits which provide the environment in which the interactions between patients, healthcare staff and family members take place. It is also the healthcare organisation which supports – or does not support – the values and beliefs of those interacting within it (Chen et al., 2007, p.S11). If there is no shared agreement about the purpose of a given system and the values it embodies, or if there is incompatibility between the beliefs and values of the individuals who make up the system, then 'interactions within the system may become confused, counterproductive or even hostile' (Chen et al., 2007, p.S12). For this reason, it is essential that both individuals and organisations respond effectively to ethical concerns (Veterans Health Administration, 2009, p.1).

Rooted in an understanding of organisations as 'systems' and emerging from the field of business ethics, organisational ethics is a relatively new discipline concerned with the way in which the values which define an organisation are articulated, applied and evaluated by and within that organisation. Spencer, Mills, Rorty and Werhane (2000), describe this in terms of a focus on the ethical dimensions of organisations: their motives, the nature and quality of their actions and the effects of these actions (p.21). Organisational ethics is generally understood in terms of an organisation's efforts to

> *define its core values and mission, identify areas in which important values come into conflict, seek the best possible resolution of those conflicts, and manage its own performance to ensure that it acts in accordance with espoused values* (Pearson, Sabin and Emanuel, 2003, p.32).

As it applies to the healthcare industry, organisational ethics addresses the ethical issues arising from the intersection of the business, financial and management interests of healthcare provision (Spencer et al., 2000, p.5). Otherwise put, organisational ethics in

healthcare is concerned with the ethical issues faced by managers and governors of healthcare organisations, and the ethical implications of organisational decisions and practices on patients, staff and the community
(Gibson, Sibbald, Connolly and Singer, 2008b, p.243).

With the emergence of a 'more explicit market approach to medicine', the ethical dimension of organisational behaviour in healthcare has become more visible in recent years (ASBH, 1998, p.24), and the growing importance of hospital accreditation has made this more pronounced. Scrutiny of the way in which ethical issues are dealt with at both clinical and organisational levels is playing an increasingly prominent role in the accreditation process. Traditionally, conflicts arising from decision making at the organisational level would have been addressed by healthcare organisations using the tools provided by business ethics; more recently, it has been recognised that a more nuanced approach is needed. With the increasing centralisation of the delivery and financing of healthcare and the emergence of cost containment as a national concern in many jurisdictions, 'the intersection between bedside, community and boardroom has become inescapable' (ASBH, 1998, p.24).

7.1.1 Organisational Ethics Issues

The kinds of issues which may be called organisational ethics issues include the following (Gibson, 2007, pp.32–3):

- Resource allocation: in an era of increasing costs, limited resources, rising consumer expectations and demands for accountability, a fair process is needed to reach publicly defensible decisions about how resources are allocated, and to maintain trust among managers, staff, patients and the community at large.

- Business development: healthcare organisations obtain funding from a number of sources, including business development, yet there is a concern that some business development opportunities may run counter to the organisation's patient care mission, either directly or indirectly (renting floor space to fast-food outlets; increasing parking fees).

- Fundraising and relationships with donors: the source of funding for healthcare organisations is coming under increased scrutiny; should charitable donations be accepted from tobacco or alcohol companies? Should individuals who have made large donations or their families receive preferential treatment or expedited access to treatment?

- Workplace ethics: the ethical climate of an organisation has a significant impact on staff attitudes, turnover rates and absenteeism, and on the prevalence of moral distress and burnout among health professionals; in organisations in which staff feel respected and fairly treated by colleagues, they report higher quality of care ratings, increased job satisfaction and greater trust in management.

- Institutional policy development: institution-wide policies governing controversial issues such as end-of-life care are needed to ensure consistency and continuity of care across the organisation, and to support health professionals and patients or families faced with difficult decisions.

- Disclosure of error, risk and unanticipated outcomes: disclosure of error or risk is seen as an important part of the fiduciary (or trust-based) relationship between the healthcare organisation and its patients, and additional guidance and support are often required to enable health professionals to implement disclosure policies in ethically challenging situations.

7.1.2 Conflicts

Just as individuals can be held morally accountable for their actions, so too can organisations; the society to which the healthcare organisation belongs has justified expectations about how it should function, and these may be tacit or explicit, morally sanctioned or legally enforced (Spencer et al., 2000, pp.20–1).

Like individuals, organisations too can face conflicts of interest and commitment, particularly in situations in which organisational demands conflict with the organisation's mission (Spencer et al., 2000, p.143). This is particularly the case in the current market-driven climate, in which the provision of healthcare is now perceived as an industry rather than as the meeting of a social need. Even a not-for-profit healthcare organisation needs to have sufficient capital to meet its operating costs and must be able to obtain funds to invest in new technology. A healthcare organisation committed to providing healthcare for a certain population is placed in a near-perpetual situation of conflict of commitment, because its resources will always be limited and therefore it will not be able to provide every kind of healthcare to each of its patients. A healthcare organisation which claims to serve patients first but prioritises profitability places itself, its managers, and often the professionals employed by it in a conflict of commitment (Spencer et al., 2000, p.143).

These are conflicts of commitment rather than conflicts of interest because healthcare organisations are complex entities with multiple responsibilities, and tensions between these responsibilities are not uncommon (Winkler and Gruen, 2005, p.110). Every healthcare organisation has to find a means of being economically viable, and this commitment will invariably clash with the commitment to provide quality healthcare, even in organisations which explicitly prioritise patient care. Yet adequate healthcare is an intrinsic social good which human beings need in order to be able to flourish, and a prerequisite for normal societal functioning (Winkler and Gruen, 2005, p.114).

Given this, businesses which provide healthcare bear special social responsibilities, irrespective of their profit-making status (Daniels and Sabin, 2002, cited in Winkler and Gruen, 2005, p.114). Although a commitment to core values is not incompatible with competitiveness in business (Spencer et al., 2000, p.145), what ultimately defines the ethical nature of the organisation are the principles according to which it sets its priorities and allocates its resources.

7.2 Ethical Leadership

Ethical values or standards adapted by organisations are generally articulated in mission statements, vision statements or codes of ethics. These statements of core organisational values represent the organisation's perception of itself as an ethical entity, the central purpose it intends to accomplish and where it wants to be at a certain point in the future. The values mentioned in the mission statement can be philosophical – for example, compassion, care, accountability, respect, trust – or 'operational' – for example, a focus on skill and knowledge, or a commitment to the provision of certain kinds of services. They also serve to distinguish that organisation from similar organisations, and influence both the structure of the organisation and the roles and behaviour of 'stakeholders' within it (Spencer et al., 2000, p.142).

7.2.1 Positive Ethical Climate

An effective organisational ethics approach involves developing and maintaining a positive ethical climate within the healthcare organisation. According to Spencer et al., the creation of a positive ethical climate involves balancing two sets of expectations:

1. it involves ensuring that the organisation's expectations for professional and managerial performance are consistent with its stated mission and goals, as they are actually implemented.

2. the organisation must embrace a set of values which reflect societal norms and expectations concerning how such organisations should operate and what goals they should prioritise (Spencer et al., 2000, p.6).

Central to the accomplishment of both is the attitude of leadership within the organisation; within any organisation committed to the development of an ethical climate, a central responsibility of leadership is to 'ensure that the organisation makes it easy for employees to "do the right thing"' (Veterans Health Administration, 2009, p.iii). According to Spencer et al., an organisation can 'impair or enhance the moral agency of the individuals employed by it' (2000, p.23). Thus, the challenge for the healthcare organisation is to create an ethical culture which enables ethical conduct, rather than a culture of compliance which enforces it (Gibson, 2007, p.33).

Organisations can be said to promote ethical conduct if leaders

- encourage and model ethical behaviour;
- reward ethical conduct;
- discipline unethical conduct;
- provide forums for discussing ethical issues; and
- emphasise fair treatment of employees (Winkler and Gruen, 2005, p.111).

In order to create a positive ethical climate in which all employees feel comfortable discussing ethical concerns, senior management must demonstrate that ethics is a priority, communicate clear expectations for ethical practice, and support and promote their institution's ethics programme (Veterans Health Administration, 2009).

Gibson lists five factors which are essential for the development of a positive ethical climate within a healthcare organisation (Gibson, 2007; Veterans Health Administration, 2009, pp.33–4):

- Senior management must play an essential role in setting the ethical tone of the organisation.
- The organisation's statement of its mission, vision and values should provide a 'moral compass' which is used in decision making within the organisation.
- Ethical guidelines and policies are essential for translating the organisation's mission, vision and values into practice and these play an important role in guiding conduct and minimising conflict.
- Processes and mechanisms for ethical decision making must be put in place and should be used in attempts to resolve value-based disagreements about how policies and guidelines are interpreted.
- Ongoing evaluation is required to ensure that organisational ethics issues are accurately identified and constructively resolved, and that the organisation's mission, vision and values are implemented, both by the organisation and at the level of individual action.

7.3 The Relationship between Clinical and Organisational Ethics

In their 1998 Task Force report, the American Society for Bioethics and Humanities (ASBH) stated that a definitive separation of the spheres of clinical ethics and organisational ethics was not possible given that many clinical ethics issues or conflicts have an organisational ethics dimension and many organisational ethics issues have implications for clinical practice (ASBH, 1998, p.24).

To take a controversial example, discussions of conflicts arising from the routine resuscitation of critically-ill patients often make reference to a shortage of ICU beds and specialist staff – clearly an organisational ethics issue which accompanies clinical ethics concerns about patient autonomy and dignity.

Yet there are clear differences between clinical ethics and organisational ethics. The former straddles the boundary between clinical practice and ethical analysis, while the latter involves the ethical analysis of the business and management practices of healthcare organisations, as well as their stewardship of public funds and the manner in which they discharge their societal and public health obligations.

Organisational ethics consultation requires additional knowledge about the business and cost-containment elements of healthcare provision and managed care, and about billing practices, marketing, resource allocation, definitions of standard or experimental care, and conflicts of interest (ASBH, 1998, p.26). Given the emerging nature of organisational ethics and the rapidly changing structure and financing of healthcare, the 'technical content' to be mastered in order to conduct such consultations often has to be learnt within the context of the consultation itself.

Consultation in relation to organisational ethics issues is usually requested by senior leaders within the organisation, and the impact of any resolution of organisational ethics issues is often much more extensive than the impact of clinical ethics consultation (ASBH, 1998, p.25). Organisational ethics is by nature much broader in scope than clinical ethics, involving as it does everyone within the healthcare organisation – payers, purchasers, visitors, the community, employees, patients and their families (Schyve, 2003, p.135).

Because the practice of organisational ethics consultation is much less well-established than clinical ethics consultation, many healthcare organisations in the US have set up organisational ethics programmes or committees in an attempt to create a process for the resolution of organisational ethics issues and to promote the development of a positive ethical climate. These initiatives are driven by the belief that, as organisational ethics evolves as a discipline, a clear separation between the function of clinical ethics services and organisational ethics services may become necessary. In their 2009 report, the ASBH Task Force draws an explicit distinction between clinical and organisational ethics consultation, claiming that, while the task of clinical ethics consultation services is to 'achieve defensible solutions to clinical ethics problems', the task of organisational ethics consultation services is to achieve defensible solutions to organisational ethics problems (ASBH, 2009, pp.12–13).

During the course of the past decade, the principal area of overlap between clinical and organisational ethics has been the sphere of policy formulation and revision. Although this continues to be part of the remit of clinical ethics committees, as organisational ethics becomes better defined, it seems likely that policy work will increasingly be carried out by organisational ethics committees or consultants. Despite differences between clinical ethics and organisational ethics, however, decision making at both clinical and organisational levels is framed against the same context of societal, institutional, communal, professional and individual values. The goal of both clinical ethics consultation and organisational ethics consultation is the same: 'to help people resolve uncertainty or conflict regarding value-laden issues' (ASBH, 1998, p.25).

Organisational ethics as a discipline has been slower to gain a foothold in the landscape of European and Irish healthcare provision than in the US and Canada. However, it seems likely that the increasing complexity of the relationship between healthcare organisations, insurance providers, healthcare systems – both public and private – and the market will sooner or later drive the creation of organisational ethics programmes in Europe, as it has done across the Atlantic. Irish healthcare organisations concerned about organisational ethics issues face a significant challenge: the difficulty of separating the spheres of clinical ethics and organisational ethics in a context in which, to date, neither is well-delineated or properly defined.

8. Module 8 Summary Learning Guides

8.1 Why the Need for Clinical Ethics?

- The provision of healthcare involves achieving a balance between promoting the well-being and best interests of patients and their right to be partners in decisions made about their treatment. This balance requires accommodating a number of different value systems, some of which may be in conflict with one another. Clinical ethics support contributes to the clarification and resolution of these value conflicts.

- Excellence in the delivery of care requires ongoing education of staff in relation to patient rights, issues of consent and confidentiality, communication methods and mediation techniques.

- Mechanisms and frameworks for ethical decision making are needed to assist health professionals in making difficult decisions.

- There is a need for a fair and reasonable process for the resolution of conflicts arising in the context of the provision of care.

- There is a need for past mistakes to be acknowledged and skilfully converted into learning opportunities for health professionals and staff, in order to prevent re-occurrence.

- There is a need for advocacy on behalf of those who do not have a voice because they lack power in the medical hierarchy (patients, members of minority populations, staff in vulnerable positions, low-paid contract employees).

8.2 Case Analysis Tool for Clinical Ethics Consultation:

- Clearly articulate the problem.
- Gather and consider all relevant information (medical and non-medical).
- Identify the various courses of action possible.
- Identify the appropriate decision makers and those who should participate in the decision-making process.
- Identify the various values and ethical principles associated with each alternative.
- Consider the consequences of each alternative – including probable harms and benefits and who will be affected.
- Select the best – or the 'least bad' – course of action.

8.3 Principles of Research Ethics

- The research must have social or scientific value.
- The research must be scientifically and methodologically valid.
- Methods of subject selection and recruitment must be fair.
- The relationship of risk to benefit must be proportionate.
- Mechanisms for independent review of the research must be observed.
- Informed consent must be obtained.
- Subjects must be respected.

8.4 Factors Essential to a Positive Ethical Climate

- Senior management play an essential role in setting the ethical tone of the organisation.
- The organisation's statement of its mission, vision and values provides a 'moral compass' for decision making within the organisation.
- Ethical guidelines and policies which operationalise or embody the organisation's mission, vision and values play an important role in guiding conduct and minimising conflict.
- Processes and mechanisms for ethical decision making help to resolve value-based disagreements about how policies and guidelines are interpreted.
- Ongoing evaluation is required to ensure that organisational ethics issues are accurately identified and constructively resolved, and that the organisation's mission, vision and values are implemented, both by the organisation and at the level of individual action.

9. Module 8 Activities

9. 1 Reflect back on the particulars of Case 1:

a. In your opinion, does it make sense to say that concepts such as 'value of life' and 'futility' are relative concepts? Document the reasons why you agree or disagree with this statement.

b. Can you think of situations in which health professionals make value judgements about patients' quality of life and these judgements may influence the treatment they receive? Can we say with certainty that existence in a persistent vegetative state – or even in intensive or long-term care – is not worth living?

c. Can you think of any (morally significant) differences between a case such as this one and a case in which health professionals are discussing discontinuing treatment for an adult in a persistent vegetative state or coma? Re-read Module 3, Case 2 in relation to the Irish Ward of Court Case (1995).

9.2 Reflect back on the particulars of Case 2:

a. In your own opinion, should the hospital have acted differently? Should the error have been disclosed to the mother, and if so, why? Would your answer be different if the neonate's body had lain undiscovered in the morgue for a longer period, say a year or more?

b. Can you think of any other exceptions to the general principle that errors should always be disclosed?

c. What do your professional guidelines have to say about the disclosure of medical errors or adverse or sentinel events?

d. Imagine that you are the clinical ethicist in this scenario and that you have to apply Harrison's framework for decision making (4.6.1 above) to the situation. Describe how this would structure your approach to the case. What information would you need? How would you weigh the demand for disclosure against the need not to harm the mother?

e. Imagine it is your task to draft the policy named after the neonate. What would be the main elements of the policy?

9.3 Reflect back on the particulars of Case 3.

a. It could be argued that, as minors suffering from a psychiatric illness, the participants in this proposed study are doubly vulnerable. Does the right to participate in research outweigh the risk posed to these participants?

b. Do you think there is a good case to be made for excluding such populations altogether from participation in research? Could it be argued that this is paternalistic or over-protective?

c. In your opinion, is there a danger that classifying a particular group as 'vulnerable' involves a form of stereotyping?

d. Is there anything missing from the list of additional protections for participants provided at the end of Case 3?

e. Take a look at Article 4 of the Clinical Trials Directive, 'Clinical Trials on Minors'. In your view, is it adequate to protect this vulnerable group of minors from exploitation? Compare this with the discussion of categories of risk presented in the US Department of Health and Human Services' Code of Federal Regulations Title 45, Part 46, and Subpart D: 'Additional Protections for Children Involved as Subjects in Research'. Which, in your opinion, offers greater protection to minors? (United States Department of Health and Human Services, 2005)

f. Can you think of any other principles which might be added to the list of principles for the ethical conduct of research provided by Emanuel et al. (2000)? Are these principles adequate to protect participants who are vulnerable in other ways, e.g. participants in developing world research?

10. Module 8 References and Further Reading

American Society for Bioethics and Humanities (ASBH) *Core Competencies for Health Care Ethics Consultation: The Report of the American Society for Bioethics and Humanities* (Glenview, IL: American Society for Bioethics and Humanities, 1998)

American Society for Bioethics and Humanities (ASBH) Clinical Ethics Task Force, *Improving Competence in Clinical Ethics Consultation: An Education Guide* (Glenview, IL: American Society for Bioethics and Humanities, 2009)

Anon., 'Nuremberg Doctor's Trial: The Nuremberg Code 1947', *British Medical Journal*, vol. 313, no. 7070, 1996, p.1448

Arnold, R.M. and Wilson Silver, M. 'Techniques for Training Ethics Consultants', in M. Aluisio (ed.), *Ethics Consultation: From Theory to Practice* (Baltimore: Johns Hopkins University Press, 2003), pp.70–87

Aulisio, M.P., Arnold, R.M. and Younger, S.J. 'Health Care Ethics Consultation: Nature, Goals, and Competencies. A Position Paper from the Society for Health and Human Values. Society for Bioethics Task Force on Standards for Bioethics Consultation', *Annals of Internal Medicine*, vol. 133, no. 1, 2000, pp.59–69

Aulisio, M.P., Arnold, R.M. and Younger, S.J. (eds), *Ethics Consultation: From Theory to Practice* (Baltimore: Johns Hopkins University Press, 2003)

Burns, J.P. and Truog, R.D. 'Futility: A Concept in Evolution', *Chest*, vol. 132, no. 6, 2007, pp.1987–93

Campbell, A.V. 'Clinical Governance: Watchword or Buzzword?' *Journal of Medical Ethics*, vol. 27, no. 2, 2001, pp.i54–i56

Chen, D.T., Werhane, P.H. and Mills, A.E. 'Role of Organization Ethics in Critical Care Medicine', *Critical Care Medicine*, vol. 35, no. 2, 2007, pp.S11–S17

College of Nurses of Ontario, 'Patient Safety: A Glossary of Terms (2006), http://www.cno.org/pubs/mag/2004/09Sept/features/patientsafety/glossary.htm [accessed 1 May 2008]

Council for International Organizations of Medical Sciences (CIOMS), *International Ethical Guidelines for Biomedical Research Involving Human Subjects* (Geneva: Council for International Organizations of Medical Sciences (CIOMS), 1982, 1993, 2002)

Council on Ethical and Judicial Affairs, American Medical Association, 'Medical Futility in End-of-Life Care: Report of the Council on Ethical and Judicial Affairs', *JAMA: Journal of the American Medical Association*, vol. 281, no. 10, 1999, pp.937–41

Curtis, J.R. and White, D.B. 'Practical Guidance for Evidence-Based ICU Family Conferences', *Chest*, vol. 134, no. 4, 2008, pp.835–43

Doyal, L. 'Clinical Ethics Committees and the Formulation of Health Care Policy', *Journal of Medical Ethics*, vol. 27, no. 2, 2001, pp.i44–i49

Dubois, J. *Ethics in Mental Health Research* (Oxford and New York: Oxford University Press, 2008)

Duval, G., Clarridge, B., Gensler, G. and Danis, M. 'A National Survey of US Internists' Experiences with Ethical Dilemmas and Ethics Consultation', *Journal of General Internal Medicine*, vol. 19, no. 3, 2004, pp.251–8

Duval, G., Sartorius, L., Clarridge, B., Gensler, G. and Danis, M. 'What Triggers Requests for Ethics Consultations?' *Journal of Medical Ethics*, vol. 27, no. 2, 2001, pp.24–9

Edwards, S.D. and Street, E. 'Clinical Ethics Committees: A Practical Response to Ethical Problems in Clinical Practice', *Clinical Child Psychology and Psychiatry*, vol. 12, no. 2, 2007, pp.253–60

Ells, C. 'Healthcare Ethics Committees' Contribution to Review of Institutional Policy', *HEC Forum*, vol. 18, no. 3, 2006, pp.265–75

Emanuel, E.J., Wendler, D. and Grady, C. 'What Makes Clinical Research Ethical?' *JAMA: Journal of the American Medical Association*, vol. 283, no. 20, 2000, pp.2701–11

European Parliament and Council of the European Union, *Directive 2001/20/EC of the European Parliament and of the Council of the European Union on the Approximation of the Laws, Regulations and Administrative Provisions of the Member States Relating to the Implementation of Good Clinical Practice in the Conduct of Clinical Trials on Medicinal Products for Human Use ('Clinical Trials Directive')* (2001), http://www.eortc. org/Services/Doc/clinical-EU-directive-04-April-01.pdf [accessed 18 August 2009]

Fiester, A. 'The Failure of the Consult Model: Why Mediation Should Replace Consultation', *American Journal of Bioethics*, vol. 7, no. 2, 2007, pp.31–2

Fletcher, J.C. and Hoffmann, D.E. 'Ethics Committees: Time to Experiment with Standards', *Annals of Internal Medicine*, vol. 120, no. 4, 1994, pp.335–8

Fletcher, J.C. and Siegler, M. 'What are the Goals of Ethics Consultations? A Consensus Statement', *Journal of Clinical Ethics*, vol. 7, no. 2, 1996, pp.122–6

Forde, R. and Vandvik, I.H. 'Clinical Ethics, Information, and Communication: Review of 31 Cases from a Clinical Ethics Committee', *Journal of Medical Ethics*, vol. 31, no. 2, 2005, pp.73–7

Fox, E., Myers, S. and Pearlman, R.A. 'Ethics Consultation in United States Hospitals: A National Survey', *American Journal of Bioethics*, vol. 7, no. 2, 2007, pp.13–25

Fox, M.D., McGee, G. and Caplan, A. 'Paradigms for Clinical Ethics Consultation Practice', *Cambridge Quarterly of Healthcare Ethics*, vol. 7, no. 3 1998, pp.308–14

General Medical Council, *Withholding and Withdrawing Life-Prolonging Treatments: Good Practice in Decision Making* (London: General Medical Council, 2002)

General Medical Council, *Consent: Patients and Doctors Making Decisions Together*, GMC/CMDT/0408 (London: General Medical Council, 2008)

Gibson, J.L. 'Organisational Ethics and the Management of Health Care Organisations', *Healthcare Management Forum*, vol. 20, no. 1, 2007, pp.38–41

Gibson, J.L., Godkin, M.D., Shawn, T.C. and MacRae, S.K. 'Innovative Strategies to Improve Effectiveness in Clinical Ethics', in P.A. Singer and A.M. Veins (eds), *The Cambridge Textbook of Bioethics* (Cambridge: Cambridge University Press, 2008), p.322

Gibson, J.L., Sibbald, R., Connolly, E. and Singer, P.A. 'Organisational Ethics', in P.A. Singer and A.M. Veins (eds), *The Cambridge Textbook of Bioethics* (Cambridge: Cambridge University Press, 2008), p.243

Gillon, R. '"Futility": Too Ambiguous and Pejorative a Term?' *Journal of Medical Ethics*, vol. 23, no. 6, 1997, pp.339–40

Gilmer, T., Schneiderman, L.J., Teetzel, H., Blustein, J., Briggs, K., Cohn, F., et al., 'The Costs of Nonbeneficial Treatment in the Intensive Care Setting', *Health Affairs*, vol. 24, no. 4, 2005, pp.961–71

Guerrier, M. 'Hospital-Based Ethics, Current Situation in France: Between 'Espaces' and Committees', *Journal of Medical Ethics*, vol. 32, no. 9, 2006, pp.503–6

Hackler, C. and Hester, M. 'What Should a HEC Look and Act Like?' in D.M. Hester (ed.), *Ethics by Committee: A Textbook on Consultation, Organization, and Education for Hospital Ethics Committees* (New York: Rowman & Littlefield, 2008), pp.1–19

Harrison, C. *Case Analysis Tool. Clinical Bioethics Service* (Toronto: Hospital for Sick Children, 2008)

Health Service Executive (HSE) Research Ethics Review Group, *Review of Research Ethics Committees and Processes in the Republic of Ireland* (Dublin: Health Service Executive, 2008)

Hester, D.M. *Ethics by Committee: A Textbook on Consultation, Organization, and Education for Hospital Ethics Committees* (New York: Rowman & Littlefield, 2008a)

Hester, D. M. 'The "What?" and "Why" of Ethics', in D.M. Hester (ed.), *Ethics by Committee: A Textbook on Consultation, Organization, and Education for Hospital Ethics Committees* (New York: Rowman & Littlefield, 2008b)

Hoop, J.G., Smyth, A.C. and Weiss Roberts, L. 'Ethical Issues in Psychiatric Research on Children and Adolescents', *Child and Adolescent Psychiatric Clinics of North America*, vol. 17, no. 1, 2008, pp.127–48

Irish Council for Bioethics, *Operational Procedures for Research Ethics Committees: Guidance* (2004), http://www.bioethics.ie/uploads/docs/guide.pdf [accessed 20 October 2009]

Jansen, L.A. 'Ethics Consultation at the End of Life', in D.M. Hester (ed.), *Ethics by Committee: A Textbook on Consultation, Organization, and Education for Hospital Ethics Committees* (New York: Rowman & Littlefield, 2008), pp.161–85

Joint Commission on the Accreditation of Healthcare Organisations, *Comprehensive Accreditation Manual for Hospitals* (Oakbrook Terrace, IL: 1992)

Jonsen, A.R., Siegler, M. and Winslade, W.J. *Clinical Ethics: A Practical Approach to Ethical Decisions in Clinical Medicine* (New York: McGraw Hill, 2006)

Kinlaw, K. 'The Hospital Ethics Committee as Educator', in D.M. Hester (ed.), *Ethics by Committee: A Textbook on Consultation, Organization, and Education for Hospital Ethics Committees* (New York: Rowman & Littlefield, 2008)

Larcher, V.F. and Lask, B. 'Paediatrics at the Cutting Edge: Do We Need Clinical Ethics Committees?' *Journal of Medical Ethics*, vol. 23, no. 4 1997, pp.245–9

Lo, B. 'Answers and Questions about Ethics Consultations', *JAMA: Journal of the American Medical Association*, vol. 290, no. 9, 2003, pp.1208–10

Lo, B. *Resolving Ethical Dilemmas: A Guide for Health Professionals* (3rd ed.) (Philadelphia: Lippincott Williams & Wilkins, 2005)

MacLean, S.A.M. 'What and Who are Clinical Ethics Committees For?' *Journal of Medical Ethics*, vol. 33, no. 9, 2007, pp.497–500

MacRae, S.K., Fox, E. and Slowther, A. 'Clinical Ethics and Systems Thinking', in P.A. Singer and A.M. Veins (eds), *The Cambridge Textbook of Bioethics* (Cambridge: Cambridge University Press, 2008), p.313

Manning, P. and Smith, D. 'The Establishment of a Hospital Ethics Committee', *Irish Medical Journal*, vol. 95, no. 2, 2002, pp.54–5

McNeill, P.M. 'A Critical Analysis of Australian Clinical Ethics Committees and the Functions they Serve', *Bioethics*, vol. 15, nos 5–6, 2001, pp.443–60

Mental Health Act No. 25/2005

Meulenbergs, T., Vermylen, J. and Schotsmans, P.T. 'The Current State of Clinical Ethics and Healthcare Ethics Committees in Belgium', *Journal of Medical Ethics*, vol. 31, no. 6, 2005, pp.318–21

Miles, S. and Purtilo, R.B. 'Institutional Support for Bioethics Committees', in M. Aluisio (ed.), *Ethics Consultation: From Theory to Practice* (Baltimore: Johns Hopkins University Press, 2003), pp.121–8

Milner, B.M. 'Implementing Hospital Accreditation: Individual Experiences of Process and Impacts', PhD thesis, Waterford Institute of Technology, 2007

Moreno, J. 'Ethics Committees: Beyond Benign Neglect', *HEC Forum*, vol. 18, no. 4, 2006, pp.368–9

Murphy, T.F. 'Hospital Ethics Committees and Research with Human Beings', in D.M. Hester (ed.), *Ethics by Committee: A Textbook on Consultation, Organization, and Education for Hospital Ethics Committees* (New York: Rowman & Littlefield, 2008), pp.215–29

National Commission for the Protection of Human Subjects of Biomedical and Behavioral Research, *Belmont Report: Ethical Principles and Guidelines for the Protection of Human Subjects of Research* (1979), http://ohsr.od.nih.gov/guidelines/belmont.html [accessed 23 April 2009]

National Institute of Health (NIH) 'National Institutes of Mental Health. Suicide in the US: Statistics and Prevention' (2009), http://www.nimh.nih.gov/health/publications/suicide-in-the-us-statistics-and-prevention/index.shtml#children [accessed 19 August 2009]

Nuffield Council on Bioethics, *Critical Care Decisions in Foetal and Neonatal Medicine: Ethical Issues* (London: Nuffield Council on Bioethics, 2006)

Oullet, D. Personal communication, 2009

Pearson, J.L., Stanley, B., King, C. and Fisher, C. 'Issues to Consider in Intervention Research with Persons at High Risk of Suicidality' (2001), http://www.nimh.nih.gov/health/topics/suicide-prevention/issues-to-consider-inintervention-research-with-persons-at-high-risk-for-suicidality.shtml [accessed 16 November 2009]

Pearson, S.D., Sabin, J.E. and Emanuel, E. *No Margin, No Mission: Healthcare Organisations and the Quest for Ethical Excellence* (Oxford and New York: Oxford University Press, 2003)

Pedersen, R., Akre, V. and Forde, R. 'What is Happening During Case Deliberations in Clinical Ethics Committees? A Pilot Study', *Journal of Medical Ethics*, vol. 35, no. 3, 2009, pp.147–52

Pharr, E. 'The Hospital Ethics Committee: Bridging the Gulf of Miscommunication and Values', *Trustee*, vol. 56, no. 3, 2003, pp.24–8

Royal College of Paediatrics and Child Health, *Withholding or Withdrawing Life-Sustaining Treatment in Children: A Framework for Practice* (London: Royal College of Paediatrics and Child Health, 2004)

Royal College of Physicians, *Ethics in Practice: Background and Recommendations for Enhanced Support* (London: Royal College of Physicians, 2005)

Schick, I.C. and Moore, F.S. 'Ethics Committees Identify Four Key Factors for Success', *HEC Forum*, vol. 10, no. 1, 1998, pp.75–85

Schneiderman, L.J. 'Ethics Consultation in the Intensive Care Unit', *Current Opinion in Critical Care*, vol. 11, no. 6, 2005, pp.600–4

Schneiderman, L.J., Gilmer, T. and Teetzel, H.D. 'Impact of Ethics Consultations in the Intensive Care Setting: A Randomized, Controlled Trial', *Critical Care Medicine*, vol. 28, no. 12, 2000, pp.3920–4

Schneiderman, L.J., Gilmer, T., Teetzel, H.D., Dugan, D.O., Blustein, J., Cranford, R., Briggs, K., Komatsu, G., Goodman-Crews, P., Cohn, F. and Young, E. 'Effect of Ethics Consultations on Non-beneficial Life-Sustaining Treatments in the Intensive Care Setting: A Randomized Controlled Trial', *JAMA: Journal of the American Medical Association*, vol. 290, no. 9, 2003, pp.1166–72

Schyve, P. 'Organisational Ethics: Promises and Pitfalls', in M. Aluisio (ed.), *Ethics Consultation: From Theory to Practice* (Baltimore: Johns Hopkins University Press, 2003)

Shelton, W. and Bjarnadottir, D. 'Ethics Consultation and the Committee', in D.M. Hester (ed.), *Ethics by Committee: A Textbook on Consultation, Organization, and Education for Hospital Ethics Committees* (New York: Rowman & Littlefield, 2008), pp.49–77

Silverman, H. 'Organizational Ethics in Healthcare Organizations: Proactively Managing the Ethical Climate to Ensure Organizational Integrity', *HEC Forum*, vol. 12, no. 3, 2000, pp.202–15

Singer, P., Pellegrino, E. and Siegler, M. 'Clinical Ethics Revisited', *BMC Medical Ethics*, vol. 2, no. 1, 2001, p.1

Slowther, A., Bunch, C., Woolnough, B. and Hope, T. *Clinical Ethics Support in the UK: A Review of the Current Position and Likely Development. Nuffield Trust Report* (London: Nuffield Trust, 2001)

Slowther, A., Hill, D. and McMillan, J. 'Clinical Ethics Committees: Opportunity or Threat?' *HEC Forum*, vol. 14, no. 1, 2002, pp.4–12

Slowther, A., Johnston, C., Goodall, J. and Hope, T. *A Practical Guide for Clinical Ethics Support* (Oxford: Ethox Centre, 2004a)

Slowther, A., Johnston, C., Goodall, J. and Hope, T. 'Development of Clinical Ethics Committees', *British Medical Journal*, vol. 328, no. 7445, 2004b, pp.950–2

Smith, M.L., Bisanz, A.K., Kempfer, A.J., Adams, B., Candelari, T.G. and Blackburn, R.K. 'Criteria for Determining the Appropriate Method for an Ethics Consultation', *HEC Forum*, vol. 16, no. 2, 2004, pp.95–113

Spencer, E.M., Mills, A.E., Rorty, M.V. and Werhane, P.H. *Organization Ethics in Health Care* (Oxford and New York: Oxford University Press, 2000)

Szeremeta, M., Dawson, J., Manning, D., Watson, A.R., Wright, M.M., Notcutt, W. and Lancaster, R. 'Snapshots of Five Clinical Ethics Committees in the UK', *Journal of Medical Ethics*, vol. 27, no. 2, 2001, pp.i9–i17

Tan, J. and Koelch, M. 'The Ethics of Psychopharmacological Research in Legal Minors', *Child and Adolescent Psychiatry and Mental Health*, vol. 2, no. 1, 2008, p.39

Tulsky, J.A. and Fox, E. 'Evaluating Ethics Consultation: Framing the Questions', *Journal of Clinical Ethics*, vol. 7, no. 2, 1996, pp.109–15

United States Department of Health and Human Services, *Code of Federal Regulations. Title 45 Public Welfare Part 46 Protection of Human Subjects* (United States Department of Health and Human Services, 2005)

van der Kloot Meijburg, H.H. and ter Meulen, R.H.J. 'Developing Standards for Institutional Ethics Committees: Lessons from the Netherlands', *Journal of Medical Ethics*, vol. 27, no. 2, 2001, pp.36–40

Veterans Health Administration, *VHA Handbook 1004.06: Integrated Ethics* (Washington DC: Veterans Health Administration, 2009)

Walker, M.U. 'Keeping Moral Space Open: New Images of Ethics Consulting', *The Hastings Center Report*, vol. 23, no. 2, 1993, pp.33–40

Williamson, L. 'The Quality of Bioethics Debate: Implications for Clinical Ethics Committees', *Journal of Medical Ethics*, vol. 34, no. 5, 2008, pp.357–60

Williamson, L., MacLean, S. and Connell, J. 'Clinical Ethics Committees in the UK: Toward Evaluation', *Medical Law International*, vol. 8, no. 3, 2007, pp.221–38

Wilson Ross, J., Bayley, C., Michel, V. and Pugh, D. *Handbook for Hospital Ethics Committees* (Chicago: American Hospital Publishing, 1986)

Winkler, E.C. and Gruen, R.L. 'First Principles: Substantive Ethics for Healthcare Organizations', *Journal of Healthcare Management*, vol. 50, no. 2, 2005, pp.109–19

World Health Organisation, *Operational Guidelines for Ethics Committees that Review Biomedical Research* (Geneva: World Health Organisation, 2000)

World Medical Association, 'Declaration of Helsinki: Ethical Principles for Medical Research Involving Human Subjects' (1964,1975, 1883, 1989, 1996, 2000, 2002, 2004, 2008), http://www.wma.net/en/30publications/10policies/b3/index.html [accessed 18 August 2009]

Zaner, R.M. 'A Comment on Community Consultation', *American Journal of Bioethics*, vol. 7, no. 2, 2007, pp.29–31

Index